Upper motor neurone syndrome and spasticity

This is a practical reference and guide for physicians, surgeons, therapists, orthotists, engineers and other health professionals involved in the management of a disabled individual with upper motor neurone syndrome and spasticity. It is a thorough review, covering all aspects of management from physiotherapy, seating and orthoses, to the use of drugs. It examines the neurophysiology of spasticity, measurement of outcome and the newer treatment techniques, such as phenol and alcohol nerve blocks and botulinum toxin injections. More invasive procedures (including intrathecal baclofen and surgical intervention for more complex and severe spasticity) are covered in detail, and the final chapter looks closely at the management of spasticity in children.

Michael P. Barnes is Professor of Neurological Rehabilitation at the University of Newcastle upon Tyne and a co-director of the Centre for Rehabilitation and Engineering Studies. He is also founder of the World Forum for Neurological Rehabilitation.

Garth R. Johnson is Professor of Rehabilitation Engineering at the University of Newcastle upon Tyne and a co-director of the Centre for Rehabilitation and Engineering Studies. He is the first Professor of Rehabilitation Engineering in Britain and is internationally known for his work in shoulder biomechanics, outcome measurement and measurement in spasticity.

CSR 1084 104 5412

Upper motor neurone syndrome and spasticity

Clinical management and neurophysiology

Edited by

Michael P. Barnes

and

Garth R. Johnson

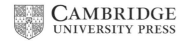

CAMBRIDGE
UNIVERSITY PRESS

PUBLISHED BY THE PRESS SYNDICATE OF THE UNIVERSITY OF CAMBRIDGE
The Pitt Building, Trumpington Street, Cambridge, United Kingdom

CAMBRIDGE UNIVERSITY PRESS
The Edinburgh Building, Cambridge CB2 2RU, UK
40 West 20th Street, New York, NY 10011–4211, USA
10 Stamford Road, Oakleigh, VIC 3166, Australia
Ruiz de Alarcón 13, 28014 Madrid, Spain
Dock House, The Waterfront, Cape Town 8001, South Africa

http://www.cambridge.org

First published 2001
Reprinted 2005

Printed in the United Kingdom at the University Press, Cambridge

Typeface Minion 10.5/14pt   *System* QuarkXPress™   [SE]

A catalogue record for this book is available from the British Library

Library of Congress Cataloguing in Publication data

Upper motor neurone syndrome and spasticity : clinical management and
neurophysiology / edited by Michael P. Barnes and Garth R. Johnson.
       p.   cm.
    Includes index.
    ISBN 0 521 79427 7 (pb)
1. Spasticity.   2. Motor neurons – Diseases.   I. Barnes, Michael P., 1952–   II. Johnson,
Garth R., 1945–
[DNLM: 1. Muscle Spasticity – physiology   2. Muscle Spasticity – therapy   3. Motor
Neuron Disease–therapy WE 550 U687 2000]
RC935.S64 U67 2001
616.8′3–dc21   00-037812

ISBN 0 521 79427 7 paperback

Contents

Contributors

Dr Louise Ada
Senior Lecturer
School of Physiotherapy
University of Sydney
Sydney
Australia

Professor A. Magid O. Bakheit
Professor of Rehabilitation Medicine
The Academic Unit
Department of Rehabilitation Medicine
Stroke Unit
Mount Gould Hospital
Plymouth PL4 7QD
UK

Dr Geoff I. Bardsley
Senior Rehabilitation Engineer
Wheelchair Service
Tayside Orthopaedic and Rehabilitation
Technology Centre
Ninewells Hospital
Dundee DD1 9SY
UK

Professor Michael P. Barnes
Professor of Neurological Rehabilitation
University of Newcastle
Hunters Moor Regional Neurorehabilitation
Centre
Hunters Road
Newcastle upon Tyne NE2 4NR
UK

Ms Roslyn N. Boyd
Senior Research Physiotherapist
The Hugh Williams Gait Laboratory
Royal Children's Hospital
Flemington Road
Parkville
Melbourne
Vic 3052
Australia

Mr Paul T. Charlton
Senior Orthotist
Peacock Medical Group Ltd
Benfield Business Park
Benfield Road
Newcastle upon Tyne NE6 4NQ
UK

Dr Elizabeth C. Davis
Specialist Registrar in Rehabilitation Medicine
Hunters Moor Regional Neurorehabilitation
Centre
Hunters Road
Newcastle upon Tyne NE2 4NR
UK

Mr Duncan W. N. Ferguson
Senior Orthotist
Peacock Medical Group
Benfield Business Park
Benfield Road
Newcastle upon Tyne NE6 4NQ
UK

Professor H. Kerr Graham
Professor of Orthopaedic Surgery
Royal Children's Hospital
Flemington Road
Parkville
Melbourne 3052
Australia

Professor Garth R. Johnson
Professor of Bioengineering
Mechanical, Materials & Manufacturing
Engineering
Stephenson Building
Newcastle upon Tyne NE1 7RU
UK

Dr Craig A. Kirkwood
Clinical Engineer (Seating)
Wheelchair Service
Tayside Orthopaedic and Rehabilitation
Technology Centre
Ninewells Hospital
Dundee DD1 9SY
UK

Dr Chit Ko Ko
Specialist Registrar in Rehabilitation
Medicine
North Staffordshire Rehabilitation Unit
The Haywood
High Lane
Burslem
Stoke-on-Trent ST6 7AG
UK

Dr Patrick Mertens
Consultant Neurosurgeon
Department of Neurosurgery
Hopital Neurologique et Neuro-Chirurgical
Pierre Wertheimer
59 Boulevard Pinel
69003 Lyon
France

Dr Marinis Pirpiris
Royal Children's Hospital
Flemington Road
Parkville
Melbourne 3052
Australia

Dr David N. Rushton
Consultant in Neurological Rehabilitation
Frank Cooksey Rehabilitation Unit
Dulwich Hospital
East Dulwich Grove
London SE22 8PT
UK

Professor Geoff Sheean
Associate Professor
Department of Neurosciences
UCSD Medical Centre
200 West Arbor Drive
San Diego
CA 92103–8465
USA

Professor Marc Sindou
Consultant Neurosurgeon
Hopital Neurologique et Neuro-Chirurgical
Pierre Wertheimer
59 Boulevard Pinel
69003 Lyon
France

Dr Anthony B. Ward
Consultant in Rehabilitation Medicine
North Staffordshire Rehabilitation Centre
The Haywood
High Lane
Burslem
Stoke-on-Trent ST6 7AG
UK

Preface

Spasticity is common, disabling and often poorly managed. We hope this book will be a practical guide and source of reference for physicians, surgeons, therapists, orthotists, engineers and other health professionals who may be involved in the management of a disabled individual with spasticity. We hope the chapters provide a thorough review of the subject yet remain readable and maintain a practical approach. We have covered all aspects of management from physiotherapy, seating, positioning and orthoses to the use of drugs, intrathecal techniques and surgery. We have also stressed the importance of adequate measurement techniques in order to determine whether desired goals have been achieved. Finally, we have not forgotten that good medicine is based on a knowledge of underlying principles and we have included a definitive review of the neurophysiology of spasticity. Overall, we hope that clinicians will find this book helpful in their own practice as well as providing a greater knowledge of the role of other professionals in the clinical management of spasticity.

M. P. Barnes and G. R. Johnson

Newcastle upon Tyne
September 1999

An overview of the clinical management of spasticity

Michael P. Barnes

Spasticity is a significant cause of disability and handicap in people with a variety of neurological disorders. It can represent a major challenge to the rehabilitation team. However, modern approaches to management, making the best use of new drugs and new techniques, can produce significant benefits for the disabled person. The details of these techniques are outlined in later chapters and each chapter has a thorough reference list. The purpose of this initial chapter is to provide a general overview of spasticity management and attempts to put the later chapters into a coherent context.

Definitions of spasticity and the upper motor neurone syndrome

Spasticity has been given a fairly strict and narrow physiologically based definition which is now widely accepted (Lance, 1980).

'Spasticity is a motor disorder characterized by a velocity-dependent increase in tonic stretch reflexes (muscle tone) with exaggerated tendon jerks, resulting from hyperexcitability of the stretch reflex, as one component of the upper motor neurone syndrome'.

This definition emphasizes the fact that spasticity is only one of the many different features of the upper motor neurone (UMN) syndrome. The UMN syndrome is a somewhat vague but nevertheless useful concept. Many of the features of the UMN syndrome are actually more responsible for disability and consequent handicap than the more narrowly defined spasticity itself. The UMN syndrome can occur following any lesion affecting some or all of the descending motor pathways. The clinical features of the UMN syndrome can be divided into two broad groups – negative phenomena and positive phenomena.

Negative phenomena of the UMN syndrome

The negative features of the UMN syndrome are characterized by a reduction in motor activity. Obviously this can cause weakness, loss of dexterity and easy fatigueability. It is often these features that are actually associated with more

Table 1.1. Features of the upper motor neurone syndrome

Negative	Positive
• Muscle weakness	• Increased tendon reflexes with radiation
• Loss of dexterity	• Clonus
• Fatigueability	• Positive Babinsky sign
	• Spasticity
	• Extensor spasms
	• Flexor spasms
	• Mass reflex
	• Dyssynergic patterns of co-contraction during movement
	• Associated reactions and other dyssynergic and stereotypical spastic dystonias

disability than the positive features. Regrettably the negative phenomena are also much less easy to alleviate by any rehabilitation strategy.

Positive phenomena of the UMN syndrome

These features can also be disabling but nevertheless are somewhat more amenable to active intervention. At the physiological level there are increased tendon reflexes often with reflex spread. There is usually a positive Babinski sign and clonus may be elicited. These may be important diagnostic signs for the physician but are of little relevance with regard to disability and handicap. The exception is sometimes the presence of troublesome clonus. This can be triggered during normal walking, such as when stepping off a kerb, or can occasionally occur with no obvious trigger, such as in bed. In these circumstances clonus can sometimes be a significant disability and occasionally needs treatment in its own right. The other positive features of the UMN syndrome cause more obvious disability.

Spasticity

A characteristic feature of spasticity is that the hypertonia is dependent upon the velocity of the muscle stretch – in other words greater resistance is felt with faster stretches (this results in the clinical sign of a 'spastic catch'). Thus, spasticity resists muscle stretch and lengthening. This has two significant consequences. First, the muscle has a tendency to remain in a shortened position for prolonged periods which in turn may result in soft tissue changes and eventually contractures (Goldspink & Williams, 1990). The second consequence is that attempted movements are obviously restricted. If, for example, the individual attempts to extend the elbow by activation of the triceps this will stretch the biceps which in turn will induce an increase in resistance and indeed may prevent full extension of the elbow. However, it is worth emphasizing that the situation is usually more complex. In the above example, relief of the spasticity in the biceps may not lead to improvement in the function of the arm as other features of the UMN syndrome, particularly muscle weakness, may have a part to play.

Soft tissue changes and contractures

Restriction of the range of movement is not always simply due to increase of tone and spasticity in the relevant muscles. The surrounding soft tissues, including tendons, ligaments and the joints themselves, can develop changes resulting in decreased compliance. It is likely that such contractures and changes in the soft tissues arise from the muscle being maintained in a shortened position. It is possible, but not absolutely proven, that maintaining a joint through a full range of movement may prevent the longer term development of soft tissue contractures. The frequency of the stretch, either actively or passively, that is required to prevent contractures is unknown. However, it is important to emphasize good posture and seating such that the muscles, as far as possible, are maintained at full stretch for at least some of every day. The recommendation is that muscles are put through a full stretch for two hours in every 24 hours (Medical Disability Society, 1988). However, more research is needed in this field to determine the degree and frequency of stretch with more certainty.

Thus, hypertonia often has both a neural component (secondary to the spasticity) and a biomechanical component (secondary to the soft tissue changes). Obviously biomechanical hypertonia is not velocity dependent and restricts movements even at slow velocities. Furthermore, biomechanical hypertonia will not respond to anti-spastic agents and the only treatment possibilities relate to physiotherapy, stretching, good positioning, splinting and casting. Ultimately surgery may be needed to relieve advancing and disabling soft tissue contracture. In practical terms there is often a mixture of neural and biomechanical hypertonia and it is very difficult clinically to determine the relative contribution of each of the components. Thus, active intervention for spasticity (e.g. by anti-spastic medication or local treatment such as phenol block or botulinum toxin injection) is worth undertaking simply to be sure of alleviating at least the neural component of the hypertonia. There is often a gratifying response even in limbs that appear to have fixed contractures.

In advanced spasticity it is often the soft tissue changes that contribute most to the disability and are resistant to treatment. Increasing deformity of the limbs will clearly lead to rapidly decreasing function and will often result in problems with regard to hygiene, positioning, transferring and feeding, and make the individual more prone to pressure sores (O'Dwyer et al., 1996).

Flexor and extensor spasms

Severe muscle spasms are often found in UMN syndrome. These can either be in a flexor pattern or an extensor pattern.

The commonest pattern of flexor spasm is flexion of the hip, knee and ankle. The spasms can sometimes occur spontaneously or more commonly in response to, often mild, stimulation. Simple movement of the legs or adjusting position in a chair can be enough to induce the spasm. The spasms themselves can be painful and are sometimes so frequent and severe that a permanent state of flexion is produced. If spasms worsen suddenly it is worth looking for aggravating factors such as pressure sores, bladder infections, irritation from a catheter or even such apparently mild stimulants as an ill-fitting orthosis or a tight-fitting catheter leg bag. Occasionally constipation or bladder retention can also produce a flexor spasm, which can then be associated with a reflex emptying (mass reflex) of the bowel or bladder.

Similar problems can occur with extensor spasms which are most common in the leg and involve extension of the hip and knee with plantar flexion and usually inversion of the ankle. Once again such spasms can be triggered by a variety of stimuli and sometimes can be so severe as to produce a permanent extensor position. Extensor spasms are probably more common than flexor spasms in incomplete spinal cord lesions and cerebral lesions but there is no clear association with any particular pathology. Occasionally a spasm can be useful from a functional point of view. Placing pressure on the base of the foot in order to stand can sometimes produce a strong extensor spasm of the leg, effectively turning it into a rigid splint which in turn aids walking. Occasionally individuals can make positive use of self-induction of spasms such as for putting on trousers. This emphasizes the importance of detailed discussion with the disabled person and their carer before assuming that the spasm will need treatment. Finally, extensor and flexor spasms can be extremely painful and even if not causing undue functional disturbance can need treatment in an attempt to relieve the acute pain associated with each spasm.

Spastic dystonia and associated reactions

Most of the previously described positive phenomena of the UMN syndrome can occur at rest. Another range of problems can occur on movement. For example, there is the classic hemiplegic posture, commonly occurring in stroke, that often occurs when the individual tries to walk. This posture consists of a flexed, adducted, internally rotated arm with pronated forearm and flexed wrist and fingers. The leg is extended, internally rotated, adducted and the ankle plantar flexed and inverted, often with toe flexion. Other patterns occurring on movement are sometimes called spastic dystonias (Denny-Brown, 1966). This is a term that probably ought to be avoided given the potential confusion with extra-pyramidal disease.

Other problems that occur on movement or attempted movement involve co-contraction of the agonist and antagonist muscles. Simultaneous contraction of agonist and antagonist muscles is a normal motor phenomenon and is required for the smooth movement of the limb. However, in the UMN syndrome agonist and antagonist muscles may co-contract inappropriately and thus disrupt normal smooth limb movement (Fellows et al., 1994). Sometimes involuntary activation of muscles remote from the muscles involved in a particular task also contract. For example, if the individual attempts to move an arm then a leg may extend or flex. Conversely the arm can flex when attempting to walk (Dickstein et al., 1996). These 'associated reactions' (Walshe, 1923) can interfere with walking by unbalancing the individual or making it impossible to do any task with the arms whilst standing. Various other patterns of dyssynergic and stereotypical contractions have been described, such as extensor thrust (Dimitrijevic et al., 1981). However, the labelling of these problems is less helpful than a prolonged period of observation and discussion with the disabled person and his or her family and carers. Simple bedside testing is usually inadequate to determine an overall treatment strategy. The pattern of spasticity and the functional consequences during attempted movement as well as at rest all need careful assessment, often over prolonged periods of time. The well-educated disabled person who can describe the problems in different circumstances is of far more value than a single examination in the out-patient clinic.

Clinical consequences

The above description of the different patterns of the UMN syndrome make it clear that there is a potentially wide range of disabilities and handicaps. In order to draw the discussion together, the major consequences can be annotated as follows.

Mobility

Probably the most common consequence of the UMN syndrome is difficulty with walking. The gait can be clumsy and unco-ordinated and falling can become a common event. Eventually walking may become impossible due to a combination of soft tissue contractures, flexor or extensor spasms, and unhelpful associated reactions. It is also worth bearing in mind that individuals with UMN syndrome may often have a whole variety of other neurological problems such as cerebellar ataxia or proprioceptive disturbance which further compounds the problem. Even if the individual cannot walk, the UMN syndrome can cause further problems with regard to difficulty maintaining a suitable seating posture. Spasticity may make it difficult to self-propel a wheelchair. Extensor spasms may constantly thrust the individual forward while sitting in the chair, giving an increased risk of shear forces causing pressure sores. Seating will often require a considerable range of bracing, supports and adjustments in order to maintain a useful and comfortable position.

Loss of dexterity

In the arm the UMN syndrome can cause further difficulties with, for example, feeding, writing, personal care and self-catheterization. Mobility in bed may be hampered and loss of dexterity in the arm may make it difficult to self-ambulate in a wheelchair. All these problems can slowly lead to decreased independence and a consequent increased reliance on a third party.

Bulbar and trunk problems

Although most of the functional consequences of spasticity occur in the arm or leg it is worth remembering that truncal spasticity can cause problems with seating and maintaining an upright posture – necessary for feeding and communication. Bulbar problems can give rise to difficulty swallowing with consequent risk of inhalation or pneumonia. Further problems can arise with communication, not only secondary to inappropriate posture, but secondary to spastic forms of dysarthria.

Pain

It is not widely recognized that spasticity and the other forms of UMN syndrome can be extremely painful. This is particularly the case with flexor and extensor spasms and sometimes treatment is needed simply for analgesia rather than improvement of function. Abnormal postures can also give rise to an increased risk of musculo-skeletal problems and osteoarthritic change in the joints. Any peripheral stimuli from problems such as ingrowing toenails or small pressure sores can in turn exacerbate the spasticity and one can enter a vicious circle of increased pain and increased spasticity.

Carers and nursing problems

Spasticity is one of the unusual conditions that can sometimes require treatment of the disabled person for the sake of the carer. Individuals, particularly with advanced spasticity, can be extremely difficult to move and nurse. Transfers from bed to toilet or bed to wheelchair can be very difficult. Hygiene can be a problem with, for example, marked adductor spasticity causing problems with perineal hygiene and catheter care. Flexion of the fingers can cause particular difficulties with hygiene in the palm of the hand. Thus, aggressive treatment of spasticity can sometimes be a factor in reducing carer stress which in turn can be the difference between the individual remaining at home or moving into an institution.

An approach to management

The previous section indicated the complexity and functional consequences of spasticity. Other chapters in this volume will outline the detail of the different approaches to the management but this section attempts to provide an overview of this process (Figure 1.1).

Aims of treatment

The first question to ask is whether treatment is needed at all. The previous section has shown that occasionally a spastic pattern can be functionally useful, such as an aid to walking or dressing. Spasticity in the UMN syndrome may be abnormal from a neurophysiological point of view but does not mean that treatment is always required. The aims of treatment will always need careful annotation and discussion with the individual. The commoner aims are to improve a specific function, reduce pain, ease the task of caring or prevent long-term problems such as soft tissue contractures. The specific aims of a particular treatment strategy always need clear explanation. This also implies that there should be an appropriate method of measuring outcome so that one knows when the aim is fulfilled. Chapter 3 discusses the topic of measurement in spasticity. Outcomes clearly need to be geared to the aim of treatment. For example, if the aim of the treatment is to improve hand function then a simple, reproducible and valid test of hand function will be required. If the outcome is a reduction of pain then perhaps use of a visual analogue scale will be helpful. The use of a global disability or ADL (activities of daily living) scale is usually inappropriate as subtle treatment effects may be masked.

It is important, particularly in people needing long-term treatment, that the aims and purpose of treatment are reviewed regularly and new goals set or old goals adjusted. This is particularly the case with the use of long-term anti-spastic medication when the side effects of treatment may at some point outweigh the benefits of intervention (see Chapter 7).

Self-management

Education of the person and their family is vital, as in all rehabilitation management. Spasticity and the UMN syndrome involve complex phenomena. The individual needs to be aware of some of the factors that may aggravate the problem such as inappropriate positioning, tight-fitting shoes or even heavy bed clothes. A detailed appraisal of the pattern of spasticity may enable the individual to relieve many of the functional problems. Both the clinician and the individual should be aware of potential aggravating factors such as the worsening effect on spasticity of bladder infection or constipation.

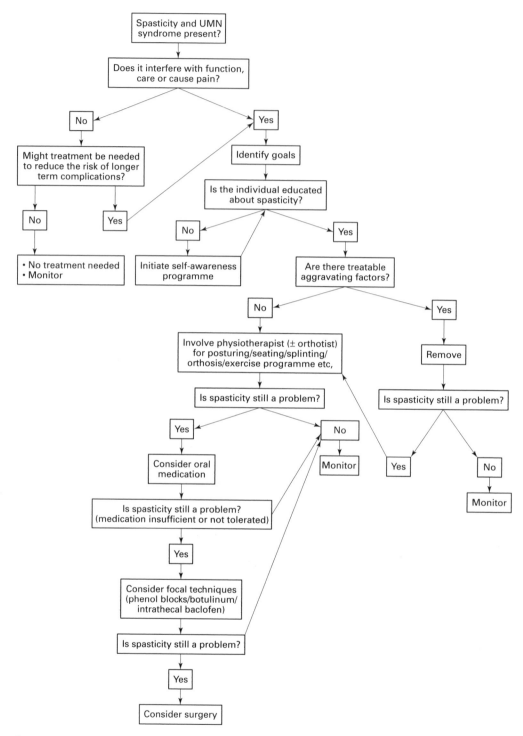

Fig. 1.1   Flow chart outlining the approach to the overall management of spasticity.

The physiotherapist and the orthotist

The early involvement of an experienced physiotherapist is invaluable. There are many potential interventions ranging from simple passive range of movement exercises to more complex anti-spastic physiotherapy approaches (see Chapters 4 and 5). The physiotherapist can also administer symptomatic treatment such as heat, advice on the use of hydrotherapy and advice on and prescription of splints and casts. At this point the input of an orthotist is essential as many situations are helped by the judicious application of a suitable orthotic device (see Chapter 6). Much can be achieved by these non-invasive techniques before resorting to medication or invasive focal treatments.

Oral medication

Chapter 7 outlines the various pharmacological possibilities of anti-spastic medication. Medication should rarely be used in isolation but usually is just part of a whole treatment strategy. Medication can provide a useful background effect which makes, for example, the fitting of an orthosis or positioning in a chair easier and more comfortable. Occasionally, particularly in mild spasticity, the use of anti-spastic medication can be sufficient in isolation to reduce a functional problem such as troublesome clonus. The problem with medication is that it is often associated with troublesome side effects. These particularly focus around increased weakness and fatigueability. Spasticity is often a focal problem and medication will clearly deliver a systemic effect. Thus, muscles that are not troublesome can be inappropriately weakened and the overall functional effect can be made worse.

Medication may reduce some of the positive effects of the UMN syndrome but at the same time make some of the negative effects worse. The purpose and goals of medication need to be carefully annotated and the use of medication constantly reviewed.

Focal techniques

The need for intervention in spasticity is often concentrated on one or a few muscle groups. Thus, a focal approach is often more appropriate than the systemic effect induced by oral medication. In recent years there has been increasing value placed on focal techniques such as phenol and alcohol nerve blocks (see Chapter 8) and the use of botulinum toxin (see Chapter 9). The latter, in particular, is a remarkably safe and useful technique but once again it is important to emphasize that it is not often a technique in isolation but is simply part of an overall treatment package. For example, the use of botulinum can facilitate positioning in physiotherapy or ease the fitting of an orthosis. Fortunately botulinum is reversible over a period of two to three months which enables reappraisal and reassessment on a regular basis. Phenol nerve blocks are equally efficacious but more difficult to administer and there is the risk of a permanent effect. However, phenol is very significantly cheaper than botulinum toxin and thus is more relevant and practical in developing countries.

Intrathecal and surgical techniques

Occasionally spasticity is very resistant to intervention and further invasive techniques need to be considered. Intrathecal baclofen (see Chapter 10) is now a well recognized and relatively safe procedure. In some centres it is used in preference to other focal techniques such as botulinum toxin. The technique is generally safe although can occasionally be associated with unwanted complications such as pump failure, infection or movement of the catheter tip.

Finally, there is the possibility of surgical intervention (see Chapter 11). There are some surgical techniques, such as rhizotomy, which relieve spasticity in their own right but often surgery is now reserved for the unwanted complications of spasticity, particularly soft tissue contracture. If soft tissue contracture is advanced and disabling then there is often no option but to resort to surgical release and repositioning of the limb. However, it is probably true that if spasticity is treated appropriately and actively at the outset then it is only the very rare individual who will need surgery.

Overall we hope that this book gives a practical and straightforward account of the various treatment approaches to spasticity as well as emphasizing the importance of setting clear goals with clear outcome measures. We trust the book makes it clear that spasticity is a highly variable and dynamic phenomenon. Treatment needs careful planning, careful monitoring and above all the input and involvement not only of the physician, physiotherapist and orthotist but also of the person with the spasticity and their carer.

REFERENCES

Denny-Brown, D. (1966). *The cerebral control of movement*, pp. 170–84. Liverpool: Liverpool University Press.

Dickstein, R., Heffes, Y. & Abulaffio, N. (1996). Electromyographic and positional changes in the elbows of spastic hemiparetic patients during walking. *Electroenceph Clin Neurophysiol*, **101**: 491–6.

Dimitrijevic, M. R., Faganel, J., Sherwood, A. M. & McKay, W. B. (1981). Activation of paralysed leg flexors and extensors during gait in patients after stroke. *Scand J Rehab Med*, **13**: 109–15.

Fellows, S. J., Klaus, C., Ross, H. F. & Thilmann, A. F. (1994). Agonists and antagonist EMG activation during isometric torque development at the elbow in spastic hemiparesis. *Electroenceph Clin Neurophysiol*, **93**: 106–12.

Goldspink, G. & Williams, P. E. (1990). Muscle fibre and connective tissue changes associated with use and disuse. In ed. A. Ada & C. Canning, *Foundations for practice. Topics in neurological physiotherapy*, pp.197–218. London: Heinemann.

Lance, J. W. (1980). Symposium synopsis. In ed. R. G. Feldman, R. R. Young & W. P. Koella, *Spasticity: disorder of motor control*. Chicago: Year Book Medical Publishers, pp 485–94.

Medical Disability Society (1988). *The management of traumatic brain injury*. London: Development Trust for the Young Disabled.

O'Dwyer, N. J., Ada, L. & Neilson, P. D. (1996). Spasticity and muscle contracture following stroke. *Brain*, **119**: 1737–49.

Walshe, F. M. R. (1923). On certain tonic or postural reflexes in hemiplegia with special reference to the so-called 'associated movements'. *Brain*, **46**: 1–37.

2

Neurophysiology of spasticity

Geoff Sheean

Introduction

The pathophysiology of spasticity is a complex subject and one frequently avoided by clinicians. Some of the difficulties relate to the definition of spasticity and popular misconceptions regarding the role of the pyramidal tracts. On a more basic level, the lack of a very good animal model has been a problem for physiologists. None the less, a clear concept of the underlying neurophysiology will give clinicians a better understanding of their patients' clinical features and provide a valuable basis upon which to make management decisions.

Definition

Some of the difficulty that clinicians experience with understanding the pathophysiology of spasticity is due to the definition of spasticity. Most textbooks launch the discussion with a definition offered by Lance (1980) and generally accepted by physiologists:

'Spasticity is a motor disorder characterized by a velocity-dependent increase in tonic stretch reflexes ("muscle tone") with exaggerated tendon jerks, resulting from hyperexcitability of the stretch reflex, as one component of the upper motor neurone syndrome.'

It may be difficult for a clinician to correlate this definition with a typical patient pictured in his or her mind. They may see instead a patient with multiple sclerosis who has increased muscle tone in the legs, more in the extensors than in the flexors, that appears to increase with the speed of the testing movements. They also recall a clasp-knife phenomenon at the knee, tendon hyperreflexia with crossed adductor reflexes, ankle clonus, extensor plantar responses, a tendency for flexor spasms and, on occasions, extensor spasms. Or perhaps they picture the stroke patient with a hemiplegic posture, similar hypertonia in the upper limbs but more in the flexors, a tendency for extension of the whole leg when weight-bearing and increasing flexion of the arm as several steps are taken.

Lance's definition has been criticized for being too narrow by describing spasticity only as a form of hypertonia (Young, 1994). However, Lance's definition points out that this form of hypertonia is simply one component of the upper motor neurone (UMN) syndrome (see Table 1.1 in Chapter 1). The clinician tends to picture the whole UMN syndrome and regard all the 'positive' features of the syndrome as 'spasticity'. For example, increasing flexor spasms is often recorded as worsening spasticity. Because these positive features do tend to occur together, the clinician often uses the presence of these other signs (tendon hyperreflexia, extensor plantar responses, etc.) to conclude that a patient's hypertonia is spasticity rather than rigidity or dystonia.

However, these positive features do not always occur together and other factors may contribute to a patient's hypertonia. Furthermore, the pathophysiology of the positive features of the UMN syndrome is not uniform, as will be explained, and their response to drug treatment may also be different. Thus, there is merit in treating each of the positive features of the UMN syndrome as separate but overlapping entities and in particular to restrict the definition of spasticity to a type of hypertonia as Lance has done.

Overview

As a chapter on spasticity, the 'negative' features of the UMN syndrome such as weakness and loss of dexterity will not be discussed. The majority of the positive features of the UMN syndrome are due to exaggerated spinal reflexes. These reflexes are under supraspinal control, but are also influenced by other segmental inputs. The spinal mechanisms or circuitry effecting these spinal reflexes may be studied electrophysiologically. This discussion of the neurophysiology of spasticity will begin then with the descending motor pathways comprising the upper motor neurones that, when disrupted, produce the UMN syndrome. Following that, the spinal reflexes responsible for the clinical manifestations will be explained. This section will include the non-reflex or biomechanical factors that are of clinical importance. The final section will deal with the spinal mechanisms that may underlie the exaggerated spinal reflexes.

Descending pathways: upper motor neurones

Spasticity and the other features, positive and negative, of the UMN syndrome (as listed in Table 1.1) arise from disruption of certain descending pathways involved in motor control. These pathways control proprioceptive, cutaneous and nociceptive spinal reflexes, which become hyperactive and account for the majority of the positive features of the UMN syndrome.

Extensive work was done, mostly on animals, in the later part of the nineteenth century and the first half of the twentieth century to discover the critical cortical areas and motor tracts. These experiments involved making lesions or electrically stimulating areas of the central nervous system and observing the results. Human observations were usually afforded by disease or trauma and occasionally by stimulation. One of the difficulties with the animal studies, especially with cats, was in translating the findings to humans. Monkey and chimpanzee experiments are thought to have greater relevance. The studies chiefly focused on which areas of the central nervous system (CNS), when damaged, would produce motor disturbances and which other areas, when ablated or stimulated, would enhance or ameliorate the signs. Lesion studies, both clinical and experimental, may also be difficult to interpret given that the lesions may not be confined to the target area; histological confirmation has not always been available.

One early model was the decerebrate cat developed by Sherrington. A lesion between the superior and inferior colliculi resulted in an immediate increase in extensor (antigravity) tone. For several reasons this is not especially satisfactory as a model of human spasticity (Pierrot-Deseilligny & Mazieres, 1985; Burke, 1988). This vast body of work was reviewed by Denny-Brown (1966) and integrated with his findings. It has been excellently summarized by Brown (1994).

The pyramidal fibres arise from both pre-central (60%) and post-central (40%) cortical areas. Those controlling motor function within the spinal cord arise from the pre-central frontal cortex, the majority from the primary motor cortex (Brodmann area 4, 40%) and pre-motor cortex (area 6, 20%). Post-central areas (primary somatosensory cortex, areas 3, 1, 2, and parietal cortex, areas 5 and 7) contribute the remainder but these are more concerned with modulating sensory function (Rothwell, 1994). At a cortical level, isolated lesions in monkeys and apes of the primary motor cortex (area 4) uncommonly produce spasticity. Rather, tone and tendon reflexes are more often reduced. It seems that lesions must also involve the premotor cortex (area 6) to produce spasticity. Such lesions made bilaterally in monkeys are associated with greater spasticity indicating a bilateral contribution to tone control. Subcortical lesions at points where the motor fibres from both areas of the cortex have converged (e.g. internal capsule) are more likely to cause spasticity. Even here, though, some slight separation of the primary motor cortex (posterior limb) and pre-motor cortex (genu) fibres allows for lesions with and without spasticity (Fries et al., 1993).

Although both cortical areas 4 and 6 must be affected to produce spasticity and both contribute to the pyramidal tracts, isolated lesions of the pyramidal tracts in the medullary pyramids (and in the spinal cord) do not produce spasticity. Hence, there are non-pyramidal UMN motor fibres arising in the cortex, chiefly in the premotor cortex (area 6), that travel near the pyramidal fibres which must also be involved for the production of spasticity. It is debatable whether these other motor pathways should be called extrapyramidal or parapyramidal. Denny-Brown (1966) preferred the former but I favour the latter, as does Burke (1988), to emphasize their close anatomical location to the pyramidal fibres and to avoid confusion with the extrapyramidal fibres from the basal ganglia that produce rigidity. This close association of pyramidal and parapyramidal fibres continues in the spinal cord where lesions confined to the lateral corticospinal tract (pyramidal fibres) produce results similar to those of the primary motor cortex and medullary pyramids, without spasticity. More extensive lesions of the lateral funiculus add spasticity and tendon hyperreflexia.

Given these findings, just what are the consequences of a pure pyramidal lesion? In primates, there is only a loss of digital dexterity (Phillips & Porter, 1977) and, in humans, mild hand and foot weakness, mild tendon hyperreflexia, normal tone and an extensor plantar response (Bucy et al., 1964; van Gijn, 1978). Although there are reports that suggest that spasticity might arise from 'pure' lesions, such as strokes, of the pyramidal tracts (Souza et al., 1988, abstract in English), there is always the concern that these lesions might really have affected adjacent parapyramidal fibres to some degree. Thus, the bulk of the UMN syndrome, both positive and negative features, is not really due to interruption of the pyramidal tracts, save perhaps for the extensor plantar response, but of the parapyramidal fibres (Burke, 1988). Although this implies that the term 'pyramidal' syndrome is a misnomer, it is so ingrained in clinical terminology that to attempt to remove it appears pedantic.

Brainstem areas controlling spinal reflexes

The following discussion is readily agreed to be somewhat simplistic but is conceptually correct. From the brainstem arise two balanced systems for control of spinal reflexes, one inhibitory and the other excitatory (Figure 2.1). These are anatomically separate and also differ with respect to suprabulbar (cortical) control.

Inhibitory system

The parapyramidal fibres arising from the premotor cortex are cortico-reticular and facilitate an important inhibitory area in the medulla, just dorsal to the pyramids, known as the ventromedial reticular formation (Brown, 1994). Electrical stimulation of this area inhibits the patella reflex of intact cats. In decerebrate cats, the previously rigid legs become flaccid (Magoun & Rhines, 1947), and muscle tone is reduced in cats that have been made spastic with chronic cerebral lesions (cited in Magoun & Rhines, 1947). In the early spastic stage of experimental poliomyelitis in monkeys, the most severe damage was found in this region (Bodian, 1946). Stimulation of this region in intact cats also inhibits the tonic vibration reflex (to be discussed later). Flexor reflex afferents are also inhibited (Whitlock, 1990) (see below). That this inhibitory centre is under cortical control was verified by the

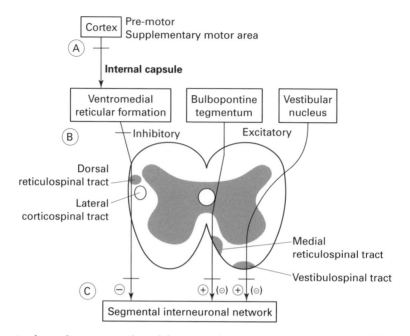

Fig. 2.1   A schematic representation of the major descending systems exerting inhibitory and
excitatory supraspinal control over spinal reflex activity. The anatomical relations and the
differences with respect to cortical control between the two systems means that
anatomical location of the upper motor neurone lesion plays a large role in the
determination of the resulting clinical pattern. (A): Lesion affecting the corticospinal fibres
and the cortico-reticular fibres facilitating the main inhibitory system, the dorsal
reticulospinal tract. (B): An incomplete spinal cord lesion affecting the corticospinal fibres
and the dorsal reticulospinal tract. (C): Complete spinal cord lesion affecting the
corticospinal fibres, dorsal reticulospinal tract and the excitatory pathways. (+) indicates
an excitatory or facilitatory pathway and (−) an inhibitory pathway. The excitatory
pathways have inhibitory effects on flexor reflexes. (From Sheean, 1998a.)

finding of potentiation of some of these effects by stimulation of the premotor
cortex or internal capsule (Andrews et al., 1973a,b). There may also be some cerebellar input (Lindsley et al., 1949). The descending output of this area is the dorsal
reticulospinal tract located in the dorsolateral funiculus (Engberg et al., 1968).

Excitatory system

Higher in the brainstem is a diffuse and extensive area that appears to facilitate
spinal stretch reflexes. Stimulation studies suggest that its origin is in the sub- and
hypothalamus (basal diencephalon), with efferent connections passing through
and receiving contributions from the central grey and tegmentum of the midbrain,
pontine tegmentum and bulbar (medullary) reticular formation (separate from the

inhibitory area above). Stimulation of this area in intact monkeys enhances the patella reflex (Magoun & Rhines, 1947) and increases reflexes and extensor tone and produces clonus in the chronic cerebral spastic cat as already discussed (see 'Inhibitory system') (Magoun & Rhines, 1947). Lesions through the bulbopontine tegmentum alleviate spasticity (Schreiner et al., 1949). Although input is said to come from the somatosensory cortex and possibly the supplementary motor area (SMA)(Whitlock, 1990), stimulation of the motor cortex and internal capsule does not change the facilitatory effects of this region (Andrews et al., 1973a,b). Thus, this excitatory area seems under less cortical control than its inhibitory counterpart. Its descending output is through the medial reticulospinal tracts in the ventromedial cord (Brown, 1994).

The lateral vestibular nucleus is another region facilitating extensor tone, situated in the medulla close to the junction with the pons. Stimulation produces disynaptic excitation of extensor motoneurones (Rothwell, 1994). Its output is via the lateral vestibulospinal tract, located in the ventromedial cord near the medial reticulospinal tract. Although long recognized as important in decerebrate rigidity, it appears less important in spasticity. An isolated lesion here has little effect on spasticity in cats (Schreiner et al., 1949) but enhances the anti-spastic effect of bulbopontine tegmentum lesions. Similarly, lesions of the vestibulospinal tracts performed to reduce spasticity had only a transient effect (Bucy, 1938).

Although both areas are considered excitatory and facilitate spinal stretch reflexes, they also inhibit flexor reflex afferents (Liddell et al., 1932; Whitlock, 1990), which mediate flexor spasms (see below). The lateral vestibulospinal tract also inhibits flexor motoneurones (Rothwell, 1994).

Other motor pathways descending from the brainstem

Rubrospinal tract

Despite its undoubted role in normal motor control in the cat, there is some doubt about the importance and even existence of a rubrospinal tract in humans (Nathan & Smith, 1955). In cats, this tract is well developed and runs close to the pyramidal fibres in the spinal cord. It facilitates flexor and inhibits extensor motoneurones (Rothwell, 1994) via interneurones. In contrast in humans, very few cells are present in the area of the red nucleus that gives rise to this tract. However, the rubro-olivary connections are better developed in humans than in the cat (Rothwell, 1994).

Coerulospinal tract

The clinical benefits of drugs such as clonidine (Nance et al., 1989) and tizanidine (Emre et al., 1994) and of therapeutic stimulation of the locus coeruleus (Feinstein et al., 1989) have refocused attention on the noradrenergic coerulospinal system. The locus coeruleus resides in the dorsolateral pontine tegmentum and gives rise to the coerulospinal tract. Coerulospinal fibres terminate in the cervical and lumbar regions and appear to facilitate presynaptic inhibition of flexor reflex afferents (Whitlock, 1990). As tizanidine reduces spasticity as well as flexor spasms, it must also modulate spinal stretch reflexes. However, there is no evidence that the coerulospinal tracts play a role in the production of spasticity or flexor spasms. Degeneration of the locus coeruleus is also seen in Parkinson's disease and Shy-Drager syndrome and neither have spasticity as a sign. Furthermore, the putative mechanism of tizanidine in spasticity is such that would be mimicked by increased coerulospinal activity. However, the coerulospinal tract appears to provide excitatory drive to alpha motoneurones (Fung & Barnes, 1986) and inhibit Renshaw cell recurrent inhibition (Fung et al., 1988), effects which would be expected to increase stretch reflexes.

Descending motor pathways in the spinal cord

As indicated above, the principal descending motor tracts within the spinal cord in the production of spasticity are the inhibitory dorsal reticulospinal tract and the excitatory median reticulospinal (MRT) and vestibulospinal tracts (VST) (Figure 2.1). As has already been discussed, isolated lesions of the lateral corticospinal (pyramidal) tract in monkeys do not produce spasticity but rather hypotonia, hyporeflexia and loss of cutaneous reflexes. Extending the lesion to involve more of the lateral funiculus (and hence the dorsal reticulospinal tract) results in spasticity and tendon hyperreflexia (Brown, 1994). Similar lesion of the dorsal half of the lateral funiculus produced similar results in humans (Putnam, 1940). Curiously though, bilateral lesions of the intermediate portion of the lateral column resulted in tendon hyperreflexia, ankle clonus and Babinski signs immediately, but rarely spasticity. Brown (1994) points out, however, that there was no histological confirmation of the extent of these lesions. In the cat, dorsolateral spinal lesions including the dorsal reticulospinal tract (DRT) produce spasticity and extensor plantar responses (Babinski sign) but not clonus or flexor spasms (Taylor et al., 1997). Furthermore, these positive UMN features appeared rapidly. These results support the idea that the DRT is critical in the production of spasticity in humans and also show that lesions in the region can result in restricted forms of the UMN syndrome, especially the dissociation of tendon hyperreflexia and spasticity.

Concerning lesions of the excitatory pathways made in an attempt to reduce spasticity, cordotomies of the anterior portions of the ventral columns to interrupt the vestibulospinal tracts were only transiently successful in reducing spasticity in the legs (Bucy, 1938). These lesions were said to spare the deeper sulcal regions where the medial reticulospinal tract resides. After more extensive cordotomies were performed, which included these tracts, and following a period of flaccidity, spasticity was markedly reduced but tendon hyperreflexia, clonus and adductor spasms persisted. These findings reinforce the more dominant role that the MRT plays and the relatively less important role of the VST, and once again illustrates that the positive feature of the UMN syndrome may occur independently. Furthermore, these findings in humans tend to support the ideas on the pathophysiology of spasticity developed from animals.

In summary, cortical lesions producing spasticity must involve both the primary motor and pre-motor cortices. Such lesions affect both pyramidal and parapyramidal cortico-reticular fibres, which run adjacent to each other in the corona radiata and internal capsule. Conceptually, there is a system of balanced control of spinal reflexes that arises within the brainstem. There is an inhibitory area in the medullary reticular formation that largely suppresses spinal reflex activity. This region receives cortical facilitation from the motor cortex (mainly pre-motor) via cortico-reticular fibres, which comprises the suprabulbar portion of the inhibitory system. The output of this medullary inhibitory centre is the DRT, which runs in the dorsolateral funiculus, adjacent to the lateral corticospinal (pyramidal) tract. Two other areas comprise the excitatory system that facilitates spinal stretch reflexes and extensor tone. The main one arises diffusely throughout the brainstem and descends as the MRT. The other is the lateral vestibular nucleus, giving rise to the VST. Both are located in the ventromedial cord, well away from the lateral corticospinal tract and the inhibitory DRT.

Thus, spasticity arises when the parapyramidal fibres of the inhibitory system are interrupted, either of the cortico-reticular fibres above the level of the medulla (cortex, corona radiata, internal capsule) or of the DRT in the spinal cord. Theoretically, isolated lesions of the inhibitory medullary reticular formation could do the same but, as Brown (1994) points out, strokes in this area tend to be fatal. It is attractive to presume that spasticity develops in this situation simply as a result of the effects of the excitatory system, which is now unbalanced by the loss of the inhibitory system, but the situation is not so simple (see 'Mechanism of the change in excitability of the spinal reflexes').

Clinico-pathological correlation

The clinical picture of the UMN syndrome seems to depend less upon the aetiology of the lesion and more upon its location in the neuraxis. It has been long recognized that the UMN syndrome following cerebral lesions is somewhat different to that of spinal lesions. Similarly, there are differences between partial or incomplete spinal lesions and complete lesions. With cerebral lesions, spasticity tends to be less severe and more often involves the extensors with a posture of lower limb extension. Flexor spasms are rare and the clasp-knife phenomenon is uncommon.

Clonus tends also to be less severe. In contrast, spinal lesions can have very severe spasticity, more often in flexors with a dominant posture of lower limb flexion (paraplegia in flexion) and prominent flexor spasms, also clasp-knife phenomenon is more common, as is clonus.

The pathophysiological substrate for these differences may reside in three factors. The existence of cortico-reticular drive to the inhibitory brainstem centre, the anatomical separateness of the inhibitory and excitatory tracts in the spinal cord and the fact that both the excitatory and inhibitory systems inhibit flexor reflex afferents, which are responsible for flexor spasms.

A suprabulbar lesion, say, in the internal capsule, would deprive the inhibitory brainstem centre of its cortical facilitation. This inhibitory centre could, however, continue to contribute some inhibition of spinal stretch reflexes and flexor reflex afferents. With a partial reduction in inhibitory drive, the excitatory system would still dominate, facilitating extensors while also inhibiting flexor reflex afferents. Hence, the whole syndrome would be milder in form and more extensor in type with few flexor spasms.

The chief clinical difference between complete and incomplete spinal cord lesions is that incomplete lesions more often show a dominant extensor tone and posture with more extensor spasms than flexor spasms, as opposed to the complete spinal lesion, which is strongly flexor (Barolat & Maiman, 1987). An incomplete cord lesion might affect the lateral columns (including the inhibitory DRT) and spare the ventral columns (along with the excitatory system). Thus, the incomplete cord lesion would abolish all inhibition of spinal stretch reflexes and leave the excitatory system unopposed to drive extensor tone but still inhibit flexor reflex afferents ('paraplegia-in-extension'). With complete spinal cord lesions, all supraspinal control is lost, and both stretch reflexes and flexor reflex afferents are completely disinhibited; a strong flexor pattern follows ('paraplegia-in-flexion').

Mechanism of the change in excitability of the spinal reflexes

The above outline of a balanced system of suprasegmental inhibitory and excitatory influences on spinal segmental reflexes could imply that the increased excitability of spinal reflexes is simply a matter of release or disinhibition. However, following acute UMN lesions there is frequently a variable period of reduced spinal reflex activity ('shock') and it is only following resolution of this that hyperactive reflexes appear. This raises the possibility that some structural and/or functional reorganization within the CNS ('plasticity') is responsible. The human CNS has been shown to be quite capable of such plasticity involving both motor and sensory pathways following limb amputation (e.g. Elbert et al., 1994; Chen et al., 1998) and brain injury (Nirkko et al., 1997). For the somatosensory pathways, reorganization occurs at cortical, brainstem and spinal levels (Florence & Kaas, 1995). Possible contributory processes include collateral sprouting of axons, receptor hypersensitivity following 'denervation' (Brown, 1994) and unmasking of previously silent synapses (Borsook et al., 1998). The idea of collateral sprouting as the basis of spasticity was first proposed by McCouch more than 40 years ago (McCouch et al., 1958), but later reports that the CNS was capable of sprouting were disputed (Noth, 1991). Subsequently, better evidence appeared that axon terminals in the mammalian spinal cord could sprout and form new synapses (Hulsebosch & Coggeshall, 1981; Krenz & Weaver, 1998). Burke (1988) believes that new synapses may simply act to reinforce existing spinal circuits rather than create entirely new circuits, a quantitative rather than a qualitative change. Thus, the positive features of the UMN syndrome involve two main mechanisms: (1) disruption of descending control of spinal pathways; and (2) structural and/or functional re-organization at the spinal level (Pierrot-Deseilligny & Mazieres, 1985).

In some patients, hyperactive reflexes appear remarkably quickly, lending some credence to the idea of a 'release' effect. In support of this, CNS plasticity has been seen within 24 hours of human limb amputation (Borsook et al., 1998); such rapidity suggests the unmasking of silent connections, rather than the formation of new ones. In addition, electrical stimulation of skin overlying the spastic biceps can produce longer lasting reductions in spasticity, indicating a therapeutically useful short-term plasticity (Dewald et al., 1996).

The mechanism of reduced spinal reflexes in spinal shock deserves some discussion in this context. It has been proposed that plasticity may play a role, involving down-regulation of receptors (Bach-y-Rita & Illis, 1993). Recovery from spinal shock could involve up-regulation of receptors, making them more sensitive to neurotransmitters (Bach-y-Rita & Illis, 1993). The supersensitivity of spinal interneurones involved in extensor reflexes to monoamines in chronic spinal rats compared with the acute preparation is an example of this (Ito et al., 1985). Non-synaptic transmission could also play a role in spinal shock and its recovery (Bach-y-Rita & Illis, 1993).

There may be some additional therapeutic relevance to understanding the underlying cellular processes behind the hyperreflexia of the UMN syndrome (Noth, 1991). If collateral sprouting is responsible, it may be possible to inhibit this process (Schwab, 1990).

Spinal segmental reflexes

Hyperexcitability of spinal reflexes forms the basis of most of the 'positive' clinical signs of the UMN syndrome, which have in common excessive muscle activity. These spinal reflexes may be divided into two groups: proprioceptive reflexes; and cutaneous and nociceptive reflexes (Table 2.1). Proprioceptive reflexes include

Table 2.1. Classification of positive features of upper motor neurone syndrome by pathophysiological mechanism

A. Afferent – disinhibited spinal reflexes
1. Proprioceptive (stretch) reflexes
      Spasticity (tonic)
      Tendon hyperreflexia and clonus (phasic)
      Clasp-knife reaction
      Positive support reaction?
2. Cutaneous and nociceptive reflexes
      (a) Flexor withdrawal reflexes
            Flexor spasms
            Clasp-knife reaction (with tonic stretch reflex)
            Babinski sign
      (b) Extensor reflexes
            Extensor spasms
            Positive support reaction

B. Efferent – tonic supraspinal drive?
      Spastic dystonia?
      Associated reactions/synkinesia?
      Co-contraction?

stretch reflexes (tonic and phasic) and the positive supporting reaction. Nociceptive/cutaneous reflexes include flexor and extensor reflexes (including the complex Babinski sign). The clasp-knife phenomenon combines features of both groups, at least in the lower limbs.

Proprioceptive stretch reflexes

Proprioception is the sensory information about movement and position of bodily parts and is mediated in the limbs by muscle spindles. Stretch of muscle spindles causes a discharge of their sensory afferents that synapse directly with and excite the motoneurones in the spinal cord innervating the stretched muscle. This stretch reflex arc is the basis of the deep tendon reflex, referred to as a phasic stretch reflex because the duration of stretch is very brief. Reflex muscle contractions evoked by longer stretches of the muscle, such as during clinical testing of muscle tone, are referred to as tonic stretch reflexes. The positive support reaction may be in part due to stretch of muscle proprioceptors in the foot (Bobath, 1990).

Phasic stretch reflexes

The clinical signs arising from hyperexcitability of phasic stretch reflexes include deep tendon hyperreflexia, irradiation of tendon reflexes and clonus. The traditional view is that percussion of the tendon causes a brief muscle stretch, a synchronous discharge of the muscle spindles and an incoming synchronized volley of Ia afferent activity that monosynaptically excites alpha motoneurones. However, Burke (1988) points out that the situation is more complex. The following summarizes his explanation. In addition to muscle stretch, the percussion of a tendon causes a wave of vibration through the limb that is also capable of stimulating muscle spindles in the muscle percussed, as well as others in the limb. This is the basis of tendon reflex 'irradiation', discussed later. Spindle activity from these other muscles could contribute to the tendon reflex. Furthermore, percussion also stimulates mechanoreceptors in the skin and other muscles. The discharge from the muscle spindles evoked by percussion is far from synchronous and spindles may fire repetitively. Finally, the reflex is unlikely to be solely monosynaptic. The rise time observed in the excitability of the soleus motoneurones following Achilles tendon percussion is around 10 ms, which is ample time for oligo- or polysynaptic pathways to be involved. These do exist for the Ia afferents and could include those from the percussed muscle as well as from other muscles in the limb excited by the percussion. Cutaneous and other mechanoreceptor afferents also have polysynaptic connections. H reflexes are commonly used to examine the phasic stretch reflex pathways in the UMN syndrome and considered equivalent to the tendon reflex. This is not the case for many of these same reasons (see 'Electrophysiological studies of spinal reflexes in spasticity').

In the UMN syndrome, percussion of one tendon often produces similar brief reflex contractions of other muscles in the limb, a phenomenon known as reflex irradiation. This is not due to the opening up of synaptic connections between various muscles in the limb (Burke, 1988) but to a simpler mechanism. As mentioned, tendon percussion sets up a wave of vibration through the limb that is capable of exciting spindles in other muscles (Lance & De Gail, 1965; Burke et al., 1983). If the stretch reflexes of those muscles are also hyperexcitable, phasic stretch reflexes will be evoked.

Clonus is a rhythmic, often self-sustaining contraction evoked by rapid muscle stretch, best seen in the UMN syndrome at the ankle, provoked by a brisk, passive dorsiflexion. It tends to accompany marked tendon hyperreflexia and responds similarly to factors which reduce hyperreflexia (Whitlock, 1990). The rhythmicity suggested a central oscillatory generator, an idea supported by the inability to modify the frequency by external factors (Walsh, 1976; Dimitrijevic et al., 1980). However, Rack and colleagues found that the frequency of the ankle clonus did vary with the imposed load, as had also been found at other joints countering the central oscillator notion (Rack et al., 1984). By changing the mechanical load, the frequency of spontaneous ankle clonus in spastic patients could vary from 2.5 Hz to 5.7 Hz. It was also possible to inhibit clonus with strong loads. Load-dependent spontaneous clonus could also be induced in normal subjects (after prolonged sinusoidal joint movements) at similar frequencies. This is no surprise as a great many normal people have experienced ankle clonus at some stage in their lives under certain conditions. The conclusion drawn by Rack et al. (1984) was that clonus is a manifestation of increased gain of the normal stretch reflex and that central mechanisms are less dominant in determining the frequency of clonus.

The mechanism underlying clonus is similar to that of tendon hyperreflexia, increased excitability of the phasic stretch reflex. A rapid dorsiflexion of the ankle by an examiner produces a brisk stretch of the gastrocnemius-soleus. A reflex contraction in the gastrocnemius-soleus is elicited, plantarflexing the ankle. This relieves the stretch, abolishing the stimulus to the stretch reflex and so the muscle relaxes. If this relaxation is sufficiently rapid while the examiner maintains a dorsiflexing force, another stretch reflex will be elicited and the ankle again plantarflexes. Thus, a rhythmic pattern of contraction and relaxation is set-up that will often continue for as long as the dorsiflexion force is maintained, referred to as sustained clonus. However, unsustained clonus can also occur in UMN lesions. Burke (1988) comments that much of the eliciting and maintaining of clonus lies in the skilled technique of the examiner and, as Rack et al. (1984) noted, it was possible to suppress clonus with stronger loads.

Tonic stretch reflexes

Muscle tone is tested clinically by passive movement of a joint with the muscles relaxed and refers to the resistance to this movement felt by the examiner. The hallmark of the UMN syndrome is a form of hypertonia, called spasticity. It had been observed clinically that slow movements would often not reveal hypertonia but faster movements would, and that thereafter this resistance increased with the speed of the passive movements. Electromyographically such resistance correlated with the reflex contraction of the stretched muscle which opposes the stretch (Herman, 1970). These contractions of stretched muscle are referred to as tonic stretch reflexes to distinguish them from the brief stretches that elicit phasic stretch reflexes. Tonic stretch reflexes have also been studied during active muscle contraction, in part to determine the role that hyperexcitability of such reflexes might play in the impairment of movement in the UMN syndrome (v.i.).

In an elegant experiment, Thilmann and colleagues (1991a) found stretch reflexes in the relaxed biceps in only half their normal subjects (Figure 2.2) and then only with very fast movements; the threshold was an angular velocity of around 200° per second. The latency of the reflex was 61–107 ms, some of which probably includes the time it takes for the mechanical displacement of the elbow to stretch the muscle and excite the spindles (Rothwell, 1994). The reflex contraction was brief and was not maintained throughout the stretching movement and is probably a phasic stretch reflex, analogous to the tendon reflex (Rothwell, 1994).

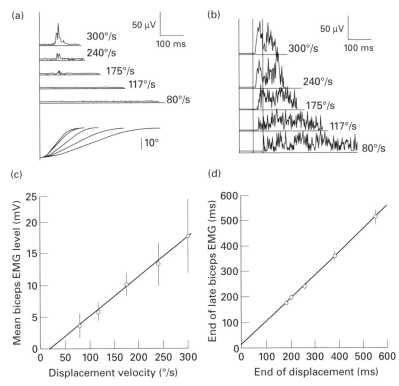

Fig. 2.2   Surface electromyography (EMG) recordings of the biceps during passive displacements of the elbow of various angular velocities. (a): Normal subjects. No EMG activity (stretch reflex) is elicited until very fast displacements are made (175°/s and faster). The reflex responses then are brief and terminate before the movement is complete (angular displacement represented below). (b): Spastic subjects show stretch reflexes, even at low angular velocities, which continue for the duration of the movement. (c): The magnitude of the EMG response increases linearly with the speed of the movement. (From Thilmann et al., 1991a.)

This was an important finding because it indicated that there is no stretch reflex at the velocities of movement usually used to test tone in normal, relaxed muscle (much slower than 200° per second). Thus, tonic stretch reflexes do not contribute to muscle tone, which therefore must come from the viscoelastic properties of the muscle. This will be discussed later in more detail.

The situation was found to be quite different in hemiparetic spastic (stroke) patients (Thilmann et al., 1991a) in whom stretch reflexes could be elicited with relatively slow movements – as slow as 35° per second. Reflex activity usually began at a relatively constant latency, at the end of the 61–107 ms window found in normal subjects. However, it continued throughout the stretching movement and usually stopped just before the end of the displacement. No electromyographic (EMG) activity was seen when the stretch was held at the end of the displacing movement. That is, there was no *static* stretch reflex. Thus, in this study, as in others (Rushworth, 1960; Burke et al., 1970; Herman, 1970; Ashby & Burke, 1971; Burke et al., 1972), spasticity was found to be an exclusively *dynamic* tonic stretch reflex. Other researchers have found otherwise (Powers et al., 1989)(see 'Static tonic reflexes' below). Some variation between patients was seen with faster rates of displacement producing shorter latency activity within the 61–107 ms 'normal' window in some and very slow velocities having much longer latencies (up to 400 ms) in others. The amount of reflex muscle contraction showed a positive linear correlation with the velocity of stretch, thus confirming that spasticity is velocity-dependent (Burke et al., 1970; Ashby & Burke, 1971; Burke et al., 1972; Powers et al., 1989). Hemiparetic patients without spasticity behaved similarly to the normal subjects.

The fact that tonic stretch reflex is not present in normal subjects raises the question of whether it is an entirely new reflex arising after an UMN lesion or an increase in excitability of an existing, dormant one. If it is the latter, is the mechanism a decrease in threshold or an increase in gain? The case for each has been argued (Powers et al., 1988, 1989; Thilmann et al., 1991a) and it has even been suggested that stretch reflex gain in spastic ankles is at the high end of the normal range (Rack et al., 1984). The absence of the reflex in normal subjects, even at rates as high as 500° per second (Ashby & Burke, 1971), would suggest an implausibly high threshold (Thilmann et al., 1991a). Against increased gain and in favour of a decreased threshold, both spastic patients and controls showed similar stretch reflex gains during active elbow flexion, a state assumed to eliminate threshold differences (Powers et al., 1989). This and similar measures of the stretch reflex during voluntary contraction are not valid assessments of spasticity however, which, by definition, requires the muscle to be at rest. Finally, arguments over the relative differences in stretch reflex gain between relaxed normal and spastic muscles may really be pointless given that such a reflex is not even present in normal subjects. As Thilmann et al. (1991a) point out, 'a qualitatively new reflex is present in the spastic subjects'.

Irrespective of whether the basic alteration is increased gain or decreased threshold, the common finding is that spasticity is due to hyperactive tonic stretch reflexes that are velocity-sensitive. There is still a threshold velocity of displacement however, as a slow movement will not elicit a reflex. Thilmann et al. (1991a) found this could be as low as 35° per second in the biceps, while a higher threshold of 100° per second has been found in the quadriceps (Burke et al., 1970). The long latency of these reflexes, even accounting for delays due to mechanical factors, suggests a polysynaptic pathway. There is good evidence that Ia afferents are linked by oligo- and polysynaptic pathways to their homonymous alpha motoneurones (Burke, 1988; Mailis

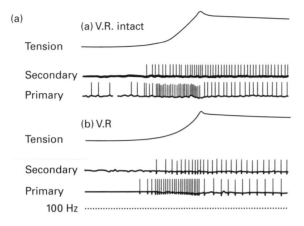

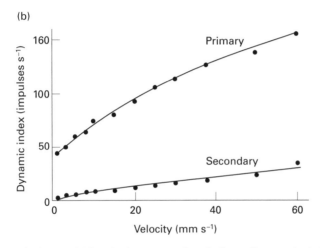

Fig. 2.3   Velocity sensitivity of primary muscle spindle endings and relative insensitivity of secondary spindle endings. (a): Spindle afferent discharges with and without fusimotor drive (V.R.=ventral root). Note the dynamic sensitivity of the primary spindle endings during the course of the stretch. Note also that both spindle endings continue to discharge in the hold phase of the stretch, particularly the secondary spindle endings, indicating that both are sensitive to length changes as well as velocity. (b): Graphic representation of the velocity-sensitivity of each spindle ending, expressed as the dynamic index. (From Matthews, 1972.)

& Ashby, 1990). Group II afferents also have polysynaptic connections and may contribute to muscle stretch reflexes (see 'Group II polysynaptic excitatory pathways').

The velocity-dependence of these stretch reflexes has been attributed to the fact that primary muscle spindles are velocity-sensitive (Herman, 1970; Dietrichson, 1971, 1973; Rothwell, 1994; Figure 2.3). In cats, fusimotor drive increases the velocity-sensitivity but fusimotor drive is not increased in human spasticity (Burke,

1983). This explanation has been challenged by results that show the velocity-sensitivity of spasticity is quite weak and non-linear (Powers et al., 1989). An alternative explanation relies upon the dependence of the motoneurone firing threshold upon the rate of change of the depolarizing current (Powers et al., 1989).

The clasp-knife phenomenon

This well-known clinical sign has as its basis a hyperexcitable tonic stretch reflex. A fast passive movement of a joint in a relaxed limb, usually knee flexion or elbow extension, encounters a gradual build-up of resistance that opposes the movement momentarily before apparently suddenly melting away, allowing continuing stretch with relative ease (Figure 2.4). The rapid build-up of resistance is spasticity, through the mechanisms already discussed. The apparently sudden decline in the stretch reflex was initially attributed to the sudden appearance of inhibition from the Golgi tendon organs (via Ib afferents), as a means to protect the muscle from dangerously high tension. It had been thought that these organs fire only at high muscle tension. However, it was later discovered that Golgi tendon organs actually have quite low tension thresholds (Houk & Henneman, 1967 cited in Rothwell, 1994). Furthermore, the inhibition of the stretch reflex extends well beyond the reduction in tension; Golgi tendon organs cease firing once the tension is relieved (Rothwell, 1994; Figure 2.5). Finally, there is evidence of *reduced* Ib inhibitory activity in some cases of spasticity (see 'Ib non-reciprocal inhibition'). It is unlikely then that Ib inhibitory activity from the Golgi tendon organs plays much of a role in the clasp-knife phenomenon (Rothwell, 1994).

The mechanism of the decline in stretch-reflex activity that gives rise to the apparently sudden release may be due to two factors. The first is the velocity-sensitivity of the stretch reflex. The resistance produced by the stretch reflex slows the movement, which reduces the stimulus responsible for it to below threshold, the reflex contraction stops and the resistance declines. Burke (1988) believes that this is all that is required for the clasp-knife phenomenon in the biceps brachii but this reasoning does not explain why the continuing movement after the 'release' does not once again evoke a stretch reflex. The clasp-knife phenomenon is seen better in the quadriceps where the second factor also applies (Burke, 1988). Here, as well as in the ankle plantarflexors (Meinders et al., 1996), the tonic stretch reflex seems not only velocity-dependent but also length-dependent, being less sensitive at longer lengths (Figure 2.4). Thus, there is not only declining velocity during the movement but also increasing length. A critical point is reached where these two factors combine to reduce the effective stimulus to the stretch reflex, which suddenly ceases. Continuing movement does not again evoke a stretch reflex because the reflex is relatively insensitive at this longer length. While the resistance seems to suddenly melt away, the mechanism is really that of a gradually declining stimulus (velocity) and

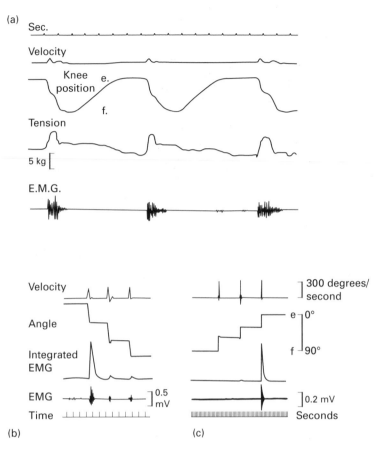

Fig. 2.4   (a): The clasp-knife phenomenon at the knee. The subject is supine and the knee is
passively flexed while surface electromyography (EMG) is recorded from the quadriceps
and force exerted by the examiner's hand at the ankle (reflecting muscle tension). Passive
flexion elicits a tonic stretch reflex, associated with a rapid build-up of tension
(resistance). This abruptly declines (clasp-knife phenomenon), coincident with the
cessation of the tonic stretch reflex. (b) and (c): Length-dependent sensitivity of the tonic
stretch reflex in the quadriceps (b) and the hamstrings (c). Muscle stretches are
performed at increasing length of the muscle. In the quadriceps (b), the maximum reflex
is elicited at the first step, with declining responses with increasing muscle length. The
opposite is seen in the hamstrings (c), where a tonic stretch reflex is not elicited until the
muscle is at nearly full stretch. (From Burke & Lance, 1973.)

stretch reflex sensitivity (length). The length-dependent sensitivity of the stretch
reflex appears to be due to length-dependent inhibition of the stretch reflex by a
group of sensory fibres known as flexor reflex afferents (FRA), which will be discussed later in more detail. In contrast to the quadriceps, stretch reflexes in the hamstrings are more sensitive at longer lengths (Figure 2.4; Burke and Lance, 1973).

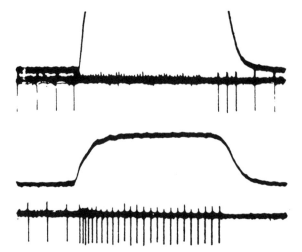

Fig. 2.5   Demonstrating the sensitivity of Golgi tendon organs to small tensions. Two recordings from stimulation of motor axons to the soleus muscle of a cat. The upper trace of each recording represents the force in the tendon, and the lower trace the tendon organ Ib afferent discharge. The lower recording shows a vigorous discharge of the tendon organ, despite the weak contraction. The upper recording, from a stronger contraction, shows an initial discharge of Golgi tendon organ afferents, with subsequent cessation due to unloading of the receptor by contraction of neighbouring motor units. (From Houk & Henneman, 1967.)

Static tonic stretch reflexes

As mentioned earlier, the stretch reflexes underlying spasticity have been regarded as dynamic, that is, present only when the joint is moving. Thilmann and colleagues (1991a) found that the stretch reflex usually declined towards the end of the movement as the velocity declined and if the muscle was held in stretch at this point, there was no EMG activity. Thus, it has been considered that there is no appreciable static component to the tonic stretch reflex of spasticity.

However, various researchers have observed clear reflex activity in the maintained phase of a ramp-and-hold stretch of elbow flexors (Figure 2.6; Denny-Brown, 1966; Powers et al., 1989; Sheean, 1998a). Several methodological reasons why such reflex activity might have been missed in previous studies have been suggested (Powers et al., 1989). One obvious reason for its absence in the quadriceps might be length-dependent inhibition responsible in part for the clasp-knife phenomenon mentioned earlier. The situation may be truly different at the ankle, where static stretch reflexes have not been seen (Herman, 1970; Berardelli et al., 1983; Hufschmidt & Mauritz, 1985).

The mechanism of static tonic stretch reflexes presumably involves receptors that are chiefly sensitive to muscle length and not velocity. The primary muscle spindles

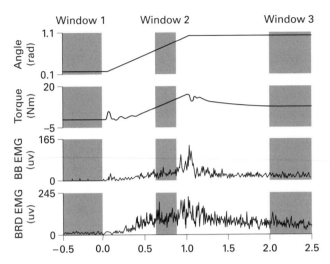

Fig. 2.6   Static tonic stretch reflexes in the spastic biceps brachii (BB) and brachioradialis (BRD).
Passive extension of the elbow (1 radian stretch at 1 radian/sec) elicits a tonic stretch
reflex during the ramp portion of the stretch (dynamic tonic stretch reflex). The rectified
surface EMG activity continues, especially in the brachioradialis, during the ramp phase of
the stretch after the movement has stopped (static tonic stretch reflex). (From Powers et
al., 1989.)

(with Ia afferents) are sensitive to both, but mainly to velocity (Rothwell, 1994).
The secondary muscle spindles, via the slower conducting group II afferents, maintain an increased firing level over baseline for as long as the muscle is held stretched
and would be suitable candidates. Some evidence from comparative therapeutic
and electrophysiological studies of baclofen and tizanidine in spinal cats suggests a
role of group II afferents in spasticity (Skoog, 1996). Both agents are equally
effective at reducing spasticity. Baclofen strongly depressed group I potentials but
had inconsistent effects on group II potentials. In contrast, tizanidine strongly
depressed the amplitude of monosynaptic field potentials in the spinal cord caused
by group II afferents with little effect on group I potentials. Additionally, L-dopa,
which depresses transmission from group II but not group I afferents, reduces spasticity, tendon hyperreflexia and clonus in humans with spinal cord injuries
(Eriksson et al., 1996). However, the depressed long-latency stretch reflexes of the
upper limb in the UMN syndrome suggests a reduced effect of group II afferents.

Burke suggests that EMG activity continuing beyond the end of a movement
must be due to some other stimulus, such as cutaneous stimulation (Burke, 1988).
Therefore, this EMG activity in the hold phase may not be a reflex due to muscle
stretch reflex. One possibility is a flexor reflex, mediated by flexor reflex afferents
(v.i.).

Tonic stretch reflexes during muscle activation

It is commonly held by clinicians that spasticity interferes with muscle function, a belief that often leads to vigorous and unhelpful attempts to reduce tone. Spasticity, however, is defined by its presence in *relaxed*, not activated, muscle. Setting aside semantics, the question is really, could hyperexcitable stretch reflexes impair function? If the tonic stretch reflex gain of activated spastic muscles were truly not increased, it would be hard to argue in favour of this. The situation is further complicated by secondary soft tissue changes that can increase tone, independent of stretch reflexes (see 'Non-reflex contributions to hypertonia').

In contrast with relaxed muscles, tonic stretch reflexes can be elicited in normal subjects while the muscle is voluntarily activated. Under these conditions, the tonic stretch reflex responses in elbow flexors between normal and spastic subjects were not significantly different (Lee et al., 1987; Powers et al., 1989). This was taken to indicate that the hyperexcitable tonic stretch reflex of spasticity was due to decreased threshold (see above) as, once threshold differences had been eliminated by voluntary activation, the stretch reflex gain was similar in the two groups. However, Nielsen (1972) had found that the stretch reflex gain of voluntarily activated spastic biceps muscles was fixed at a high level, compared with normal subjects in whom gain was strongly dependent upon the degree of voluntary activation. Given this, and the fact that the experimental paradigm is difficult to control (Noth, 1991), it is possible that differences in activated tonic stretch reflex gain between the two groups might have been missed.

A variation on this theme is the modulation of stretch reflexes during more complex movements such as gait. Short-latency stretch reflexes of soleus in normal subjects show substantial phase-dependent modulation during walking, probably through Ia presynaptic inhibition (Dietz et al., 1990) (see 'Ia presynaptic inhibition'). That as much as 30–60% of the soleus EMG activity during the stance phase of walking is due to stretch reflexes (Yang et al., 1991b) demonstrates their importance in normal gait. It has been argued that this impairment of stretch reflex modulation, because of disrupted supraspinal control (Fung & Barbeau, 1994), could contribute to the gait disorder in spasticity (Boorman et al., 1992), by failure of the appropriate pattern of reflex suppression. In support of this idea, defective stretch reflex modulation in spastic subjects with multiple sclerosis has been reported (Sinkjaer et al., 1996) and hyperactive soleus stretch reflexes during active dorsiflexion were found that impaired movement (Corcos et al., 1986). Soleus (Yang & Whelan, 1993; Stein, 1995) and quadriceps (Dietz et al., 1990) H reflexes are also normally modulated during gait and cycling (Boorman et al., 1992) and impaired soleus H reflex modulation has also been found in spastic patients (Yang et al., 1991a; Boorman et al., 1992; Sinkjaer et al., 1995). There was, however, a poor correlation between impaired soleus H reflex modulation and the degree of walking difficulty in spastic patients with spinal cord lesions (Yang et al., 1991a).

However, Ada et al. (1998) found that although abnormal tonic stretch reflexes were present at rest in the gastrocnemius of spastic subjects (post-stroke), the action tonic stretch reflexes present during simulated gait were no different to those of controls. They concluded that spasticity would not contribute to walking difficulties after stroke. Other researchers agree (Sinkjaer et al., 1993) and add that non-reflex (soft tissue) hypertonia is more important in impairing ankle movement during walking (Dietz et al., 1981; Dietz & Berger, 1983; Hufschmidt & Mauritz, 1985). The issue is clearly an important one. Attempts to reduce spasticity in order to improve function, especially gait, may be futile.

The physiological mechanisms underlying stretch reflex hyperexcitability

For a long time, the analogy was drawn between the stretch reflex hyperexcitability of the decerebrate cat and that of human spasticity. In the decerebrate cat, stretch reflexes are hyperexcitable because of increased fusimotor drive (via gamma motoneurones) to the muscle spindles making them more sensitive to stretch. Consequently, Ia afferent activity is proportionately increased. A similar mechanism was assumed to be operating in human spasticity, but by the early 1980s it had become evident that fusimotor activity was not increased. The evidence for this conclusion was eloquently summarized and discussed by Burke (1983). Thus, if excessive proprioceptive afferent input was not the explanation, what could explain the enhanced reflex responses to normal afferent input? Could it be that the alpha motoneurones themselves are hyperexcitable, ready to overreact in response to the normal and appropriate afferent input? Or, given that the reflex circuits activated by the clinical stimuli (e.g. tendon tap, passive stretch) are complex, involving interneurones that are under strong supraspinal control, is it possible that either the gain of these circuits is increased or the threshold is lowered?

The latter is the prevailing view, although it is difficult to investigate the possibility of hyperexcitable alpha motoneurones without using spinal reflexes, as will be discussed later. Thus, the basis of stretch reflex hyperexcitability, which underlies the clinical signs of enhanced tendon reflexes and reflex irradiation, clonus and spasticity, is abnormal processing of proprioceptive information within the spinal cord. A similar mechanism operates in the exaggerated nociceptive and cutaneous reflexes, also an important component of the UMN syndrome. As has been mentioned, there has been some argument as to whether this abnormal processing arises from an increased gain or from a reduced threshold.

Non-reflex contributions to hypertonia: biomechanical factors

Contractures are a well-known and feared complication of the UMN syndrome reducing the range of motion of a joint. There has been a recent investigation of the relationship between the stretch reflex hyperexcitability of spasticity and contractures (O'Dwyer et al., 1996), which will be discussed later. However, contractures are not the only soft tissue changes to occur in the UMN syndrome. Muscles and tendons may become stiff and less compliant, resisting passive stretch and manifesting as increased tone. The passive range of movement might still remain normal if there is no fixed shortening or contracture. As we saw earlier, normal subjects do not exhibit stretch reflexes at normal rates of passive limb movement. Thus, it is the visco-elastic properties of the soft tissues alone that produce normal muscle tone. In other words, normal muscle tone is entirely biomechanical with no neural contribution (Burke, 1988). Thus, there can be no real 'hypotonia' due to neurological disease (van der Meche & van Gijn, 1986; Burke, 1988). In the UMN syndrome, both neural and biomechanical factors may contribute to increased muscle tone.

This is an important concept, mainly because the treatment approaches to each type of hypertonia are different. Increased neural tone might respond to anti-spasticity medications or injections of botulinum toxin or phenol, whereas biomechanical tone would not. Increased biomechanical tone is best treated by physical measures, for example, passive stretching, splinting and serial casting.

The important role that soft tissue changes play in muscle tone and posture has been highlighted by Dietz and colleagues (1981) and confirmed by others (Hufschmidt & Mauritz, 1985; Thilmann et al., 1991b; Sinkjaer et al., 1993, 1996; Sinkjaer & Magnussen, 1994; Nielsen & Sinkjaer, 1996; Becher et al., 1998). Plantarflexion of the ankle during gait is a common sequelae of the UMN syndrome. It was generally assumed that this was produced by a combination of overactivity of the plantarflexors (referred to as spasticity) and underactivity of the ankle dorsiflexors. The latter would occur because of weakness from the UMN lesion and possibly reciprocal inhibition of these muscles by the presumed overactive plantarflexors. However, they found that despite the plantarflexed ankle, the plantarflexors were actually underactive rather than overactive and that there was excessive activity in the dorsiflexors, presumably in an attempt to correct the posture (Figure 2.7). The purpose of the research (Dietz et al., 1981) had been to investigate the suggestion that 'spasticity' played a role in the gait disturbance of the UMN syndrome but found that, at least at the ankle, that soft tissue changes were more important.

Similar experiments have been performed in the upper limb, correlating EMG activity of the elbow flexors, as a measure of stretch reflex hyperexcitability (spasticity), and resistance to passive movement, measured as torque (Lee et al., 1987; Dietz et al., 1991; Ibrahim et al., 1993; O'Dwyer et al., 1996). Higher than normal torque/EMG ratios indicate a significant soft tissue contribution to muscle hypertonia.

In clinical practice it can be difficult to distinguish between neural and biomechanical hypertonia. Velocity-dependent hypertonia and the clasp-knife phenomena would suggest a neural cause. Hypertonia with slow stretches would

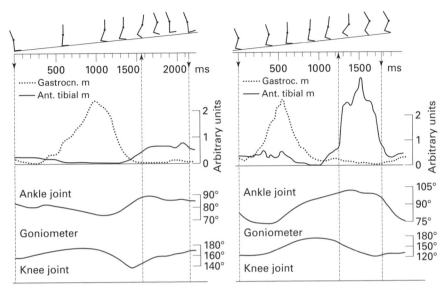

Fig. 2.7   Electromyographic (EMG) activity (rectified and averaged) during walking of tibialis
anterior (ant.tibial m) and gastrocnemius (gastrocn. m) of a normal subject (left side) and
a spastic patient (right side). Vertical lines indicate lift off and touch down of the foot on
the treadmill. Note that in the spastic subject, the foot remains plantarflexed during the
swing phase, in the absence of significant EMG activity in gastrocnemius and despite
greater than normal EMG activity in tibialis anterior. This indicates that the plantarflexed
posture is not due to weakness of tibialis anterior, or to excessive contraction of
gastrocnemius, either from stretch or co-contraction. Biomechanical factors in the triceps
surae must be causing the resistance to ankle dorsiflexion. (From Dietz et al., 1981.)

suggest reduced soft tissue compliance (Malouin et al., 1997). The distinction often
can be made with electromyography or, less practically, by examination under
anaesthesia. In many cases, both components are present (Sinkjaer et al., 1996;
Malouin et al., 1997).

The mechanism underlying reduced soft tissue compliance is probably the same
as the presumed mechanism of contracture formation, that is, prolonged immobilization of muscles and tendons at short length. This situation may arise because of
spasticity (e.g. elbow flexors resisting straightening), spasms or poor positioning of
weak muscles. Thus, neural hypertonia (spasticity) could result in secondary biomechanical hypertonia (Figure 2.8). Such soft tissue changes can occur quite
rapidly, as early as two months after stroke (O'Dwyer et al., 1996; Malouin et al.,
1997). The stiffness could reside in either the passive connective tissue of the
muscles, tendons and even joints (reviewed in Herbert, 1988; Sinkjaer &
Magnussen, 1994) or in the muscle fibres themselves, where histochemical changes
resembling denervation have been found (Dietz et al., 1986). Muscles immobilized

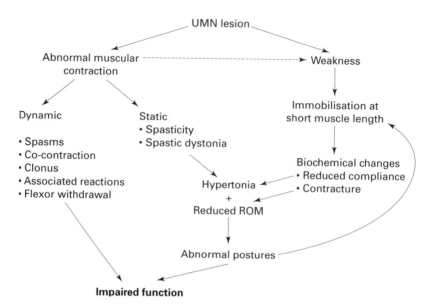

Fig. 2.8   A model of the interaction between neural and biomechanical components of hypertonia in the upper motoneurone syndrome.

at short-length develop altered length–tension relationships that make them shorter and stiffer (Figure 2.9; see Herbert, 1988, for review). The number of sarcomeres is also reduced, in proportion to the reduced length, which appears to be designed to maintain optimal myofilament overlap. Chronic active muscle shortening, that is, actively contracting muscles, appears to accelerate the loss of sarcomeres. Thus, spasticity and the flexor and extensor spasms of the UMN syndrome could rapidly result in reduced soft tissue compliance and muscle shortening. Fortunately, these changes are reversible if the muscle is lengthened but timing must be important; prolonged immobilization at short-length can result in permanent shortening, or contractures.

It has been assumed that stretch hyperreflexia, spasticity, could result in prolonged muscle shortening, eventually leading to contracture. This assumption has provided an additional reason for treating spasticity in order to avoid this outcome (Brown, 1994). However, the relationship between spasticity and contracture has been challenged (O'Dwyer et al., 1996). Contractures develop from prolonged muscle shortening, irrespective of whether there is active muscle contraction or not (O'Dwyer & Ada, 1996), and result in a reduced range of joint motion. They are frequently accompanied by increased muscle stiffness and therefore clinical hypertonia, which may also contribute to a reduced range of motion (O'Dwyer & Ada, 1996). However, fixed muscle shortening (i.e. contracture) can occur without hypertonia – there is a reduced range of joint motion but the tone within the avail-

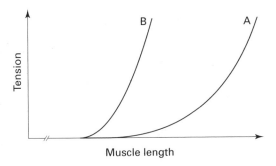

Fig. 2.9   The effects of prolonged immobilization on muscle length and stiffness. Curve A is from a normal mouse soleus and curve B from a soleus muscle immobilized in a shortened position for three weeks. The length of the muscle is naturally shorter but the length-tension curve is steeper indicating that it is also stiffer. (From Herbert, 1988, and adapted from Williams & Goldspink, 1978).

able range of motion is normal. In a study of stroke patients, contracture without spasticity was more common than with spasticity in elbow flexors (O'Dwyer et al., 1996). These authors proposed that the muscle shortening produced by contracture may actually aggravate spasticity by shortening intrafusal fibres as well as extrafusal, thus activating them earlier in the stretch than usual. An additional hypothesis that this shortening might also make the spindles more sensitive to stretch (Vandervoot et al., 1992) can be discounted for the same reasons as the increased fusimotor drive theory of spasticity (Burke, 1983).

One possible contribution to stiffness of the muscle fibres in spasticity is increased thixotropy. Thixotropy is a form of resistance to muscle stretch due to intrinsic stiffness of the muscle fibres resulting from cross-linking of actin and myosin filaments and is dependent upon the history of the movement (Walsh, 1992; Proske et al., 1993). Thixotropic stiffness has been found to be increased in spasticity (Carey, 1990) but others have found it to be normal (Brown et al., 1987). Thixotropy also affects intrafusal fibres (primary muscle spindles), altering their sensitivity to stretch (e.g. Hagbarth et al., 1985; Proske et al., 1993), but this has yet to be studied in spasticity.

Nociceptive/cutaneous reflexes

Included in this category are the clinical phenomena of flexor spasms, extensor spasms and the extensor plantar response (Babinski sign). These are exteroceptive reflexes, defined as those mediated by non-proprioceptive afferents from skin, subcutaneous and other tissues that subserve the sensory modalities of touch, pressure, temperature and pain. The clasp-knife phenomenon will also be discussed again here briefly.

Flexor withdrawal reflexes and flexor spasms

Flexor reflex afferents

In the cat, electrical stimulation of a group of sensory afferents arising from a variety of sources were found to have the effect of ipsilateral excitation of flexor and inhibition of extensor muscles (Rothwell, 1994). The result is a 'triple flexion' response of ankle dorsiflexion, knee flexion and hip flexion. Sensory afferents that evoke this flexion reflex are functionally defined as flexor reflex afferents (FRA). These include afferents from secondary muscle spindles (group II), non-encapsulated muscle (groups II, III and IV), joint mechanoreceptors and the skin (Figure 2.10). Stimulation of FRAs exerts a weaker, opposite effect on the contralateral limb, with inhibition of flexors and excitation of extensors, resulting in limb extension (the 'crossed extensor reflex'). One purpose of such a reflex would be to withdraw the limb from the stimulus (flexion) while supporting the animal on the other extended limb. FRAs have actions other than that described and may also be involved in the so-called 'stepping generator' through their ipsilateral flexion/contralateral extension action (Rothwell, 1994).

FRA reflexes are polysynaptic and generally polysegmental, the latter suggesting involvement of the propriospinal pathways. The word 'flexor' implies that this is their only action but FRAs have access to alternative pathways with differing effects, including extensor facilitation and flexor inhibition (Burke, 1988). FRAs are under strong supraspinal control, both excitatory and inhibitory. The flexor reflex is facilitated in the spinal cat but suppressed in the mid-collicular (decerebrate) cat (Rothwell, 1994). The supraspinal control presumably determines which of the available pathways are activated by the FRAs according to the particular task (Burke, 1988). The dorsal reticulospinal tract (DRT) is generally accepted to inhibit FRAs (Whitlock, 1990). However, flexor spasms were not produced by dorsolateral spinal lesions in cats involving the DRT (Taylor et al., 1997). In another study though, a similar lesion enhanced spinal transmission from group II and III afferents (Cavallari & Pettersson, 1989). Inhibition also comes from the MRTs and VSTs (Brown, 1994). The effects of L-dopa and tizanidine indicate that the FRA activity is strongly suppressed by dopaminergic (Schomburg & Steffens, 1998) and noradrenergic (Delwaide & Pennisi, 1994) pathways, respectively. The corticospinal and rubrospinal tracts facilitate FRAs (Burke, 1988). Evidence from animal studies suggests that serotonergic pathways facilitate flexor reflexes (Maj et al., 1985). Supraspinal centres receive input from the FRAs via ascending tracts, including the spinocerebellar pathways. Such input keeps them appraised of the state of the spinal interneuronal networks and no doubt helps in their decision as to which of the FRA actions to facilitate. The quality of the peripheral stimulus also may be important. Gentle pressure on the cat hindfoot produces an extension response (plantarflexion) whereas a noxious pin-prick evokes a flexion response

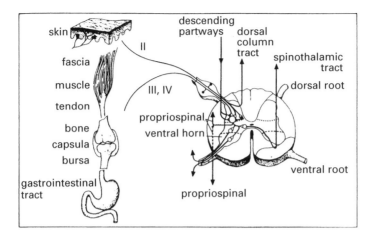

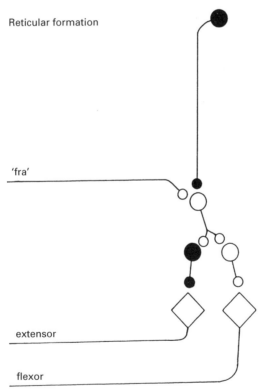

Fig. 2.10.   (a): Illustrating the multi-modal (skin, muscle, joint) nature of the group II, III, and IV fibres that comprise the flexor reflex afferents (FRAs) and some of their central connections. (b): FRAs converge on a polysynaptic spinal network that excites flexor and inhibits extensor motoneurones. The interneurones involved are inhibited by the dorsal reticulospinal tract (DRT) that arises in the pontomedullary reticular formation. Thus, afferent stimuli, both nociceptive and non-nociceptive, from a wide variety of sources, can excite FRAs and produce a flexor withdrawal reflex. In spasticity, these are exaggerated and manifest as flexor spasms. ((a): From Benecke et al., 1987; (b): from Burke, 1988.)

(dorsiflexion) (Rothwell, 1994). When facilitated in the spinal cat, less than noxious stimuli can elicit a flexion withdrawal response. FRAs are suppressed by opiates (Schomburg & Steffens, 1998).

Flexor withdrawal reflexes

Electrophysiologically, the flexor withdrawal reflex in the cat has two components (Rothwell, 1994). The short latency component has a central delay of only a few milliseconds while the delay for the long latency component is 30–50 ms. The short latency component appears to inhibit the later one.

Flexor withdrawal reflexes can be demonstrated in humans by noxious stimulation of the foot. A 10–20 ms train of electrical stimuli delivered to the sole at low intensity produces a short latency response in tibialis anterior at around 50–60 ms. At higher stimulus intensities, a later, stronger response appears at around 110–40 ms. It is this late component that dorsiflexes the foot and produces the withdrawal (Shahani & Young, 1971). The earlier response acts as a priming movement. At higher stimulus intensities, the latency of both components decreases (with larger reductions in the later component) and the amplitude and duration of the responses increases (Shahani & Cros, 1990). The latency of the late response would allow time for a cortical component but the reflex persists in total spinal cord transection indicating its spinal origin. The situation in humans is therefore similar to that in the cat. The latency of these electrically-evoked reflexes suggests they are mediated by group II afferents, which conduct at around 40 ms, and not the very slowly conducting C fibres that conduct pain sensation (Rothwell, 1994). Others have suggested the group III afferents are responsible (Roby-Brami & Bussel, 1993). In the UMN syndrome, the early component disappears (Shahani & Young, 1980) while the late component is preserved but desynchronized (Meinck et al., 1985).

Meinck and colleagues investigate this reflex in detail (Meinck et al., 1985; Figure 2.11). Tibialis anterior had the lowest threshold of all the physiological leg flexors. Tonic activation of the muscles shortened the latency of both the early and late components and eliminated the threshold differences. This suggested supraspinal modulation of the reflex. Changing stimulus characteristics could also enhance the reflex. In the UMN syndrome, they found an impaired early component, a net increase in reflex activity, desynchronization, an abnormal sensitivity to facilitation, and irradiation to muscles not normally involved. Similar findings were found irrespective of the site of the UMN lesion, spinal cord, brainstem or cerebrum. On the other hand, Shahani & Young (1980) observed electrophysiological differences in the flexor withdrawal reflexes following spinal cord transection and cerebral hemisphere lesions.

Flexor spasms

In the UMN syndrome, patients may suffer from spasms of the legs that resemble those of the flexor withdrawal reflex. These flexor spasms may occur in response to

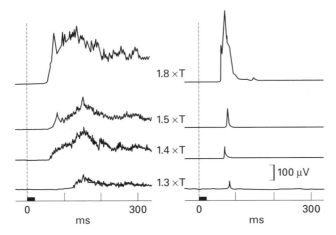

Fig. 2.11   Tibialis anterior flexor withdrawal reflexes elicited in a spastic subject by medial plantar nerve stimulation. The hemiplegic side is shown on the left and the normal side on the right. As stimulus intensity is increased (expressed as a multiple of motor threshold, T), the amplitude of the reflex on both sides increases. The hemiplegic side shows an absence of the early phase until higher stimulus intensities and a prolonged late phase. Furthermore, the latency of the response from the hemiplegic side is highly dependent upon stimulus intensity, whereas the normal side is not. (From Meinck et al., 1985.)

a variety of sensory stimuli or apparently spontaneously. Common stimuli include nociceptive (bed-sores) and non-nociceptive cutaneous stimuli, visceral stimuli such as bladder or bowel distension or bladder irritation (cystitis, in-dwelling catheters). Apparently spontaneous spasms are probably due to occult stimuli (Whitlock, 1990). It is likely that flexor spasms represent disinhibited and distorted flexor withdrawal reflexes. Differences in the occurrence of flexor spasms in partial spinal, complete spinal and cerebral lesions have been discussed earlier.

Flexor spasms are clearly separate from spasticity, as defined at the beginning of this chapter. However, they often accompany spasticity, especially in spinal cord lesions, and can be painful and debilitating.

The extensor plantar response

The extensor plantar response, or Babinski sign, is discussed here following flexor spasms as it is really best considered a disinhibited flexion withdrawal reflex. Toe extension or dorsiflexion is regarded physiologically as flexion. In the spinal cat, the flexion withdrawal reflex includes dorsiflexion of the hallux, in addition to the foot. Stroking the sole of infants also produces this response until the age of one. Thereafter, this response is modified so that the toes and ankle plantarflex while knee flexion and hip flexion are unchanged. This response still withdraws the stimulated part from the stimulus (sole) by arching the foot while at the same time maintaining contact with the ground through the toes. Such a modification is seen as an adaptation to the upright walking posture (Rothwell, 1994). In the UMN syndrome, the full flexion reflex returns with dorsiflexion of all the toes and the ankle. This is the only sign of the UMN syndrome that is unequivocally linked to the pyramidal tracts (Burke, 1988; Nathan, 1994; van Gijn, 1996).

However, Burke (1988) points out that the situation is actually quite complex. The plantar response is usually evoked by a stroke along the lateral border of the sole and over the ball of the foot, producing the normal response of toe plantarflexion. However, stimulation of the nearby base of the toes and pad of the hallux normally produces the opposite response of toe dorsiflexion. Cutaneous fields often overlap and the examiner could stray more towards this latter area. The normal plantar response would then be the product of two opposing reflexes, with the plantarflexor reflex tending to dominate. However, should there be, in addition, contraction of the pre-tibial muscles (a frequent occurrence in anticipation of an unpleasant stroking of the sole), sufficient reciprocal inhibition could be produced to suppress the plantarflexor muscles, leaving the dorsiflexor response unopposed and so the great toe dorsiflexes. The reflex response also depends upon the stimulus. Non-nociceptive sural nerve stimulation produces great toe plantarflexion but nociceptive stimulation produces the full flexor withdrawal reflex, including great toe dorsiflexion.

Thus, the direction of great toe movement when testing the plantar response may depend upon the exact placement of the stimulus and its intensity and upon the degree of pre-tibial activation. Burke (1988) would view as definitely pathological an extensor plantar response from a non-nociceptive stimulus given to the mid-portion of the sole and would be suspicious of such a response to a nociceptive stimulus, particularly if accompanied by the typical 'triple flexion' response described earlier. Medical students are frequently under the misconception that the plantar stimulus should be painful. Furthermore, many neurologists examine with the patient sitting on the side of the bed, with the legs suspended. This could lead to a slight activation of pre-tibial muscles against gravity.

An extensor plantar response is a flexion withdrawal response, mediated by FRAs, which are facilitated by the pyramidal tracts (Lundberg & Voorhoeve, 1962). Somewhat paradoxically, the extensor plantar response is a firm sign of pyramidal tract injury, which would be expected to reduce FRA activity, not enhance it (Burke, 1988). The explanation lies in the complexity of the FRA circuits alluded to earlier, in which there may exist alternative pathways with opposing actions. The action of the pyramidal tracts on FRAs from the plantar surface is facilitation of a reflex of toe plantarflexion (physiological extension). Loss of this facilitation in a pyramidal lesion allows the alternative reflex pathway of great toe dorsiflexion to act unopposed. Despite being an exaggerated flexion reflex, the Babinski sign is not always associated with increases in other flexor reflex activity (van Gijn, 1978).

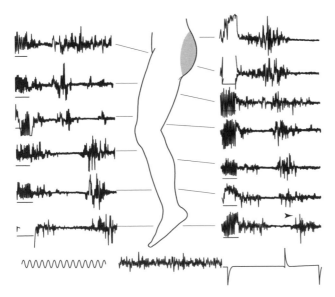

Fig. 2.12   Extensor reflexes in the normal lower limb. Recordings from gluteus maximus performing a mild background contraction in response to noxious stimuli presented to the skin on different parts of the ventral and dorsal leg. Immediate strong contraction was produced by stimulation over the gluteal region, whereas most other areas produced a brief period of inhibition. (From Hagbarth, 1960.)

Extensor reflexes and spasms

In a similar way to flexion withdrawal reflexes, non-nociceptive cutaneous stimulation in cats (Hagbarth, 1952) and humans (Hagbarth, 1960; Kugelberg, 1962) can evoke extension responses in the stimulated limbs. Similar to flexion reflexes, extension reflexes are protective, serving to move the area stimulated away from the stimulus. Whether a stimulus evokes a flexion or extension response is in part dependent upon the location of the stimulus. Extension responses in humans may be evoked from such areas as the groin, buttock and posterior leg (Figure 2.12). Similar extension responses occur with abrupt iliopsoas stretch and as the 'crossed extension' component of a contralateral flexion withdrawal reflex (see above). The positive support reaction, to be described later, is another extensor reflex and may be both proprioceptive and exteroceptive in nature. As already mentioned, such flexion and extension reflexes are built into the spinal stepping generator subserving locomotion. Thus both flexor and extensor spasms are simply exaggerated and usually inappropriate manifestations of existing spinal reflexes (Burke, 1988). Extensor spasms and an extensor posture could also be viewed as functionally advantageous by providing a rigid supporting limb for stance and gait.

Following complete spinal cord transection, patients often experience both flexor and extensor spasms, understandable as both reflex pathways would be completely disinhibited by the loss of supraspinal control. Patients may after several months settle into a state of predominant extensor spasms (Hagbarth, 1960; Kugelberg, 1962) but paraplegia-in-flexion is also common. Perhaps the dominant posture is a matter of the net effect of the many afferent (exteroceptive and proprioceptive) inputs at the time. A bedsore on the heel or urinary infection could transform paraplegia-in-extension into paraplegia-in-flexion. For reasons outlined earlier, partial spinal cord lesions tend to have fewer flexor spasms and take on a more dominant extensor tone (Barolat & Maiman, 1987).

Other UMN phenomena

Associated reactions

In the UMN syndrome, physical activity in one part of the body may be accompanied by unnecessary involuntary activity in another. A typical example would be the progressive elbow flexion seen in a hemiparetic stroke patient during walking and is a familiar component of the 'hemiplegic posture'. Generally the part showing the associated reaction, the elbow flexors in the example given, are also affected by the UMN syndrome and usually display some degree of spasticity. The extent of the associated reaction seems to depend upon both the degree of motor effort (e.g. the effort of walking) and the degree of hypertonia in the limb showing the associated reaction. Thus, physiotherapists have used the associated reaction as a gauge of the patient's spasticity and overall motor function and has even been treated directly (Bobath, 1990). The phenomenon of associated reaction was first reported by Walshe in 1923 and has been described variously as, 'released postural reactions deprived of voluntary control' (Walshe, 1923), 'synkinesia' (Bourbonnais et al., 1995) and 'stereotypic flexor synergy' (Bobath, 1990).

Dickstein and colleagues (1996) have investigated the associated reaction of elbow flexion in hemiparetic subjects during walking. They found a rapid increase in elbow flexion during the first four steps and a gradual increase thereafter (Figure 2.13). Confirming previous notions, the degree of elbow flexion correlated with the Ashworth score of elbow flexor tone. However, there was a poor correlation between the EMG activity of the elbow flexors and the degree of elbow flexion. They concluded that non-reflex, soft tissue changes played an important role in this associated reaction.

Clearly though, there is also a neural component involving motoneurone activity. The mechanism of this is uncertain but thought to be multifactorial (Dewald & Rymer, 1993). Dewald & Rymer (1993) concluded that enhanced flexion withdrawal reflexes probably do not play the primary role but that disturbed descending supraspinal commands may be involved. Their hypothesis is that unaffected bulbospinal motor pathways with more diffuse, polysegmental motoneurone

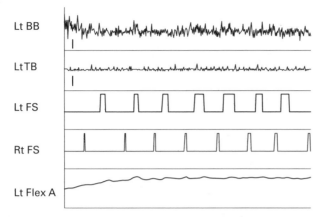

Fig. 2.13   Associated reactions studied in the upper limb. A patient with a left hemiplegia exhibited
progressive left elbow during gait with each successive step (time along the x-axis; total
sweep about 54 seconds). Surface electromyography (EMG) was recorded from the left
(Lt) biceps (BB) and triceps (TB) brachii. Traces labelled left (Lt) and right (Rt) FS
represent successive foot steps. Flexion angle (Flex A) of the left elbow is shown in the
bottom trace. Note increasing elbow flexion but a stable level of biceps EMG activity,
indicating biomechanical factors in the elbow flexion. (From Dickstein et al., 1996.)

connections may assume the role of the damaged UMN tracts in transmission of
descending voluntary commands. These older bulbospinal pathways are less
focused than the pyramidal tracts. They have substantial connections to motoneurones of the axial and proximal limb musculature and could result in the synergic
patterns observed. Propriospinal pathways could also be involved. Compatible with
the pattern of tone in the hemiparetic UMN syndrome, descending motor drive
may favour flexors rather than extensors, through increased excitability of flexor
motoneurones and the interneurones of the flexor reflex pathways.

A further contributing factor could be vestibulospinal reflexes. Assumption of
the upright posture, as in walking, enhances excitability of 'anti-gravity' motoneurones. Disinhibition of this pathway could generate sufficient descending motor
drive to produce elbow flexion (and leg extension). Such a mechanism could contribute to the so-called hemiplegic posture, a form of spastic dystonia (Burke,
1988). Alternatively, it could simply contribute to an increased excitability of the
elbow flexor motoneurones such that non-focused descending voluntary commands would favour these flexors.

Co-contraction

Co-contraction refers to the simultaneous contraction of both agonist and antagonist muscles. In normal postnatal motor development, extensive co-contraction
is a normal feature, associated with heteronymous, monosynaptic Ia projections

from biceps to triceps and to regional synergists and antagonists (O'Sullivan et al., 1998). Normally these connections become restricted to primary synergists in the first four years of life (O'Sullivan et al., 1998).

Controlled co-contraction thereafter is an important feature of normal motor function providing postural stability or fixation of a body part, for example, to stabilize the wrist when hitting a tennis ball. In these situations it is considered appropriate and functional, and a manifestation of normal reciprocal innervation. Normal co-contraction is initiated and modulated as the movement demands. Co-contraction is dysfunctional when it is inappropriate or excessive and impairs agonist function, also making the agonist appear weaker than it is. Dysfunctional or pathological co-contraction is a common feature of dystonia and has been demonstrated more in cerebral palsy (Crenna, 1998) than in adult brain injury (O'Sullivan et al., 1998). Furthermore, the contribution of pathological co-contraction in adult spasticity to impaired movement is controversial (Conrad et al., 1985), with both protagonists (Yanagisawa & Tanaka, 1978; Corcos et al., 1986; el-Abd et al., 1993) and antagonists (Mizrahi & Angel, 1979; Dietz et al., 1981; Dietz & Berger, 1983; Fellows et al., 1994; Davies et al., 1996). This is particularly so for movements of the ankle, where some researchers believe that biomechanical factors may be more important (Dietz et al., 1981; Dietz & Berger, 1983; Becher et al., 1998). These results have been challenged (Conrad et al., 1985). The question of the existence and importance of co-contraction has therapeutic relevance. Inappropriate antagonist contraction could be reduced, focally by botulinum toxin injections (Sheean, 1998b) or phenol nerve blocks, or by other anti-spasticity agents such as baclofen (Latash & Penn, 1996).

The pathophysiological substrate of co-contraction in dystonia is impairment of Ia reciprocal inhibition (Berardelli et al., 1998) in the spinal cord. Normally, agonist Ia activity exerts an inhibitory effect on the antagonist motoneurones via an interneurone (see Figure 2.16). This activity is influenced by supraspinal inputs (co-contraction is activated and de-activated at a cortical level (Humphrey & Reed, 1983) and by other segmental afferents (Delwaide & Olivier, 1987). Abnormalities of Ia reciprocal inhibition have been reported in spasticity and could contribute to co-contraction (Crone et al., 1994; Okuma & Lee, 1996). Impaired spinal Ia reciprocal inhibition in dystonia probably arises from disordered supraspinal modulation and a similar mechanism in spasticity is plausible. In spastic cerebral palsy the heteronymous Ia connections of infancy mentioned earlier are persistent, but this is not the case in adult hemiparesis due to stroke (O'Sullivan et al., 1998). Further discussion of reciprocal inhibition is presented below.

Co-contraction should be differentiated from a hyperactive stretch reflex in the antagonist muscle that is elicited by the lengthening produced by the agonist action. For example, active elbow extension by triceps will lengthen the biceps and may elicit a stretch response. This will appear as simultaneous contraction of both muscles but is fundamentally different to co-contraction produced by simultaneous motor drive to both muscles, a 'diffusion of descending commands' (Fellows et al., 1994). Both situations could arise from similar pathophysiological mechanisms, however, that is, defects of Ia reciprocal inhibition (Delwaide & Olivier, 1987). The distinction could be made by isometric contraction of triceps that does not stretch biceps; the presence of biceps activity would indicate true co-contraction. One difficulty in interpreting isometric studies is the normal occurrence of co-contraction in isometric movements (Flanders & Cordo, 1987). Thus, in one study (Fellows et al., 1994), there was no greater co-contraction of elbow flexors and extensors during isometric contractions in hemiparetic patients than with normal controls.

Intact Ia reciprocal inhibition in the UMN syndrome may also cause problems. The ankle plantarflexors are frequently overactive and could inhibit the ankle dorsiflexors through preserved (Yanagisawa et al., 1976) or even increased (Ashby & Wiens, 1989) Ia reciprocal inhibition, contributing to their apparent weakness and foot drop. Furthermore, local anaesthetic injections into the triceps surae to block afferent fibres led to increased strength of the ankle dorsiflexors (Yanagisawa & Tanaka, 1978). Dietz and colleagues (1981) have challenged this whole concept, however, finding minimal plantarflexor EMG activity and *excessive* activation of ankle dorsiflexors during walking, despite a plantarflexed posture and hypertonia at the ankle. They concluded that soft tissue changes were responsible, rather than neural causes.

Spastic dystonia

Dystonia is a condition characterized by 'sustained muscle contractions, frequently causing twisting and repetitive movements, or abnormal postures' (Fahn et al., 1987). This definition usually refers to conditions arising from basal ganglia disorders. Patients suffering an UMN syndrome frequently adopt an abnormal posture, well known to most clinicians as the 'hemiplegic' or 'decorticate' posture. The hemiplegic posture involves flexion of the elbow, wrist and fingers, with adduction of the shoulder and pronation of the forearm. The leg is extended at the hip and knee, plantarflexed and inverted at the ankle, with adduction of the hip. This may be loosely described as 'dystonia' but the term is confusing when used in the context of the UMN lesion and spasticity.

Although frequently accompanied by spasticity, the hemiplegic posture of spastic dystonia is fundamentally different. Spasticity is velocity dependent and mediated by hyperactive proprioceptive stretch reflexes. The continuous muscle contraction maintaining spastic dystonia is present without limb movement. Furthermore, it is not dependent upon afferent input from the limb, as it persists after dorsal root section (Denny-Brown, 1966). It probably arises from continuous suparspinal drive to the spinal motoneurones and is altered by postural changes (Denny-Brown, 1966), presumably through proprioceptive or vestibular mechanisms (Burke, 1988). The phenomenon of associated reactions (v.s.) indicates that the hemiplegic posture is also subject to other influences.

Thus, unlike most of the other positive features of the UMN syndrome, the motor drive behind spastic dystonia is not a spinal reflex; it is *efferent* mediated rather than *afferent* mediated. This distinction has important therapeutic implications. Spastic dystonia would not be expected to respond well to traditional antispastic therapies such as diazepam and baclofen, which suppress spinal reflex activity, nor to dorsal rhizotomy. However, it would still respond to treatments that modify motor nerve or muscle activity, such as dantrolene, botulinum toxin and phenol injections and peripheral nerve section. It should be noted that some sustained abnormal postures in the UMN are reflex-mediated, such as the continuous leg flexion of paraplegia-in-flexion following total spinal cord section (already discussed). Soft tissue and joint pathology may also contribute to sustained abnormal postures.

Positive support reaction

This term is more commonly used by physiotherapists than physicians to describe a pattern of plantarflexion and inversion of the ankle of a patient with an UMN syndrome, upon attempted weight bearing (Bobath, 1990). Others have termed this phenomenon the tonic ambulatory foot response (Manfredi et al., 1975). There may be extension of the knee, producing a pattern of extensor thrust of the lower limb (Schomburg, 1990). A positive support reaction can be extremely debilitating and prevent standing and walking. It is presumed to be a reflex involving a proprioceptive stimulus elicited by stretch of the intrinsic foot muscles and an exteroceptive stimulus elicited by contact of the foot with the ground (Bobath, 1990). A similar physiological spinal extensor reflex exists in infants (Rothwell, 1994) and is normally suppressed. Analogous to the Babinski sign, this reflex is presumably disinhibited by the UMN lesion.

The suparspinal control of this reflex in humans is not known. However, a positive support reaction appeared in the cat following a lesion of the dorsolateral funiculus containing the (inhibitory) reticulospinal pathways, accompanied by spasticity (Taylor et al., 1997).

Electrophysiological studies of spinal reflexes in spasticity

It is well established that spinal phasic and tonic stretch, flexor withdrawal and other reflexes are hyperexcitable in the UMN syndrome, following interruption of the descending UMN pathways. However, the actual spinal circuitry responsible for the production of these effects is less well established. A number of the spinal reflex mechanisms involved in motor control already mentioned have been studied electrophysiologically in an attempt to understand the basis of the hyperexcitable proprioceptive reflexes and other phenomena of the UMN syndrome (Table 2.2). Most attention has been given to inhibitory mechanisms, with the expectation of finding decreased inhibition. However, excitatory mechanisms and the level of excitability of alpha motoneurones have also been examined. Flexor withdrawal reflexes, the basis of flexor spasms in the UMN syndrome, have already been discussed.

Spinal inhibitory mechanisms

The four main spinal inhibitory activities that have been studied are Ia presynaptic inhibition, Ia reciprocal inhibition, Ib non-reciprocal inhibition and Renshaw cell inhibition. Most techniques are based upon modulation of H reflexes, which will be discussed briefly.

H reflexes

These were first discovered in the triceps surae by Hoffman in 1926, hence the name, H reflex. Low intensity electrical stimulation of the tibial nerve in the popliteal fossa elicits a reflex contraction of triceps surae without direct activation of the motor axons in the nerve (Figure 2.14). By selecting appropriate stimulus parameters, the Ia afferents could be stimulated selectively. The latency of the reflex is around 30 ms. For a long time the H reflex was incorrectly thought to be equivalent to the tendon reflex (T reflex), except that the spindle is bypassed. It had considered that comparison of H and T reflex amplitudes would reflect muscle spindle sensitivity (and thus fusimotor drive) and that both are monosynaptic reflexes involving only Ia afferents. Burke (1985) has discussed this, and several associated myths. H reflexes involve both oligo- and polysynaptic pathways (and thus interneurones) that are under supraspinal control as well as subject to other segmental influences. Thus, in addition to being a useful test in routine clinical neurophysiology, it is also a powerful tool in the study of spinal reflex pathways.

Ia presynaptic inhibition

Collaterals of muscle spindle Ia afferents form axo-axonal synapse with the Ia afferent terminals and inhibit the release of neurotransmitter. This inhibitory activity is GABA-ergic and under supraspinal control. Presynaptic inhibition is important in normal motor control and exhibits task-dependent modulation by both CNS pattern generators and afferent feedback from the periphery (Stein, 1995). Muscle belly vibration, a potent stimulus of muscle spindles Ia afferents, elicits both

Table 2.2. The neurophysiology and neuropharmacology of spasticity

Spinal segmental activity	Electrophysiological test	Abnormality	Neurotransmitter	Medication effect
Ia Pre-synaptic inhibition	Vibratory inhibition of H reflex	Reduced	GABA (−)	Diazepam (+) Baclofen (−) Tizanidine (+)
Ia Reciprocal inhibition	Conditioning of H reflex	Reduced	? Glycine (−)	Tizanidine (+)
Ib Non-reciprocal inhibition	Conditioning of H reflex	Reduced	Glycine (−)	Tizanidine (+)
Recurrent inhibition	Conditioning of H reflex	Increased and decreased		Baclofen (−)
Flexor withdrawal reflexes	Foot stimulation	Increased	Glutamate (+)	Tizanidine (−) Baclofen (−) L-Dopa (−)
α motoneurone excitability	H_{max}/M_{max}	Increased	?	Tizanidine (−) Baclofen (−)
	F wave amplitude	Increased	?.	Tizanidine (−)
Other polysynaptic	H reflex recovery	Increased	EAAs	Diazepam (−) Baclofen (+)
Ia excitatory	TVR	Decreased	EAA?	Diazepam (−) Baclofen (−)
Group II excitatory	Long latency reflexes	Decreased and increased	EAA?	Tizanidine (−) L-Dopa (−)
				Baclofen weak (−)

Notes:

TVR: tonic vibration reflex; GABA: gamma-aminobutyric acid.

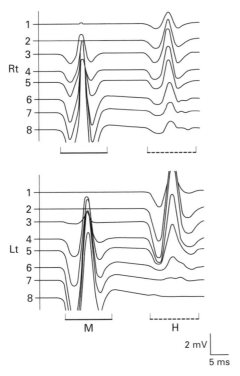

Fig. 2.14   H reflexes elicited from the left and right soleus muscle of a normal subject by stimuli of increasing intensity delivered to the tibial nerve in the popliteal fossa. Note the appearance of the H reflex at around 30 ms latency before an M wave has appeared. Increasing stimulus intensity (from trace 1 to 8) results initially in an increased H reflex amplitude, followed by a decline and replacement by an F wave. (Kimura, 1989.)

excitatory and inhibitory responses. The excitatory response is contraction of the vibrated muscle, the tonic vibration reflex (see below), while at the same time tendon and H reflexes are inhibited (de Gail et al., 1966; Figure 2.15). Vibratory inhibition of H reflexes is one of several methods available to evaluate presynaptic inhibition (Stein, 1995). Another is to examine the modulation of H or stretch reflexes during movement, thought to be effected via presynaptic. It is conceivable that reduction in presynaptic inhibition could result in increased tendon reflexes and possibly spasticity (Delwaide, 1993).

Vibratory inhibition of H reflexes is reduced in spastic subjects (Burke & Ashby, 1972; Calancie et al., 1993; Milanov, 1994), and task-dependent modulation is impaired (Schieppati et al., 1985; Iles & Roberts, 1986; Yang et al., 1991a; Boorman et al., 1992; Toft & Sinkjaer, 1993; Stein, 1995; Sinkjaer et al., 1996). Other methods of evaluating presynaptic inhibition have also revealed impairment in spastic patients (Nielsen et al., 1995). There may be differences in presynaptic inhibition

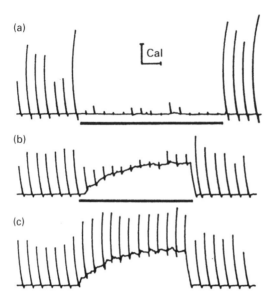

Fig. 2.15   The tonic vibration reflex (TVR) and suppression of knee jerks by vibration in the human quadriceps. Knee jerks are elicited every 5 seconds and are depressed during the vibration of the muscle (black bar) both without (a) and with (b) the development of a TVR. In (c), the subject is mimicking a TVR with voluntary contraction but knee jerks are not inhibited. Vibration is a powerful stimulus of primary muscle spindle endings. This phenomenon illustrates the apparently paradoxical combination of simultaneous motoneurone excitation (TVR) and inhibition (knee-jerk suppression) by Ia afferent activity. Calibration: Vertical 0.4 kg for (a), 0.6 kg for (b) and (c). Horizontal 10 seconds. (From de Gail et al., 1966.)

between spasticity of spinal and cerebral origins (Faist et al., 1994). The effect of afferent feedback from the periphery on presynaptic inhibition is revealed by the prolonged reduction of vibratory inhibition and spasticity by transcutaneous electrical nerve stimulation (TENS) (Levin & Hui-Chan, 1992).

Could impaired Ia presynaptic inhibition be a major contributor to spasticity? Some weak correlation with the degree of spasticity measured clinically by the Ashworth scale (Ashworth, 1964) has been found by some (Harburn et al., 1995), but not by others (Faist et al., 1994). A better correlation exists between reduced presynaptic inhibition and tendon hyperreflexia (Delwaide & Pennisi, 1994). Yang et al. (1991a) found marked variability in the degree of impaired H-reflex modulation, a function of presynaptic inhibition, during walking among spastic spinal patients, and the degree of impaired modulation seemed poorly related to the severity of difficulty walking. Presynaptic inhibition is also reduced in Parkinson's disease (Roberts et al., 1994; Hayashi et al., 1997), a condition characterized by rigidity rather than spasticity; hence, additional factors must be operating to produce the spastic state.

Indirect evidence also suggests a role for impaired presynaptic inhibition in spasticity. Increased vibratory inhibition is a feature of 'spinal shock', suggesting increased presynaptic inhibition, followed by spasticity and reduced presynaptic inhibition (Calancie et al., 1993). The clinical anti-spastic effects of diazepam (Verrier et al., 1975; Delwaide, 1985a), baclofen (Milanov, 1992), tizanidine (Delwaide & Pennisi, 1994; Milanov & Georgiev, 1994), clonidine (Nance et al., 1989), TRH (Morin & Pierrot-Deseilligny, 1988) and TENS (Levin & Hui-Chan, 1992) are accompanied by improvements in measures of presynaptic inhibition. As tizanidine reduces presynaptic inhibition (Delwaide & Pennisi, 1994; Milanov & Georgiev, 1994), clonus was expectedly reduced in one study (Delwaide & Pennisi, 1994) but tendon reflexes were unchanged in another (Milanov & Georgiev, 1994). This discrepancy casts some doubt upon the conclusion presented earlier that impaired presynaptic inhibition correlates better with tendon hyperreflexia than with muscle hypertonia.

The supraspinal control of presynaptic inhibition is unclear. Studies in humans using transcranial magnetic stimulation reveal conflicting results in the lower limb, indicating both facilitation (Meunier & Pierrot-Deseilligny, 1998), and depression (Valls-Sole et al., 1994; Iles, 1996) of presynaptic inhibition by the corticospinal tracts. Vestibulospinal connections to interneurones mediating presynaptic inhibition are also known (Iles & Pisini, 1992) and might partly explain the modulation of presynaptic inhibition with changes in body position; presynaptic inhibition is normally reduced when going from supine to standing (Mynark et al., 1997)

Ia reciprocal inhibition

The Ia afferents of an agonist muscle inhibit, via Ia interneurones, the alpha motoneurones of its antagonist (Figure 2.16). The Ia inhibitory interneurone receives both segmental (including Renshaw cells) and supraspinal afferents, including facilitation from corticospinal fibres (Delwaide, 1993). Ia reciprocal inhibition is readily studied in upper and lower limb muscles. One method (Figure 2.16) involves threshold conditioning electrical stimuli that are applied to the nerve supplying antagonist muscles (e.g. peroneal nerve at the knee innervating ankle dorsiflexors) while observing the effect on the H reflex obtained from the agonists (ankle plantarflexors). Two main inhibitory effects are seen, distinguished by timing. The first is a short-latency, short duration inhibition attributed to disynaptic mechanisms and the second is a later, long-lasting inhibition attributed to presynaptic mechanisms.

Abnormalities have been reported in the early, di-synaptic phase of inhibition in spasticity involving the lower (Crone et al., 1994; Okuma & Lee, 1996) and upper limbs (Nakashima et al., 1989; Artieda et al., 1991; Panizza et al., 1995). Okuma & Lee (1996) report reduced di-synaptic inhibition by the ankle dorsiflexors on the plantarflexors in some hemiplegic patients with marked plantarflexor (extensor)

(a)

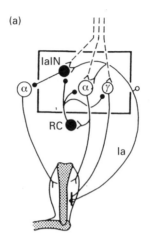

(b)

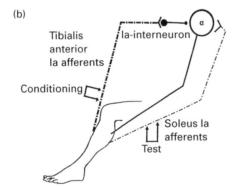

(c)

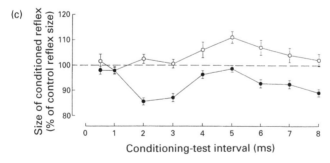

Fig. 2.16   Reciprocal inhibition. (a): Illustrates the spinal circuitry of Ia reciprocal inhibition between agonist and antagonist muscles and the involvement of Renshaw cells and supraspinal connections (b): Experimental technique for studying reciprocal inhibition in the lower limb. A conditioning shock is given to the peroneal nerve (from tibialis anterior) and the effect on the tibial nerve H reflex from soleus is observed for different time intervals between the two stimuli. (c): Responses in normal (closed circles) and spastic patients (open circles). The normal subjects demonstrate an early (1–4 ms), and a late period inhibition (6–8 ms) that is absent in spastic patients and replaced by facilitation. ((a) from Hultborn et al., 1979; (b) and (c) from Crone et al., 1994.)

spasticity but normal results in others. Patients with only mild spasticity actually had *increased* inhibition and patients with improving spasticity, studied serially, showed increasing inhibition. Crone and colleagues (1994) studied the lower limbs of patients with multiple sclerosis and found that most often the di-synaptic phase of inhibition was abolished and in some cases replaced by a facilitatory phase of slightly longer latency (Figure 2.16). Yanagisawa & Tanaka (1978) studied patients with both capsular and spinal lesions and also found impairment of reciprocal inhibition from ankle dorsiflexors to plantarflexors, but preserved and strong reciprocal inhibition in the reverse direction. The late inhibitory phase is less well studied, but impairment has also been reported in human spasticity (Nakashima et al., 1989; Artieda et al., 1991; Panizza et al., 1995) which is less well correlated with the presence of spasticity (Okuma & Lee, 1996).

In contrast, Boorman and colleagues (1991) found weak inhibition of the soleus H reflexes in patients with spinal cord lesions that was not present in normal controls. Studies of cats subjected to spinal hemisection reveal *greater* facilitation of this reflex on the side of the lesion (Hultborn & Malmsten, 1983). Methodological factors may underlie the different results.

Impaired Ia reciprocal inhibition has been implicated in the abnormal co-contraction of the UMN syndrome. However, a potential criticism of the reflex studies cited is that they were performed at rest and therefore did not mimic the clinical situation where co-contraction occurs during voluntary movement. Boorman and colleagues (1996) studied 'natural reciprocal inhibition' by observing the inhibitory effect of voluntary ankle dorsiflexion on the soleus H reflex in spastic patients with incomplete spinal cord lesions. Reciprocal inhibition was impaired and correlated with the degree of co-contraction.

Thus, abnormalities of Ia reciprocal inhibition may contribute to co-contraction of agonist and antagonist muscle pairs and possibly impaired voluntary activation, but its role in the production of spasticity is unclear. This is partially so because spasticity is a sign elicited by passive stretch of muscles at rest so that the antagonist pair of the stretched muscle should be relaxed and therefore not providing any stimulus for reciprocal inhibition. None the less, some correlation has been found between the degree of impaired reciprocal inhibition and the severity of clinical spasticity in the upper limbs (Panizza et al., 1995).

Ib non-reciprocal (autogenic) inhibition

Golgi tendon organs give rise to Ib afferents that project to inhibitory interneurones (Ib interneurones), which in turn exert an inhibitory effect on extensor and a facilitatory effect on flexor motoneurones (Delwaide, 1993). Like most spinal interneurones, the Ib interneurones receive input from descending spinal pathways as well as segmental afferents. The corticospinal tract may facilitate and the dorsal reticulospinal tract may inhibit this reflex activity (Fine et al., 1998). Impaired Ib non-reciprocal inhibition contributes to extensor hypertonia decerebrate rigidity in the cat (Eccles & Lundberg, 1959) and so it was postulated that it may play a similar role in the UMN syndrome in humans.

A method to study Ib non-reciprocal inhibition was devised by Pierrot-Deseilligny (Pierrot-Deseilligny et al., 1981). Stimulation of the medial gastrocnemius group I afferents inhibits the soleus H reflex, an effect thought to be mediated by Ib non-reciprocal inhibition (Figure 2.17). Delwaide found that this inhibitory reflex activity was essentially absent on the hemiplegic side of spastic patients and replaced by facilitation (Figure 2.17a,b; Delwaide & Olivier, 1988). In contrast, Ib inhibition was found to be normal in patients with spinal cord lesions (Figure 2.17c), suggesting there may be pathophysiological differences between spinal and cerebral spasticity (Downes et al., 1995). Ib inhibition is diminished during walking in normal human subjects, similar to the cat where inhibition is replaced by excitation (Stephens & Yang, 1996). This has not yet been investigated in spastic patients, but as Ib inhibition is already reduced at rest further reduction during walking could account for the increased extensor activity observed. Ib non-reciprocal inhibition is reduced by nociceptive discharges from muscle (Rossi & Decchi, 1997). This might provide a basis for the clinical observation of increased spasticity, as opposed to flexor spasms, in the presence of noxious limb lesions.

Interestingly, abnormalities of Ib non-reciprocal inhibition have also been observed in the rigidity syndromes of Parkinson's disease (Delwaide et al., 1991) and progressive supranuclear palsy (Fine et al., 1998). Despite good correlation between impaired Ib inhibition and clinical hypertonia in the UMN syndrome (Delwaide & Pennisi, 1994), other factors must be operating as there is no spasticity in these syndromes. There is some indirect evidence that the Ib inhibition interneurones are not glycinergic (Floeter et al., 1996).

Recurrent (Renshaw) inhibition

Renshaw cells are spinal interneurones that are activated by a collateral of the alpha motoneurone axon. They inhibit not only the homologous motoneurone from which they receive the collateral (recurrent inhibition) but also its paired gamma motoneurone and the Ia inhibitory interneurones that mediate reciprocal inhibition of antagonist motoneurones (Figure 2.18). Thus, Renshaw cells provide negative feedback on agonist motoneurones and facilitate (disinhibit) antagonist motoneurones. Similar to other spinal reflexes, Renshaw cell activity, or recurrent inhibition, may be studied electrophysiologically by an H reflex conditioning technique (Bussel & Pierrot-Deseilligny, 1977). As with most spinal interneurones, Renshaw cell activity is influenced by descending motor pathways demonstrated by changes in recurrent inhibition during voluntary or postural movements (Rossi et al., 1992). The reticulospinal pathways may exert a tonic facilitatory effect and

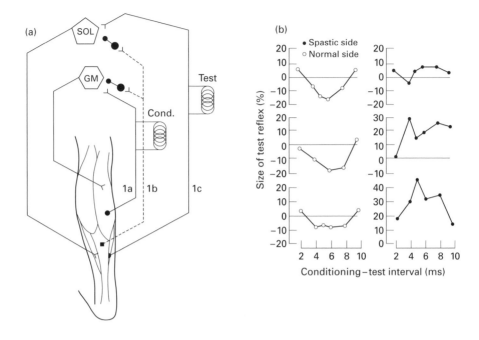

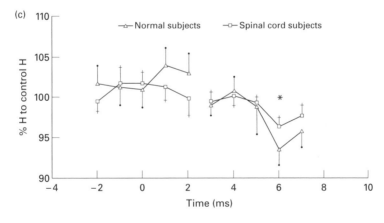

Fig. 2.17   Ib non-reciprocal inhibition. (a): Technique after Pierrot-Deseilligny et al. (1981). Conditioning stimulus given to the nerve to medial gastrocnemius (GM) and the test stimulus to the tibial nerve at varying interstimulus intervals, recording the H reflex from soleus (SOL). (b): The soleus H reflex in three hemiplegic subjects (normal side shown on left, spastic on right of diagram, average of 20 responses). The H reflex is modulated on the normal side with an initial period of facilitation followed by a period of inhibition. On the spastic hemiplegic side, there is little or no inhibition but rather, facilitation. (c): In contrast, results of Ib non-reciprocal inhibition in the soleus H reflex of normal (diamond symbol) and spastic (square symbol) subjects with spinal cord lesions. The spastic subjects showed an impairment of inhibition at the 6 ms test interval similar to that of normal controls. ((a) and (b) from Delwaide and Olivier, 1988; (c) from Downes et al., 1995.)

(a)

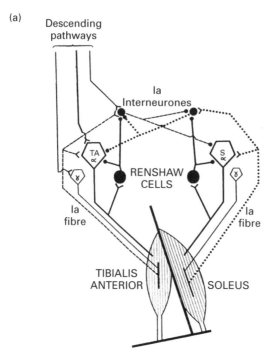

(b)

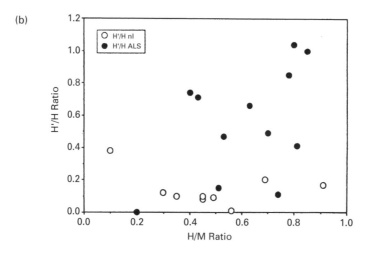

Fig. 2.18   Renshaw cell recurrent inhibition. (a): Renshaw cells provide negative feedback on their alpha motoneurone partner and the Ia inhibitory interneurone mediating reciprocal inhibition of the antagonist muscle. (b) Recurrent inhibition studied in patients (closed circles) with amyotrophic lateral sclerosis (ALS) and spasticity and in normal (nl) subjects (open circles). Generally elevated H'/H ratios in the patient group indicates reduced recurrent inhibition. (From Raynor & Shefner, 1994.)

themselves receive branches from the corticospinal tracts (Mazzocchio & Rossi, 1997). There are also vestibular inputs (Rossi & Mazzocchio, 1988). The coerulospinal tracts have direct contacts onto Renshaw cells and inhibit recurrent inhibition (Fung et al., 1988). Renshaw cells are thus important modulators of motoneurone excitability and diminished recurrent inhibition could contribute to reflex hyperexcitability in the UMN syndrome. The modulation by vestibular input suggests a possible role in the changes in reflex activity associated with posture in the UMN syndrome.

It was therefore surprising to find *increased* recurrent inhibition at rest in chronic spinal cats (Hultborn & Malmsten, 1983). Recurrent inhibition is also increased in humans with spasticity from spinal lesions (Mazzocchio & Rossi, 1989; Shefner et al., 1992) and there is some correlation with the degree of clinical spasticity (Shefner et al., 1992). Patients showing improvement in spasticity were associated with decreases in recurrent inhibition towards normal (Shefner et al., 1992). Interestingly, in one study, only those with hereditary spastic paraparesis and spinal cord transection showed reduced recurrent inhibition; two out of three patients with spastic paraparesis due to cord compression were normal (Mazzocchio & Rossi, 1989). Recurrent inhibition is reportedly normal at rest in hemiplegic patients (Katz & Pierrot-Deseilligny, 1982) but reduced in patients with amyotrophic lateral sclerosis (ALS) and spasticity (Figure 2.18b; Raynor & Shefner, 1994). In the ALS patients, there was a correlation between the impairment of recurrent inhibition and the Achilles tendon reflex. In a mixed group of spastic patients with spinal and cerebral lesions, recurrent inhibition was found to be normal in half the patients and reduced or absent in the other half (Mazzocchio & Rossi, 1997). Thus, recurrent inhibition in the UMN syndrome is variable and again, the abnormalities of spinal physiology associated with spasticity may depend upon the type and location of the lesion causing the UMN syndrome.

Some of the spastic paraparetic patients studied by Mazzocchio & Rossi (1989) failed to modulate recurrent inhibition during voluntary contraction of soleus. This subgroup included subjects with both normal and reduced Renshaw cell activity at rest. Katz & Pierrot-Deseilligny (1982) also found impairment of the normal modulation during voluntary contraction but slightly increased recurrent inhibition at rest. This finding suggests that separate descending motor pathways may modulate recurrent inhibition at rest and during voluntary activity. For mentally retarded patients without spasticity but who had rigidity, their other movement disorders also showed failure of supraspinal modulation of recurrent inhibition (Rossi et al., 1992). This could suggest that the descending motor pathways that were disordered in those subjects are different to those responsible for spasticity.

The role that abnormal recurrent inhibition plays in the hyperexcitability of stretch reflexes and production of spasticity is therefore uncertain. Disordered recurrent inhibition might, however, contribute to disturbed movement synergies seen in the UMN syndrome (Mazzocchio & Rossi, 1997). Disturbed Renshaw activity could also lead to dysfunction of other spinal reflex circuits. A lesion of the facilitatory reticulospinal tracts could make Renshaw cells less sensitive to other supraspinal influences, which could result in increased Ia reciprocal inhibition (Mazzocchio & Rossi, 1997). Generally though, Ia reciprocal inhibition is reduced in spasticity (see above).

Excitatory spinal activity

Alpha motoneurone excitability

If, following an UMN lesion, the alpha motoneurones become intrinsically more excitable as a result of a change in their biophysical properties, their response to afferent stimuli might be greater. This could account for motor overactivity that characterizes the positive features of the UMN syndrome, such as hyperexcitable spinal reflexes and the 'efferent' mediated phenomena.

Studies of spinal cats have generally not supported this hypothesis (Delwaide, 1993). However, some work on motoneurone membrane properties has kept the issue alive. Alpha motoneurones have the property of bistability, the ability to fire stably at two different frequencies and to jump between the two states. Long-lasting periods of increased motoneurone excitability, called plateau potentials, are thought to be responsible for bistability. Plateau potentials can be initiated and terminated by short-lasting synaptic excitation and inhibition respectively, and are dependent upon activity in descending noradrenergic and serotonergic systems. They have been recorded in chronic spinal cats (Eken et al., 1989). The possible role of plateau potentials in spasticity has been discussed elsewhere (Nielsen & Hultborn, 1993).

The two main measures studied in humans are F wave amplitudes and persistence, and H reflex amplitudes (often expressed as a ratio of the maximum M wave, the H_{max}/M_{max} ratio). The F wave represents the recurrent discharge of a small percentage of the motoneurone pool activated antidromically by electrical stimulation of a motor nerve. The reproducibility of the H/M ratio has been demonstrated (Levin & Hui-Chan, 1993). Studies of both F waves (Schiller & Stalberg, 1978; Eisen & Odusote, 1979; Uncini et al., 1990; Bischoff et al., 1992; Milanov, 1994) and the H_{max}/M_{max} ratio (Shemesh et al., 1977; Little & Halar, 1985; Ongerboer de Visser et al., 1989; Koelman et al., 1993) have indicated increased alpha motoneurone excitability in spasticity. However, these indirect means of evaluating alpha motoneurone excitability do not readily distinguish intrinsic motoneurone excitability and the effect of altered synaptic inputs (net increase in excitation) and the results are likely to reflect the latter (Delwaide, 1993; Milanov, 1994).

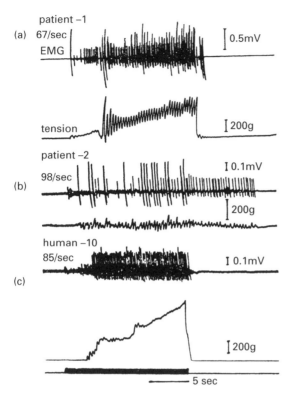

Fig. 2.19   Tonic vibration reflexes (TVR) in spasticity. Electromyography (EMG) recorded from wire
electrodes in the quadriceps muscles while force is measured during a period of vibration
(black bar). (a): The well-preserved TVR of a spastic subject demonstrating vibratory
clonus. (b): An impaired TVR in a spastic subject showing only vibratory clonus. (c) TVR of
a normal subject; note no vibratory clonus. (From Kanda et al., 1973.)

Excitatory interneurone hyperexcitability

Both Ia and group II afferents have excitatory polysynaptic connections to the alpha
motoneurones that have been studied in spasticity (Delwaide & Olivier, 1987).

Ia polysynaptic excitatory pathways

Sustained high-frequency vibration of a relaxed muscle produces a slowly rising
contraction, known as a tonic vibration reflex (TVR), that gradually declines after
the cessation of the vibration (Figure 2.19; Delwaide & Olivier, 1987). Vibration is
a potent stimulus of muscle spindles and the reflex is believed to involve polysynaptic Ia afferent pathways. This pathway receives supraspinal facilitation originat-
ing in the brainstem, based on its persistence in the decerebrate cat and abolition
by cervical cord section (Matthews, 1972). The TVR is present in humans but

rather than being exaggerated, it is impaired in spastic patients (Figure 2.19b; Hagbarth & Eklund, 1966; Kanda et al., 1973; Dimitrijevic et al., 1977). There may be superimposed vibratory clonus (Kanda et al., 1973). It would seem then that the Ia polysynaptic excitatory pathways play no role in the production of spasticity. However, the TVR has some value in spasticity. The anti-spasticity agents diazepam (Verrier et al., 1977) and baclofen (McLellan, 1973) suppress the TVR, which can therefore act as a non-specific gauge of the effect of these medications on polysynaptic reflexes.

Group II polysynaptic excitatory pathways

The role of group II muscle spindle afferents, as one of the flexor reflex afferents (FRA), in the polysynaptic flexor withdrawal reflex has already been mentioned. It had been assumed, therefore, that because the FRAs facilitate flexors and inhibit extensors, muscle spindle group II afferents would not be important in spasticity of the extensors. However, these afferents from the extensors were later discovered to be excitatory (Matthews, 1972) and were postulated to contribute to the M_2 phase of the stretch reflex (Matthews, 1984), also known as the long latency stretch reflex (LLR). A small stretch applied to a tonically contracting muscle produces a short latency response (SLR) and a response of longer latency (LLR). Additional evidence was provided that group II spindle afferents were involved in the enhanced extensor stretch reflexes of the decerebrate cat (McGrath & Matthews, 1973; Kanda & Rymer, 1977; Pierrot-Deseilligny & Mazieres, 1985).

Thus, it was reasonable to suppose that group II afferents could play a role in the hyperexcitable stretch reflexes of human spasticity. As mentioned earlier pharmaco-physiological studies involving L-dopa (Eriksson et al., 1996), tizanidine (Skoog, 1996) and, to a lesser extent, baclofen (Skoog, 1996), support the idea. However, LLRs are often reduced in spastic patients (Deuschl & Lucking, 1990), arguing against increased group II excitatory activity (Cody et al., 1987). The LLR is a trans-cortical reflex (Deuschl & Lucking, 1990) and so perhaps this is not surprising. Others, however, report increased LLR amplitude and duration in the triceps surae that correlates with the degree of clinical hypertonia (Berardelli et al., 1983). In addition, serotonin agonists depress transmission from group II afferents (Jankowska et al., 1994) but serotonergic drugs reportedly *aggravate* spasticity (Stolp-Smith & Wainberg, 1993; del Real et al., 1996) and increase motoneurone excitability (Bedard et al., 1987), while serotonin antagonists such as cyprohepti-dine improve spasticity (Wainberg et al., 1990).

Irrespective of the behaviour of LLRs in spasticity, there is a more fundamental disagreement over the importance of group II afferents in the LLR in humans, with some claiming no role (Deuschl & Lucking, 1990). Hence, at present the role of group II spindle afferents in human spasticity is controversial.

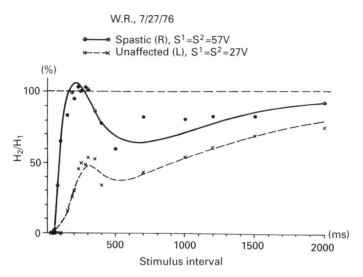

Fig. 2.20   Soleus H reflex recovery curves in a hemiplegic subject showing the normal and spastic sides. Note the general enhancement of the recovery curve on the spastic side. (From Sax & Johnson, 1980.)

H-reflex recovery curves

A soleus H reflex recovery curve is produced by paired stimulation of the tibial nerve in the popliteal fossa. The amplitude of the second H reflex (H_2) is compared with the first H reflex (H_1) and the H_2/H_1 amplitude ratio plotted against interstimulus time interval (Figure 2.20; Sax & Johnson, 1980). The first stimulus is the conditioning stimulus and may be either weaker (subliminal or subthreshold) or equal to the second 'test' stimulus. As shown in Figure 2.20, following the conditioning stimulus there are periods of early suppression and facilitation, and a later period of suppression with a gradual recovery to normal. The H reflex recovery involves polysynaptic pathways and has been used to investigate disorders of muscle tone, such as rigidity and spasticity, as a measure of polysynaptic influences on spinal motoneurone excitability (Kagamihara et al., 1998). The facilitatory and inhibitory effects are probably mediated by circuits involving Ia afferents within the spinal cord, the facilitatory effects of which seem under supraspinal control, but not the inhibitory (Rossi et al., 1988).

The results in human spasticity suggest facilitation of the recovery curve compared with normal subjects or the unaffected limb (Figure 2.20; Sax & Johnson, 1980; Koelman et al., 1993; Panizza et al., 1995). Some correlation with the severity of spasticity has been reported (Panizza et al., 1995). However, the methodology of these studies has been criticized making their results difficult to interpret and their value questionable (Ashby, 1980; Lance, 1980; Kagamihara et al., 1998) and they have largely gone out of favour (Delwaide, 1985b). H reflex recovery curves have featured in pharmacological studies of anti-spasticity agents (Delwaide et al., 1980) with effective medications showing differing effects. As with other tests of spinal reflexes, similar abnormalities of the H reflex recovery curve are also present in Parkinson's disease (Sax & Johnson, 1980) and dystonia (Koelman et al., 1995).

Conclusion regarding spinal mechanisms in the UMN syndrome

Despite the wealth of research, clear correlations between individual spinal interneuronal circuits and the clinical features of the UMN syndrome are lacking, except in the case of flexor spasms. The results are plagued by inconsistencies in the basic finding of the presence or absence of abnormality between individual patients and between studies, particularly for recurrent inhibition. Furthermore, many of the abnormalities described are also found in patients with dystonia and Parkinson's disease, where spasticity, tendon hyperreflexia, flexor and extensor spasms are absent. Despite some association with existence of spasticity, the electrophysiological abnormalities described do not always correlate with clinical measures of the degree of spasticity (Shemesh et al., 1977; Cody et al., 1987; Levin & Hui-Chan, 1993), raising doubt about their pathophysiological role in spasticity. An exception might be flexor withdrawal reflexes and flexor spasms, but in any case these are separate from spasticity (hyperactive tonic stretch reflexes). Hence, it is fair to say that no one test accurately reflects the basic pathophysiological substrate of spasticity and it is quite probable that the condition is a heterogeneous one. Perhaps the strongest association exists between Ia presynaptic inhibition and tendon hyperreflexia.

None the less, these electrophysiological tests often become more normal with anti-spastic medication, sometimes coincident with a reduction in clinical measures of spasticity (e.g. Mondrup & Pedersen, 1984; Macdonell et al., 1989; Nance et al., 1989; Delwaide & Pennisi, 1994), and sometimes not (Martinelli, 1990). For example, the H/M ratio, reciprocal Ia inhibition and recurrent inhibition were unchanged following protirelin tartrate administration, despite clear reduction in hypertonia and tendon hyperreflexia (Martinelli, 1990). Such a finding might lead to the conclusion that abnormalities of these spinal reflex activities in these patients (post-stroke) were not important in the production of the clinical signs. Thus, the spinal reflex changes may simply be epiphenomena. One potential problem when attempting to correlate electrophysiological findings with the clinical signs is that hypertonia may be due to both (neural) stretch hyperreflexia and biomechanical factors (Nielsen & Sinkjaer, 1996). Thus, a patient with minimal spasticity but marked hypertonia due to soft tissue changes may have only minimally abnormal spinal electrophysiological studies.

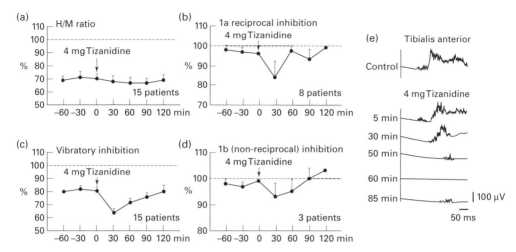

Fig. 2.21   A battery of electrophysiological tests of spinal interneuronal pathways in spastic subjects before and after a single oral dose of tizanidine, 4 mg. Note an effect on Ia reciprocal inhibition (b), vibratory inhibition ((c), representing Ia presynaptic inhibition), Ib non-reciprocal inhibition (d) and flexor withdrawal reflexes from tibialis anterior elicited by sural nerve stimulation (e). The H/M ratio ((a), representing alpha motoneurone excitability) was unchanged. (From Delwaide & Pennisi, 1994.)

One beneficial product of these electrophysiological studies has been the ability to observe and quantify the effects of anti-spastic drugs. Effective drugs often have completely different electrophysiological effects, despite similar clinical efficacy (Figure 2.21; Delwaide & Pennisi, 1994). Combined drug and electrophysiological studies may also help elucidate the pathophysiological mechanisms responsible for spasticity. It has even been suggested that the prescription of anti-spastic agents should be based more scientifically upon the results of electrophysiological tests, such as those outlined above (Delwaide & Pennisi, 1994) and could even provide a logical basis for combination drug therapy (Delwaide, 1985b).

Neuropharmacology of the UMN syndrome

This subject has been dealt with in other reviews (Noth, 1991; Young, 1994; Gracies et al., 1997). However, from the foregoing discussion, the neurotransmitters GABA, glycine, noradrenaline, dopamine, serotonin and excitatory amino acids (glutamate) seem to play a role. Much of this information has come from observations of the clinical and electrophysiological effects of anti-spasticity agents, their agonists and antagonists. Caution must therefore be exerted before drawing the conclusion that these neurotransmitters are important in the production of spasticity and the other positive UMN features, as opposed to their ability to ameliorate these signs.

REFERENCES

Ada L., Vattanasilp, W., O'Dwyer, N. J., & Crossbie, J. (1998). Does spasticity contribute to walking dysfunction after stroke? *J Neurol Neurosurg Psychiatry*, **64**: 628–35.

Andrews, C. J., Knowles, L. & Hancock J. (1973a). Control of the tonic vibration reflexes by the brain-stem reticular formation in the cat. *J Neurol Sci*, **18**: 217–26.

Andrews, C. J., Neilson, P. D. & Knowles, L. (1973b). Electromyographic study of the rigido-spasticity of athetosis. *J Neurol Neurosurg Psychiatry*, **36**: 94–103.

Artieda, J., Quesada, P. & Obeso, J. A. (1991). Reciprocal inhibition between forearm muscles in spastic hemiplegia. *Neurology*, **41**: 286–9.

Ashby, P. (1980). Discussion. In *Spasticity: Disordered Motor Control*, ed. RG Feldman, R.R. Young & W. P. Koella, p. 332. Chicago: Year Book Medical Publishers.

Ashby, P. & Burke, D. (1971). Stretch reflexes in the upper limb of spastic man. *J Neurol Neurosurg Psychiatry*, **34**: 765–71.

Ashby, P. & Wiens, M. (1989). Reciprocal inhibition following lesions of the spinal cord in man. *J Physiol*, **414**: 145–57.

Ashworth, B. (1964) Preliminary trial of carisoprodol in multiple sclerosis. *Practitoner*, **192**: 540–2.

Bach-y-Rita, P. & Illis, L. S. (1993). Spinal shock: possible role of receptor plasticity and non synaptic transmission. *Paraplegia*, **31**: 82–7.

Barolat, G. & Maiman, D. J. (1987). Spasms in spinal cord injury: a study of 72 subjects. *J Am Paraplegia Soc*, **10**: 35–9.

Becher, J. G., Harlaar, J., Lankhorst, G. J. & Vogelaar, T. W. (1998). Measurement of impaired muscle function of the gastrocnemius, soleus, and tibialis anterior muscles in spastic hemiplegia: a preliminary study. *J Rehabil Res Dev*, **35**: 314–26.

Bedard, P. J., Tremblay, L. E., Barbeau, H., Filion, M., Maheux, R., Richards, C. L. & DiPaolo, T. (1987). Action of 5–hydroxytryptamine, substance P, thyrotropin-releasing hormone and clonidine on motoneurone excitability. *Can J Neurol Sci*, **14** (Suppl. 3): 506–9.

Benecke, R. (1990). Spasticity/spasms: clinical aspects and treatment. In *Motor Disturbances*, vol. II, ed. A. Berardelli, R. Benecke, M. Manfield & C. D. Marsden, pp. 169–77. London: Academic Press.

Berardelli, A., Rothwell, J. C., Hallett, M., Thompson, P. D., Manfredi, M. & Marsden, C. D. (1998). The pathophysiology of primary dystonia. *Brain*, **121**, 1195–212.

Berardelli, A., Sabra, A. F., Hallett, M., Berenberg, W. & Simon, S. R. (1983). Stretch reflexes of triceps surae in patients with upper motor neuron syndromes. *J Neurol Neurosurg Psychiatry*, **46**, 54–60.

Bischoff, C., Schoenle, P. W. & Conrad, B. (1992). Increased F-wave duration in patients with spasticity. *Electromyogr Clin Neurophysiol*, **32**: 449–453.

Bobath, B. (1990). *Adult Hemiplegia: Evaluation and Treatment*, 3rd edn., pp. 11–12. London: Butterworth-Heinemann.

Bodian, D. (1946). Experimental evidence on the cerebral origin of muscle spasticity in acute poliomyelitis. *Proc Soc Exp Biol Med*, **61**: 170–5.

Boorman, G., Becker, W. J., Morrice, B. L. & Lee, R. G. (1992). Modulation of the soleus H-reflex during pedalling in normal humans and in patients with spinal spasticity. *J Neurol Neurosurg Psychiatry*, **55**: 1150–6.

Boorman, G., Hulliger, M., Lee, R. G., Tako, K. & Tanaka, R. (1991). Reciprocal Ia inhibition in patients with spinal spasticity. *Neurosci Lett*, **127**: 57–60.

Boorman, G. I., Lee, R. G., Becker, W. J. & Windhorst, U. R. (1996). Impaired 'natural reciprocal inhibition' in patients with spasticity due to incomplete spinal cord injury. *Electroencephalogr Clin Neurophysiol*, **101**: 84–92.

Borsook, D., Becerra, L., Fishman, S., Edwards, A., Jennings, C. L., Stojanovic, M., Papinicolas, L., Ramachandran, V. S., Gonzalez, R. G. & Breiter, H. (1998). Acute plasticity in the human somatosensory cortex following amputation. *Neuroreport*, **9**: 1013–17.

Bourbonnais, D., Boissy, P., Gravel, D., Arsenault, B., Brule, N. & Kaegi, C. (1995). Quantification of upper limb synkinesis in hemiparetic subjects. *Rehabilitation R and D Progress Report 1994, Department of Veterans Affairs*, No. 32, pp. 118–19.

Brown, J. K., van Rensburg, F., Walsh, G., Lakie, M. & Wright, G. W. (1987). A neurological study of hand function of hemiplegic children. *Dev Med Child Neurol*, **29**: 287–304.

Brown, P. (1994). Pathophysiology of spasticity (editorial). *J Neurol Neurosurg Psychiatry*, **57**: 773–7

Bucy, P. C. (1938). Studies on the human neuromuscular mechanism. II. Effect of ventromedial cordotomy on muscular spasticity in man. *Arch Neurol Psychiatry*, **40**: 639–62.

Bucy, P. C., Keplinger, J. E. & Siqueira, E. B. (1964). Destruction of the 'pyramidal tract' in man. *J Neurosurg*, **21**: 385–98.

Burke, D. (1983). Critical examination of the case for or against fusimotor involvement in disorders of muscle tone. In *Motor Control Mechanisms in Health and Disease*, ed. J. E. Desmedt, pp. 133–50. New York: Raven Press.

Burke, D. (1985). Mechanisms underlying the tendon jerk and H-reflex. In *Clinical Neurophysiology in Spasticity*, ed. P. J. Delwaide & R. R. Young, pp. 55–62. Amsterdam: Elsevier Science Publishers BV.

Burke, D. (1988). Spasticity as an adaptation to pyramidal tract injury. In *Functional Recovery in Neurological Disease, Advances in Neurology*, ed. S. G. Waxman, vol 47, pp. 401–23. New York: Raven Press.

Burke, D. & Ashby, P. (1972). Are spinal 'presynaptic' inhibitory mechanisms suppressed in spasticity? *J Neurol Sci*, **15**: 321–6.

Burke, D., Gandevia, S. C. & McKeon, B. (1983). The afferent volleys responsible for spinal proprioceptive reflexes in man. *J Physiol (Lond)*, **339**: 535–52.

Burke, D., Gillies, J. D. & Lance, J. W. (1970). The quadriceps stretch reflex in human spasticity. *J Neurol Neurosurg Psychiatry*, **33**: 216–23.

Burke, D., Knowles, L., Andrews, C. & Ashby, P. (1972). Spasticity, decerebrate rigidity and the clasp knife phenomenon. An experimental study in the cat. *Brain*, **95**: 31–48.

Burke, D. & Lance, J. W. (1973). Studies of the reflex effects of primary and secondary spindle endings in spasticity. In *New Developments in Electromyography and Clinical Neurophysiology*, ed. J. E. Desmedt, vol 3, pp. 475–95. Basel: Karger.

Bussel, B. & Pierrot-Diseilligny, E. (1977). Inhibition of human motoneurons, probably Renshaw origin, elicited by an orthodromic motor discharge. *J Physiol (Lond)*, **269**: 319–39.

Calancie, B., Broton, J. G., Klose, K. J., Traad, M., Difini, J. & Ayyar, D. R. (1993). Evidence that alterations in presynaptic inhibition contribute to segmental hypo- and hyperexcitability after spinal cord injury in man. *Electroencephalogr Clin Neurophysiol*, **89**: 177–86.

Carey, J. R. (1990). Manual stretch: effect on finger movement control in stroke subjects with spastic extrinsic finger flexor muscles. *Arch Phys Med Rehabil*, **71**: 888–94.

Cavallari, P. & Pettersson, L. G. (1989). Tonic suppression of reflex transmission in low spinal cats. *Exp Brain Res*, **77**: 201–12.

Chen, R., Corwell, B., Yaseen, Z., Hallett, M. & Cohen, L. G. (1998). Mechanisms of cortical reorganization in lower-limb amputees. *J Neurosci*, **18**: 3443–50.

Cody, F. W., Richardson, H. C., MacDermott, N. & Ferguson, I. T. (1987). Stretch and vibration reflexes of wrist flexor muscles in spasticity. *Brain*, **110**: 433–50.

Conrad, B., Benecke, B. & Meinck, H. M. (1985). Gait disturbances in paraspastic patients. In *Clinical Neurophysiology in Spasticity*, ed. P. J. Delwaide & R. R. Young, pp. 155–74. Amsterdam: Elsevier Science Publishers BV.

Corcos, D. M, Gottleib, G. L., Penn, R. D., Myklebust, B. & Agarwal, G. C. (1986). Movement deficits caused by hyperexcitable stretch reflexes in spastic humans. *Brain*, **109**: 1043–58.

Crenna, P. (1998). Spasticity and 'spastic' gait in children with cerebral palsy. *Neurosci Neurobehav Rev*, **22**: 571–8.

Crone, C., Nielsen, J., Petersen, N., Ballegaard, M. & Hultborn, H. (1994). Disynaptic reciprocal inhibition of ankle extensors in spastic patients. *Brain*, **117**: 1161–8.

Davies, J. M., Mayston, M. J. & Newham, D. J. (1996). Electrical and mechanical output of the knee muscles during isometric and isokinetic activity in stroke and healthy adults. *Disabil Rehabil*, **18**: 83–90.

de Gail, Lance, J. W. & Nielsen, P. D. (1966). Differential effects on tonic and phasic reflex mechanisms produced by vibration of muscle in man. *J Neurol Neurosurg Psychiatry*, **29**: 1–11.

del Real, M. A., Hernandez, A., Vaamonde, J. & Gudin, M. (1996). Exacerbation of spasticity induced by serotonin reuptake inhibitors. *Neurologia*, **11**: 272 (letter).

Delwaide, P. J. (1985a). Electrophysiological analysis of the mode of action of muscle relaxants in spasticity. *Ann Neurol*, **17**: 90–5.

Delwaide, P. J. (1985b). Electrophysiological testing of spastic patients: its potential usefulness and limitations. In *Clinical Neurophysiology in Spasticity*, ed. P. J. Delwaide & R. R. Young, pp. 185–203. Amsterdam: Elsevier Science Publishers BV.

Delwaide, P. J. (1993). Pathophysiological mechanisms of spasticity at the spinal cord level. In *Spasticity: Mechanisms and Management*, ed. A. F. Thilmann, D. J. Burke & W. Z. Rymer, pp. 296–308. Berlin: Springer-Verlag.

Delwaide, P. J., Martinelli, P. & Crenna, P. (1980). Clinical neurophysiological measurement of spinal reflex activity. In *Spasticity: Disordered Motor Control*, ed. R. G. Feldman, R. R. Young & W. P. Koella, pp. 345–71. Chicago: Year Book Medical Publishers.

Delwaide, P. J. & Olivier, E. (1987). Pathophysiological aspects of spasticity in man. In *Motor Disturbances I*, ed. R. Benecke, B. Conrad & C. D. Marsden, pp. 153–68. London: Academic Press.

Delwaide, P. J. & Olivier, E. (1988). Short-latency autogenic inhibition (IB inhibition) in human spasticity. *J Neurol Neurosurg Psychiatry*, **51**: 1546–50.

Delwaide, P. J. & Pennisi, G. (1994). Tizanidine and electrophysiologic analysis of spinal control mechanisms in humans with spasticity. *Neurology*, **44**(Suppl. 9): S21–S28.

Delwaide, P. J., Pepin, J. L. & Maertens de Noordhout, A. (1991). Short-latency autogenic inhibition in patients with Parkinsonian rigidity. *Ann Neurol*, **30**: 83–9.

Denny-Brown, D. (1966). *The Cerebral Control of Movement*. Liverpool: Liverpool University Press.

Deuschl, G. & Lucking, C. H. (1990). Physiology and clinical applications of hand muscle reflexes. *Electroencephalogr Clin Neurophysiol*, **41**(Suppl): 84–101.

Dewald, J. P., Given, J. D. & Rymer, W. Z. (1996). Long-lasting reductions of spasticity induced by skin electrical stimulation. *IEEE Trans Rehabil Eng*, **4**: 231–42.

Dewald, J. P. A. & Rymer, W. Z. (1993). Factors underlying abnormal posture and movement in spastic hemiparesis. In *Spasticity: Mechanisms and Management*, ed. A. F. Thilmann, D.J. Burke & W. Z. Rymer, pp. 123–38. Berlin: Springer-Verlag.

Dickstein, R., Heffes, Y. & Abulaffio, N. (1996). Electromyographic and positional changes in the elbows of spastic hemiparetic patients during walking. *Electroenceph Clin Neurophysiol*, **101**: 491–6.

Dietrichson, P. (1971). Phasic ankle reflex in spasticity and Parkinsonian rigidity. The role of the fusimotor system. *Acta Neurol Scand*, **47**: 22–51.

Dietrichson, P. (1973). The role of the fusimotor system in spasticity and parkinsonian rigidity. In *New Developments in Electromyography and Clinical Neurophysiology*, ed. J. E. Desmedt, vol 3, pp. 496–507. Basel: Karger.

Dietz, V. & Berger, W. (1983). Normal and impaired regulation of muscle stiffness in gait: a new hypothesis about muscle hypertonia. *Exp Neurol*, **79**: 680–7.

Dietz, V., Faist, M. & Pierrot-Deseilligny, E. (1990). Amplitude modulation of the quadriceps H-reflex in the human during the early stance phase of gait. *Exp Brain Res*, **79**: 221–4.

Dietz, V., Ketelsen, U. P., Berger, W. & Quintern, J. (1986). Motor unit involvement in spastic paresis. Relationship between leg muscle activation and histochemistry. *J Neurol Sci*, **75**: 89–103.

Dietz, V., Quintern, J. & Berger, W. (1981). Electrophysiological studies of gait in spasticity and rigidity. Evidence that altered mechanical properties of muscle contribute to hypertonia. *Brain*, **104**: 431–49.

Dietz, V., Trippel, M. & Berger, W. (1991). Reflex activity and muscle tone during elbow movements in patients with spastic paresis. *Ann Neurol*, **30**: 767–79.

Dimitrijevic, M. R., Nathan, P. W. & Sherwood, A. M. (1980). Clonus: the role of central mechanisms. *J Neurol Neurosurg Psychiatry*, **43**: 321–32.

Dimitrijevic, M. R., Spencer, W. A., Trontelj, J. V. & Dimitrijevic, M. (1977). Reflex effects of vibration in patients with spinal cord lesions. *Neurology*, **27**: 1078–86.

Downes, L., Ashby, P. & Bugaresti, J. (1995). Reflex effects from Golgi tendon organ (Ib) afferents are unchanged after spinal cord lesions in humans. *Neurology*, **45**: 1720–4.

Eccles, R. M. & Lundberg, A. (1959). Supraspinal control of interneurones mediating spinal reflexes. *J Physiol*, **147**: 565–84.

Eisen, A. & Odusote, K. (1979). Amplitude of the F wave: a potential means of documenting spasticity. *Neurology*, **29**: 1306–9.

Eken, T., Hultborn, H. & Kiehn, O. (1989). Possible functions of transmitter-controlled plateau potentials in alpha motoneurones. *Prog Brain Res*, **80**: 257–67.

el-Abd, M. A., Ibrahim, I. K. & Dietz, V. (1993). Impaired activation pattern in antagonistic elbow muscles of patients with spastic hemiparesis: contribution to movement disorder. *Electromyogr Clin Neurophysiol*, 33: 247–55.

Elbert, T., Flor, H., Birbaumer, N., Knecht, S., Hampson, S., Larbig, W. & Taub, E. (1994). Extensive reorganization of the somatosensory cortex in adult humans after nervous system injury. *Neuroreport*, 5: 2593–7.

Emre, M., Leslie, G. C., Muir, C., Part, N. J., Pokorny, R. & Roberts, R. C. (1994). Correlations between dose, plasma concentrations, and antispastic action of tizanidine (Sirdalud). *J Neurol Neurosurg Psychiatry*, 57: 1355–9.

Engberg, I., Lundberg, A. & Ryall, R. W. (1968). Reticulospinal inhibition of transmission in reflex pathways. *J Physiol*, 194: 201–23.

Eriksson, J., Olausson, B. & Jankowska, E. (1996). Antispastic effects of L-dopa. *Exp Brain Res*, 111: 296–304.

Fahn, S., Marsden, C. D. & Calne, D. B. (1987). Classification and investigation of dystonia. In *Movement Disorders 2*, ed. C. D. Marsden & S. Fahn, pp. 332–58, London: Butterworths.

Faist, M., Mazevet, D., Dietz, V. & Pierrot-Deseilligny, E. (1994). A quantitative assessment of presynaptic inhibition of Ia afferents in spastics. Differences in hemiplegics and paraplegics. *Brain*, 117: 1449–55.

Feinstein, B., Gleason, C. A. & Libet, B. (1989). Stimulation of locus coeruleus in man. Preliminary trials for spasticity and epilepsy. *Stereotact Funct Neurosurg*, 52: 26–41.

Fellows, S. J., Klaus, C., Ross, H. F. & Thilmann, A. F. (1994). Agonist and antagonist EMG activation during isometric torque development at the elbow in spastic hemiparesis. *Electroenceph Clin Neurophysiol*, 93: 106–12.

Fine, E. J., Hallett, M., Litvan, I., Tresser, N. & Katz, D. (1998). Dysfunction of Ib (autogenic) spinal inhibition in patients with progressive supranuclear palsy. *Mov Disord*, 13: 668–72.

Flanders, M. & Cordo, P. J. (1987). Quantification of peripherally induced reciprocal activation during voluntary muscle contraction. *Electroencephalogr Clin Neurophysiol*, 67: 389–94.

Floeter, M. K., Andermann, F., Andermann, E., Nigro, M. & Hallett, M. (1996). Physiological studies of spinal inhibitory pathways in patients with hereditary hyperplexia. *Neurology*, 46: 766–72.

Florence, S. L. & Kaas, J. H. (1995). Large-scale reorganization at multiple levels of the somatosensory pathway follows therapeutic amputation of the hand in monkeys. *J Neurosci*, 15: 8083–95.

Fries, W., Danek, A., Scheidtman, K. & Hamburger, C. (1993). Motor recovery following capsular stroke. Role of descending pathways from multiple motor areas. *Brain*, 116: 369–82.

Fung, J. & Barbeau, H. (1994). Effects of conditioning cutaneomuscular stimulation on the soleus H-reflex in normal and spastic paretic subjects during walking and standing. *J Neurophysiol*, 72: 2090–104.

Fung, S. J., & Barnes, C. D. (1986). Increased efficacy of antidromic and orthodromic activation of cat alpha motoneurons upon arrival of coerulospinal volleys. *Arch Ital Biol*, 124: 229–43.

Fung, S. J., Pompeiano, O. & Barnes, C. D. (1988). Coerulospinal influence on recurrent inhibition of spinal motonuclei innervating antagonistic hindleg muscles of the cat. *Pflugers Arch*, 412: 346–53.

Gracies, J. M., Nance, P., Elovic, E., McGuire, J. & Simpson, D. M. (1997). Traditional pharmacological treatments for spasticity. Part II: General and regional treatments. *Muscle Nerve*, (Suppl 6): S92–S120.

Hagbarth, K. E. (1952). Excitatory and inhibitory skin areas for flexor and extensor motoneurones. *Acta Physiol Scand*, 26(Supl. 94): 1–58.

Hagbarth, K. E. (1960). Spinal withdrawal reflexes in the human lower limb. *J Neurol Neurosurg Psychiatry*, 23: 222–7.

Hagbarth, K. E. & Eklund, G. (1966). Tonic vibration reflexes (TVR) in spasticity. *Brain Res*, 2: 201–3.

Hagbarth, K. E., Hagglund, J. V, Nordin, M. & Wallin, E. U. (1985). Thixotropic behaviour of human finger flexor muscles with accompanying changes in spindle and reflex responses to stretch. *J Physiol (Lond)*, 368: 323–42.

Harburn, K. L, Vandervoort, A. A., Helewa, A., Goldsmith, C. H., Kertesz, A., Teasell, R. W. & Hill, K. M. (1995). A reflex technique to measure presynaptic inhibition in cerebral stroke. *Electromyogr Clin Neurophysiol*, 35: 149–63.

Hayashi, R., Tokuda, T., Tako, K. & Yanagisawa, N. (1997). Impaired modulation of tonic muscle activities and H-reflexes in the soleus muscle during standing in patients with Parkinson's disease. *J Neurol Sci*, 153: 61–7.

Herbert, R. (1988). The passive mechanical properties of muscle and their adaptations to altered patterns of use. *Aust J Physiotherap*, 34: 141–9.

Herman, R. (1970). The myotatic reflex: clinicophysiological aspects of spasticity and contraction. *Brain*, 93: 272–312.

Houk, J. C. & Henneman, E. (1967). Responses of golgi tendon organs to active contractions of the soleus muscle in the cat. *J Neurophysiol*, 330: 466–81.

Hufschmidt, A. & Mauritz, K. H. (1985). Chronic transformation of muscle in spasticity: a peripheral contribution to increased tone. *J Neurol Neurosurg Psychiatry*, 48: 676–85.

Hulsebosch, C. E. & Coggeshall, R. E. (1981). Sprouting of dorsal root axons. *Brain Res*, 224: 170–4.

Hultborn, H. & Malmsten, J. (1983). Changes in segmental reflexes following chronic spinal cord hemisection in the cat. II. Conditioned monosynaptic test reflexes. *Acta Physiol Scand*, 119: 423–33.

Hultborn, H., Lindstrom, S. & Wigstrom, H. (1979). On the function of recurrent inhibition in the spinal cord. *Exp Brain Res*, 37: 399–403.

Humphrey, D. R. & Reed, D. J. (1983). Separate cortical systems for control of joint movement and joint stiffness: reciprocal activation and coactivation of antagonist muscles. In *Motor Control Mechanisms in Health and Disease*, ed. J. E. Desmedt, pp. 347–72. New York: Raven Press.

Ibrahim, I. K., Berger, W., Trippel, M. & Dietz, V. (1993). Stretch-induced electromyographic activity and torque in spastic elbow muscles. Differential modulation of reflex activity in passive and active motor tasks. *Brain*, 116: 971–89.

Iles, J. F. (1996). Evidence for cutaneous and corticospinal modulation of presynaptic inhibition of Ia afferents from the human lower limb. *J Physiol (Lond)*, 491: 197–207.

Iles, J. F. & Pisini, J. V. (1992). Vestibular-evoked postural reactions in man and modulation of human locomotion. *Rev Neurol (Paris)*, **143**: 241–54.

Iles, J. F. & Roberts, R. C. (1986). Presynaptic inhibition of monosynaptic reflexes in the lower limbs of subjects with upper motoneuron disease. *J Neurol Neurosurg Psychiatry*, **49**: 937–44.

Ito, T., Furukawa, K., Karasawa, T., Kadokawa, T. & Shimizu, M. (1985). Functional change in the rat spinal cord by chronic spinal transection and possible roles of monoamine neurons. *Jpn J Pharmacol*, **38**: 243–51.

Jankowska, E., Lackberg, Z. S. & Dyrehag, L. E. (1994). Effects of monoamines on transmission from group II muscle afferents in sacral segments in the cat. *Eur J Neurosci*, **6**: 1058–61.

Kagamihara, Y., Hayashi, A., Okuma, Y., Nagaoka, M., Nakajima, Y. & Tanaka, R. (1998). Reassessment of H-reflex recovery curve using the double stimulation procedure. *Muscle Nerve*, **21**: 352–60.

Kanda, K. & Rymer, W. Z. (1977). An estimate of the secondary spindle receptor afferent contribution to the stretch reflex in extensor muscles of the decerebrate cat. *J Physiol (Lond)*, **264**: 63–87.

Kanda, K., Homma, S. & Watanabe, S. (1973). Vibration reflex in spastic patients. In *New Developments in Electromyography and Clinical Neurophysiology*, ed. J. E. Desmedt, vol. 3, pp. 469–74. Basel: Karger.

Katz, R. & Pierrot-Deseilligny, E. (1982). Recurrent inhibition of alpha-motoneurons in patients with upper motor neuron lesions. *Brain*, **105**: 103–24.

Kimura, J. (1989). *Electrodiagnosis in Diseases of Nerve and Muscle: Principles and Practice*, 2nd edn. Philadelphia: F A Davis.

Koelman, J. H., Bour, L. J., Hilgevoord, A. A., van Bruggen, G. J. & Ongerboer de Visser, B. W. (1993). Soleus H-reflex tests and clinical signs of the upper motor neuron syndrome. *J Neurol Neurosurg Psychiatry*, **56**: 776–81.

Koelman, J. H., Willemse, R. B., Bour, L. J., Hilgevoord, A. A., Speelman, J. D. & Ongerboer de Visser, B. W. (1995). Soleus H-reflex tests in dystonia. *Mov Disord*, **10**, 44–50.

Krenz, N. R. & Weaver, L. C. (1998). Sprouting of primary afferent fibers after spinal cord transection in the rat. *Neuroscience*, **85**: 443–58.

Kugelberg, E. (1962). Polysynaptic reflexes of clinical importance. *Electroenceph Clin Neurophysiol*, (Suppl. 22): 103–11.

Lance, J. W. (1980) Symposium synopsis. In *Spasticity: Disordered Motor Control*, ed. R. G. Feldman, R. R. Young & W. P. Koella, pp. 485–94. Chicago: Year Book Medical Publishers.

Lance, J. W. & de Gail, P. (1965). Spread of phasic muscle reflexes in normal and spastic subjects. *J Neurol Neurosurg Psychiatry*, **28**: 328–34.

Latash, M. L. & Penn, R. D. (1996). Changes in voluntary motor control induced by intrathecal baclofen in patients with spasticity of different etiology. *Physiother Res Int*, **1**: 229–46.

Lee, W. A., Boughton, A. & Rymer, W. Z. (1987). Absence of stretch reflex gain enhancement in voluntarily activated spastic muscle. *Exp Neurol*, **98**: 317–35.

Levin, M. F. & Hui-Chan, C. W. (1992). Relief of hemiparetic spasticity by TENS is associated with improvement in reflex and voluntary motor functions. *Electroencephalogr Clin Neurophysiol*, **85**: 131–42.

Levin, M. F. & Hui-Chan, C. (1993). Are H and stretch reflexes in hemiparesis reproducible and correlated with spasticity? *J Neurol*, **240**: 63–71.

Liddell, E. G. T., Matthes, K., Oldberg, E. & Ruch, T. C. (1932). Reflex release of flexor muscles by spinal transection. *Brain*, **55**: 239–45.

Lindsley, D. B., Schreiner, L. M. & Magoun, W. (1949). An electromyographic study of spasticity. *J Neurophysiol*, **12**: 197–205.

Little, J. W. & Halar, E. M. (1985). H-reflex changes following spinal cord injury. *Arch Phys Med Rehabil*, **66**: 19–22.

Lundberg, A. & Voorhoeve, P. (1962). Effects from the pyramidal tract on spinal reflex arcs. *Acta Physiol Scand*, **56**: 201–19.

Macdonell, R. A, Talalla, A., Swash, M. & Grundy, D. (1989). Intrathecal baclofen and the H-reflex. *J Neurol Neurosurg Psychiatry*, **52**: 1110–12.

Magoun, H. W. & Rhines, R. (1947). *Spasticity. The Stretch Reflex and Extrapyramidal Systems.* Springfield: Thomas.

Mailis, A. & Ashby, P. (1990). Alterations in group Ia projections to motoneurons following spinal lesions in humans. *J Neurophysiol*, **64**: 637–47.

Maj, J., Chojnacka-Wojcik, E., Lewandowska, A. & Tatarczynska, E. (1985). Central antiserotonin action of fluperlapine. *Pol J Pharmacol Pharm*, **37**: 517–24.

Malouin, F., Bonneau, C., Pichard, L. & Corriveau, D. (1997). Non-reflex mediated changes in plantarflexor muscles early after stroke. *Scand J Rehabil Med*, **29**: 147–53.

Manfredi, M., Sacco, G. & Sideri, G. (1975). The tonic ambulatory foot response. A clinical and electromyographic study. *Brain*, **98**: 167–80.

Martinelli, P. (1990). Use of TRH-T for the symptomatic treatment of the pathology of the upper motoneurons and electrophysiologic evaluation of its efficacy. *Ann Ital Med Int*, **5**: 262–9.

Matthews, P. B. (1984). Evidence from the use of vibration that the human long-latency stretch reflex depends upon spindle secondary afferents. *J Physiol (Lond)*, **348**: 383–415.

Matthews, P. B. C. (1972). *Mammalian Muscle Receptors and their Central Actions.* London: Edward Arnold.

Mazzocchio, R. & Rossi, A. (1989). Recurrent inhibition in human spinal spasticity. *Ital J Neurol Sci*, **10**: 337–47.

Mazzocchio, R. & Rossi, A. (1997). Involvement of spinal recurrent inhibition in spasticity. Further insight into the regulation of Renshaw cell activity. *Brain*, **120**: 991–1003.

McCouch, G. P., Austin, G. M. Liu, C. N. & Liu, C. Y. (1958). Sprouting as a cause of spasticity. *J. Neurophysiol*, **21**: 205–16.

McGrath, G. J. & Matthews, P. B. (1973). Evidence from the use of vibration during procaine nerve block that the spindle group II fibres contribute excitation to the tonic stretch reflex of the decerebrate cat. *J Physiol (Lond)*, **235**: 371–408.

McLellan, D. L. (1973). Effect of baclofen upon monosynaptic and tonic vibration reflexes in patients with spasticity. *J Neurol Neurosurg Psychiatry*, **36**: 555–60.

Meinck, H-M., Benecke, R. & Conrad, B. (1985) Spasticity and the flexor reflex. In *Clinical Neurophysiology in Spasticity*, ed. P. J. Delwaide & R. R. Young, pp. 41–54. Amsterdam: Elsevier Science Publishers BV.

Meinders, M., Price, R., Lehmann, J. F. & Questad, K. A. (1996). The stretch reflex response in the normal and spastic ankle: effect of ankle position. *Arch Phys Med Rehabil*, **77**: 487–92.

Meunier, S. & Pierrot-Deseilligny, E. (1998). Cortical control of presynaptic inhibition of Ia afferents in humans. *Exp Brain Res*, **119**: 415–26.

Milanov, I. G. (1992). Mechanisms of baclofen action on spasticity. *Acta Neurol Scand*, **85**: 305–10.

Milanov, I. (1994). Examination of the segmental pathophysiological mechanisms of spasticity. *Electromyogr Clin Neurophysiol*, **34**: 73–9.

Milanov, I. & Georgiev, D. (1994). Mechanisms of tizanidine action on spasticity. *Acta Neurol Scand*, **89**: 274–9.

Mizrahi, E. M. & Angel, R. W. (1979). Impairment of voluntary movement by spasticity. *Ann Neurol*, **5**: 594–95.

Mondrup, K. & Pedersen, E. (1984). The effect of the GABA-agonist, progabide, on stretch and flexor reflexes and on voluntary power in spastic patients. *Acta Neurol Scand*, **69**: 191–9.

Morin, C. & Pierrot-Deseilligny, E. (1988). Spinal mechanism of the antispastic action of TRH in patients with amyotrophic lateral sclerosis. *Rev Neurol (Paris)*, **144**: 701–3.

Mynark, R. G., Koceja, D. M. & Lewis, C. A. (1997). Heteronymous monosynaptic Ia facilitation from supine to standing and its relationship to the soleus H-reflex. *Int J Neurosci*, **92**: 171–86.

Nakashima, K., Rothwell, J. C., Day, B. L., Thompson, P. D., Shannon, K. & Marsden, C. D. (1989). Reciprocal inhibition between forearm muscles in patients with writer's cramp and other occupational cramps, symptomatic hemidystonia and hemiparesis due to stroke. *Brain*, **112**: 681–97.

Nance, P. W., Shears, A. H. & Nance, D. M. (1989). Reflex changes induced by clonidine in spinal cord injured patients. *Paraplegia*, **27**: 296–301.

Nathan, P. W. (1994). Effects on movement of surgical incisions into the human spinal cord. *Brain*, **117**: 337–46.

Nathan, P. W. & Smith, M. C. (1955). Long descending tracts in man. I. Review of present knowledge. *Brain*, **78**: 248–303.

Nielsen, J. & Hultborn, H. (1993). Regulated properties of motoneurons and primary afferents: new aspects on possible spinal mechanisms underlying spasticity. In *Spasticity: Mechanisms and Management*, ed. A. F. Thilmann, D. J. Burke & W. Z. Rymer, pp. 177–92. Berlin: Springer-Verlag.

Nielsen, J., Petersen, N. & Crone, C. (1995). Changes in transmission across synapses of Ia afferents in spastic patients. *Brain*, **118**: 995–1004.

Nielsen, J. F. & Sinkjaer, T. (1996). A comparison of clinical and laboratory measures of spasticity. *Mult Scler*, **1**: 296–301.

Nielsen, P. D. (1972). Interaction between voluntary activation and tonic stretch reflex transmission in normal and spastic patients. *J Neurol Neurosurg Psychiatry*, **35**: 853–60.

Nirkko, A. C, Rosler, K. M., Ozdoba, C., Heid, O., Schroth, G. & Hess, C. W. (1997). Human cortical plasticity: functional recovery with mirror movements. *Neurology*, **48**: 1090–3.

Noth, J. (1991). Trends in the pathophysiology and pharmacotherapy of spasticity. *J Neurol*, **238**: 131–9

O'Dwyer, N. J. & Ada, L. (1996). Reflex hyperexcitability and muscle contracture in relation to spastic hypertonia. *Curr Opin Neurol*, 9: 451–5.

O'Dwyer, N. J., Ada, L. & Neilson, P. D. (1996). Spasticity and muscle contracture following stroke. *Brain*, 119: 1737–49.

Okuma, Y. & Lee, R. G. (1996). Reciprocal inhibition in hemiplegia: correlation with clinical features and recovery. *Can J Neurol Sci*, 23: 15–23.

Ongerboer de Visser, B. W., Bour, L. J., Koelman, J. H. & Speelman, J. D. (1989). Cumulative vibratory indices and the H/M ratio of the soleus H-reflex: a quantitative study in control and spastic subjects. *Electroencephalogr Clin Neurophysiol*, 73: 162–6.

O'Sullivan, M. C., Miller, S., Ramesh, V., Conway, E., Gilfillan, K., McDonough, S. & Eyre, J. A. (1998). Abnormal development of biceps brachii phasic stretch reflex and persistence of short latency heteronymous reflexes from biceps to triceps brachii in spastic cerebral palsy. *Brain*, 121: 2381–95.

Panizza, M., Balbi, P., Russo, G. & Nilsson, J. (1995). H-reflex recovery curve and reciprocal inhibition of H-reflex of the upper limbs in patients with spasticity secondary to stroke. *Am J Phys Med Rehabil*, 74: 357–63.

Phillips, C. G. & Porter, R. (1977). *Corticospinal Neurones. Their Role in Movement.* New York: Academic Press.

Pierrot-Deseilligny, E. & Mazieres, L. (1985). Spinal mechanisms underlying spasticity. In *Clinical Neurophysiology in Spasticity*, ed. P. J. Delwaide & R. R. Young, pp. 63–76. Amsterdam: Elsevier Science Publishers BV.

Pierrot-Deseilligny, E., Morin, C., Bergego, C. & Tankov, N. (1981). Pattern of group I fibre projections from ankle flexor and extensor muscles in man. *Exp Brain Res*, 42: 337–50.

Powers, R. K., Campbell, D. L. & Rymer, W. Z. (1989). Stretch reflex dynamics in spastic elbow flexors. *Ann Neurol*, 25: 32–42.

Powers, R. K., Marder-Meyer, O. T. & Rymer, W. Z. (1988). Quantitative relations between hypertonia and stretch reflex threshold in spastic hemiparesis. *Ann Neurol*, 23: 115–24.

Proske, U., Morgan, D. L., Gregory, J. E. (1993). Thixotropy in skeletal muscle and in muscle spindles: a review. *Prog Neurobiol*, 41: 705–21.

Putnam, T. J. (1940). Treatment of unilateral paralysis agitans by section of the lateral pyramidal tract. *Arch Neurol Psychiatry*, 44: 950–76.

Rack, P. M. H., Ross, H. F. & Thilmann, A. F. (1984). The ankle stretch reflexes in normal and spastic subjects: the response to sinusoidal movement. *Brain*, 107: 637–54.

Raynor, E. M. & Shefner, J. M. (1994). Recurrent inhibition is decreased in patients with amyotrophic lateral sclerosis. *Neurology*, 44: 2148–53.

Roberts, R. C., Part, N. J., Farquhar, R. & Butchart, P. (1994). Presynaptic inhibition of soleus Ia afferent terminals in Parkinson's disease. *J Neurol Neurosurg Psychiatry*, 57: 1488–91.

Roby-Brami, A. & Bussel, B. (1993). Late flexion reflex in paraplegic patients: evidence for a spinal stepping generator. In *Spasticity: Mechanisms and Management*, ed. A. F. Thilmann, D. J. Burke & W. Z. Rymer, pp. 333–43. Berlin: Springer-Verlag.

Rossi, A., Chi, B, & Vecchione, V. (1992). Supraspinal influences on recurrent inhibition in humans. Paralysis of descending control of Renshaw cells in patients with mental retardation. *Electroencephalogr Clin Neurophysiol*, 85: 419–24.

Rossi, A. & Decchi, B. (1997). Changes in Ib heteronymous inhibition to soleus motoneurons during cutaneous and muscle nociceptive stimulation in humans. *Brain Res*, **774**: 55–61.

Rossi, A. & Mazzocchio, R. (1988). Influence of different static head-body positions on spinal lumbar interneurons in man: the role of the vestibular system. *ORL J Otorhinolaryngol Relat Spec*, **50**: 119–26.

Rossi, A., Mazzocchio, R. & Schieppati, M. (1988). The H reflex recovery curve reinvestigated: low-intensity conditioning stimulation and nerve compression disclose differential effects of presumed group Ia fibres in man. *Hum Neurobiol*, **6**: 281–8.

Rothwell, J. C. (1994). *Control of Human Voluntary Movement*, 2nd edn. London: Chapman and Hall.

Rushworth, G. (1960). Spasticity and rigidity: an experimental study and review. *J Neurol Neurosurg Psychiatry*, **23**: 99–118.

Sax, D. S. & Johnson, T. L. (1980). Spinal reflex activity in man. In *Spasticity: Disordered Motor Control*, ed. R. G. Feldman, R. R. Young & W. P. Koella, pp. 301–3. Chicago: Year Book Medical Publishers.

Schieppati, M., Poloni, M. & Nardone, A. (1985). Voluntary muscle release is not accompanied by H-reflex inhibition in patients with upper motoneuron lesions. *Neurosci Lett*, **61**: 177–81.

Schiller, H. H. & Stalberg, E. (1978). F responses studied with single fibre EMG in normal subjects and spastic patients. *J Neurol Neurosurg Psychiatry*, **41**: 45–53.

Schomburg, E. D. (1990). Spinal sensorimotor systems and their supraspinal control. *Neurosci Res*, **7**: 265–340.

Schomburg, E. D. & Steffens, H. (1998). Comparative analysis of L-DOPA actions on nociceptive and non-nociceptive spinal reflex pathways in the cat. *Neurosci Res*, **31**: 307–16.

Schreiner, L. M., Lindsley, D. B. & Magoun, W. (1949). Role of brain stem facilitatory systems in maintenance of spasticity. *J Neurophysiol*, **12**: 207–16.

Schwab, M. E. (1990). Myelin-associated inhibitors of neural growth. *Exp Neurol*, **109**: 2–5.

Shahani, B. T. & Cros, D. (1990). Neurophysiological testing in spasticity. In *The Practical Management of Spasticity in Children and Adults*, ed. M. B. Glen & J. Whyte, pp. 34–43. Philadelphia: Lea and Febiger.

Shahani, B. T. & Young, R. R. (1971). Human flexor reflexes. *J Neurol Neurosurg Psychiatry*, **34**: 616–27.

Shahani, B. T. & Young, R. R. (1980). The flexor reflex in spasticity. In *Spasticity: Disordered Motor Control*, ed. R. G. Feldman, R. R. Young & W. P. Koella, pp. 287–95. Chicago: Year Book Medical Publishers.

Sheean, G. L. (1998a). Pathophysiology of spasticity. In *Spasticity Rehabilitation*, ed. G. Sheean., pp. 17–38. London: Churchill Communications Europe Ltd.

Sheean, G. L. (1998b). The treatment of spasticity with botulinum toxin. In *Spasticity Rehabilitation*, ed. G. Sheean., pp. 109–26. London: Churchill Communications Europe Ltd.

Shefner, J. M., Berman, S. A., Sarkarati, M. & Young, R. R. (1992). Recurrent inhibition is increased in patients with spinal cord injury. *Neurology*, **42**: 2162–8.

Shemesh, Y., Rozin, R. & Ohry, A. (1977). Electrodiagnostic investigation of motor neuron and spinal reflex arch (H-reflex) in spinal cord injury. *Paraplegia*, **15**: 238–44.

Sinkjaer, T., Andersen, J. B. & Nielsen, J. F. (1996). Impaired stretch reflex and joint torque modulation during spastic gait in multiple sclerosis patients. *J Neurol*, 243: 566–74.

Sinkjaer, T. & Magnussen, I. (1994). Passive, intrinsic and reflex-mediated stiffness in the ankle extensors of hemiparetic patients. *Brain*, 117: 355–63.

Sinkjaer, T., Toft, E. & Hansen, H. J. (1995). H-reflex modulation during gait in multiple sclerosis patients with spasticity. *Acta Neurol Scand*, 91: 239–46.

Sinkjaer, T., Toft, E., Larsen, K., Andreassen, S. & Hansen, H. J. (1993). Non-reflex and reflex mediated ankle joint stiffness in multiple sclerosis patients with spasticity. *Muscle Nerve*, 16: 69–76.

Skoog, B. (1996). A comparison of the effects of two antispastic drugs, tizanidine and baclofen, on synaptic transmission from muscle spindle afferents to spinal interneurones in cats. *Acta Physiol Scand*, 156: 81–90.

Souza, R. de O., Gusmao, D. L., de Figueiredo, W. M. & Duarte, A. C. (1988). Pure spastic hemiplegia of pyramidal origin. *Arq Neuropsiquiatr*, 46: 77–87.

Stein, R. B. (1995). Presynaptic inhibition in humans. *Prog Neurobiol*, 47: 533–44.

Stephens, M. J. & Yang, J. F. (1996). Short latency, non-reciprocal group I inhibition is reduced during the stance phase of walking in humans. *Brain Res*, 743: 24–31.

Stolp-Smith, K. A. & Wainberg, M. (1993). Antidepressant aggravation of spasticity. (Abstract.) *J Am Paraplegia Soc*, 16: 140.

Taylor, J. S., Friedman, R. F., Munson, J. B. & Vierck Jr., C. J. (1997). Stretch hyperrreflexia of triceps surae muscles in the conscious cat after dorsolateral spinal lesions. *J Neurosci*, 17: 5004–15.

Thilmann, A. F., Fellows, S. J. & Garms, E. (1991a). The mechanism of spastic muscle hypertonus. *Brain*, 114: 233–44.

Thilmann, A. F., Fellows, S. J. & Ross, H. F. (1991b). Biomechanical changes at the ankle joint after stroke. *J Neurol Neurosurg Psychiatry*, 54: 134–9.

Toft, E. & Sinkjaer, T. (1993). H-reflex changes during contractions of the ankle extensors in spastic patients. *Acta Neurol Scand*, 88: 327–33.

Uncini, A., Cutarella, R., Di Muzio, A., Assetta, M., Lugaresi, A. & Gambi, D. (1990). F response in vascular and degenerative upper motor neuron lesions. *Neurophysiol Clin*, 20: 259–68.

Valls-Sole, J., Alvarez, R. & Tolosa, E. S. (1994). Vibration-induced presynaptic inhibition of the soleus H reflex is temporarily reduced by cortical magnetic stimulation in human subjects. *Neurosci Lett*, 170: 149–52.

van der Meche, F. G. & van Gijn, J. (1986). Hypotonia: an erroneous clinical concept? *Brain*, 109: 1169–78.

Vandervoort, A. A., Chesworth, B. M., Cunningham, D. A., Rechnitzer, P.A., Paterson, D. H. & Koval, J. J. (1992). An outcome measure to quantify passive stiffness of the ankle. *Can J Public Health*, 83 (Suppl. 2): S19–S23.

van Gijn, J. (1978). The Babinski sign and the pyramidal syndrome. *J Neurol Neurosurg Psychiatry*, 41: 865–73.

van Gijn, J. (1996). The Babinski sign: the first hundred years. *J Neurol*, 243: 675–83.

Verrier, M., Ashby, P. & MacLeod, S. (1977). Diazepam effect on reflex activity in patients with complete spinal lesions and in those with other causes of spasticity. *Arch Phys Med Rehabil*, **58**: 148–53.

Verrier, M., MacLeod, S. & Ashby, P. (1975). The effect of diazepam on presynaptic inhibition in patients with complete and incomplete spinal cord lesions. *Can J Neurol Sci*, **2**: 179–84.

Wainberg, M., Barbeau, H. & Gauthier, S. (1990). The effects of cyproheptadine on locomotion and on spasticity in patients with spinal cord injuries. *J Neurol Neurosurg Psychiatry*, **53**: 754–63.

Walsh, E. G. (1976). Clonus: beats provoked by application of a rhythmic force. *J Neurol Neurosurg Psychiatry*, **39**: 266–74.

Walsh, E. G. (1992). Muscles, masses and motion: the physiology of normality, hypotonicity, spasticity and rigidity. In *Clinics in Developmental Medicine*, No. 125, pp. 78–102. Oxford: Blackwell Scientific/Mac Keith Press.

Walshe, F. M. R. (1923). On certain tonic or postural reflexes in hemiplegia, with special reference to the so-called 'associated movements'. *Brain*, **46**: 1–37.

Whitlock, J. A. (1990) Neurophysiology of spasticity. In *The Practical Management of Spasticity in Children and Adults*, ed. M. B. Glen & J. Whyte, pp. 8–33. Philadelphia: Lea and Febiger.

Williams, P. E. & Goldspink, G. (1978). Changes in sarcomere length and physiological properties in immobilized muscle. J Anat, **127**: 459–68.

Yanagisawa, N. & Tanaka, R. (1978). Reciprocal Ia inhibition in spastic paralysis in man. *Electroenceph Clin Neurophysiol*, **34** (Suppl): 521–6.

Yanagisawa, N., Tanaka, R. & Ito, Z. (1976). Reciprocal Ia inhibition in spastic hemiplegia of man. *Brain*, **99**: 555–74.

Yang, J. F. & Whelan, P. J. (1993) Neural mechanisms that contribute to cyclical modulation of the soleus H-reflex in walking in humans. *Exp Brain Res*, **95**: 547–56.

Yang, J. F., Fung, J., Edamura, M., Blunt, R., Stein, R. B. & Barbeau, H. (1991a). H-reflex modulation during walking in spastic paretic subjects. *Can J Neurol Sci*, **18**: 443–52.

Yang, J. F., Stein, R. B. & James, K. B. (1991b) Contribution of peripheral afferents to the activation of the soleus muscle during walking in humans. *Exp Brain Res*, **87**: 679–87.

Young, R. R. (1994). Spasticity: a review. *Neurology*, **44** (Suppl. 9): S12–S20.

3

Measurement of spasticity

Garth R. Johnson

Introduction

Even today, while there are a number of validated techniques for the measurement of associated disability, the measurement of spasticity at the level of impairment is probably in its infancy. Because of the relative lack of treatment or therapy to reduce spasticity, there has been limited development of methods for its measurement. However, with the relatively recent advent of treatments for spasticity such as botulinum toxin, there is now a considerable incentive to develop new methods.

One particular barrier to reliable measurement relates to the need for a precise definition. The measurement of any physical phenomenon is impossible in the absence of a definition, and this is equally true in the case of spasticity. At the clinical level, there is almost certainly a wide variety of assumed definitions concerning stiffness and the lack or difficulty of movement. A relatively precise statement has been provided by Lance (1980). Spasticity, which is directly equated with spastic hypertonia, is a motor disorder that is 'characterized by a velocity-dependent increase in the tonic stretch reflexes (muscle tone) with exaggerated tendon jerks, resulting from the hyperexcitability of the stretch reflex, as one component of the upper motor neurone syndrome' following a lesion at any level of the corticofugal pathways – cortex, internal capsule, brainstem or spinal cord. Furthermore, spastic hypertonia is the exaggeration of the spinal proprioceptive reflexes resulting from a loss of descending inhibitory control (Burke, 1988).

While these definitions would appear to be reasonably precise, there is a need to ask whether current clinical testing procedures are consistent with the model which underlies them and whether the model itself is sufficiently representative to allow reliable testing. Essentially, the contributions to increased tone are likely to be alpha motor neurone activity, and tonic and phasic reflexes. However, the presence or absence of reflex activity is likely to be a function of both muscle length and velocity of stretch, and the gain in the reflex loops is a further variable. It therefore appears that, at minimum, there are five variables which may account for the level of spasticity. The measurement challenge, therefore, is to develop a procedure which is broadly consistent with the clinical definition and perception of the impairment,

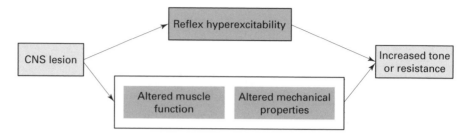

Fig. 3.1   The major contributions to resistance to passive motion result from changes in both the reflex behaviour and in the passive mechanical properties of the muscle.

but which is sensitive to the important variables. For instance, do the assessment procedures commonly in use always distinguish between spasticity, contracture or other abnormal tone such as the rigidity encountered in Parkinson's disease?

Approaches to measurement

Probably because of neurophysiological complexity and the lack of rigid definitions discussed above, there has been a variety of approaches to the measurement of spasticity. While the majority of clinicians probably rely on validated scales, there have been several attempts to use physical or biomechanical approaches. However, the common element of all these methods is that they are concerned with the quantification of resistance to passive motion, and it must be remembered that this can result from a combination of the neurophysiological effects discussed above together with biomechanical changes to the muscle(s), tendon(s) and capsule. This is summarized in Figure 3.1.

While the primary theme of this chapter is to consider methods for the measurement of the impairment associated with spasticity, it is important to note that techniques of both impairment and disability may be used clinically. While one particular approach to the measurement of disability, gait analysis, will be discussed later, it is important to stress that the relationships between disability and spasticity are poorly understood and have yet to be explored fully.

Use of scales to measure spasticity

Requirements of measurement scales

Since most measurement of spasticity is performed using clinical scales, it is useful first to examine the properties of these instruments. A prerequisite for the use of any measurement scale is a knowledge of its performance characteristics and limitations, as these play a key part in interpreting the data and determining the appropriate

Table 3.1. The properties of scales

Type of scale	Mutually exclusive	Logical order	Scaled to perceived quantity	Intervals of equal length	True zero point
Nominal (e.g. type of stroke)	X				
Ordinal (e.g. strength measured on MRC scale)	X	X	X		
Interval (e.g. range of movement)	X	X	X	X	
Ratio (e.g. absolute strength)	X	X	X	X	X

method of statistical analysis. The key aspects of measurement scales will be considered before going on to examine the attributes of instruments for the measurement of spasticity.

Level of measurement

There are four distinct levels of measurement that can be identified hierarchically: nominal (categorical); ordinal; interval; and ratio levels. These are described in Table 3.1 with examples.

The Ashworth scales

In the clinical setting, the most commonly used technique of measurement is the Ashworth scale (Ashworth, 1964) developed originally for the assessment of patients with multiple sclerosis. The Ashworth test is based upon the assessment of the resistance to passive stretch by the clinician who applies the movement. However, although this would appear to be broadly in conformity with the Lance definition, its reliability might be expected to depend upon the ability of the observer both to control the rate of stretch and to assess the resistance. However, despite its widespread use and further development (Bohannon & Smith, 1987), there are relatively few data available on the reliability of this scale. The properties of these scales have been reviewed in detail by Pandyan and colleagues (Pandyan et al., 1999), and the major points are discussed in Table 3.2.

Ashworth and modified Ashworth scales – level of measurement

Since the Ashworth scale does not measure the resistance to passive movement objectively, it cannot be treated as either a ratio or an interval level measure. The

Table 3.2. Definitions of the Ashworth and modified Ashworth scales

Score	Ashworth scale (Ashworth, 1964)	Modified Ashworth scale (Bohannon & Smith, 1987)
0	No increase in tone	No increase in muscle tone
1	Slight increase in tone giving a catch when the limb was moved in flexion or extension	Slight increase in muscle tone, manifested by a catch and release or by minimal resistance at the end of the range of motion when the affected part(s) is moved in flexion or extension.
1+		Slight increase in muscle tone, manifested by a catch, followed by minimal resistance throughout the remainder (less than half) of the ROM (range of movement).
2	More marked increase in tone but limb easily flexed.	More marked increase in muscle tone through most of the ROM, but affected part(s) easily moved.
3	Considerable increase in tone – passive movement difficult.	Considerable increase in muscle tone, passive movement difficult.
4	Limb rigid in flexion or extension.	Affected part(s) rigid in flexion or extension.

originator has proposed that the scale should be treated as an ordinal level measure of resistance to passive movement. Although it is not possible to give a clear guideline as to what would define a slow passive stretch, evidence suggests that a maximum angular velocity of 80°/s (Hufschmidt & Mauritz, 1985; Lamontagne et al., 1998) is permissible before reflex activity influences the muscle resistance. However, further investigation of this is almost certainly required.

The modified Ashworth scale, proposed by Bohannon & Smith (1987), contains an additional level of measurement (1+) and contains a revised definition of the lower end of the Ashworth scale. However, this modification may have introduced an ambiguity in the scale which reduces it to a nominal level measure of resistance to passive movement. The reasons for this are the lack of clear clinical or biomechanical definitions for the terms 'catch' and 'release' and an assumption that 'catch and release' at end range of movement is the same as 'minimal resistance to passive movement'. In particular, the differentiation between grades 1 and 1+ depends upon the presence or absence of either release or minimal resistance to passive movement at end range of movement, the latter of which is probably influenced by the viscoelastic properties. Since there is no published evidence supporting either an ordinal relationship between the grades 1 and 1+ or a relationship between the catch and release, minimal resistance to passive movement, increased resistance to passive movement, and spasticity, it is not possible to treat the modified Ashworth scale as an ordinal measure of resistance to passive movement.

Published data support the use of the original Ashworth scale as an ordinal level measure of resistance to passive movement. However, the modified Ashworth scale could be considered to be an ordinal level measure of resistance to passive movement if the ambiguity between the 1 and 1+ categories could be resolved.

Reliability of the Ashworth scales

Original Ashworth scale

Two studies have investigated the reliability of the original Ashworth scale (Lee et al., 1989; Nuyens et al., 1994), and a further four have studied the reliability of the modified Ashworth scale (Bohannon & Smith, 1987; Bodin & Morris, 1991; Sloan et al., 1992; Allison et al., 1996). One further study has compared the reliability of the two scales (Hass et al., 1996). There appears to be conflicting evidence on the reliability of the Ashworth scales.

In the original paper, the Ashworth scale was used as one of several clinical observations to classify spasticity (Ashworth, 1964) although, surprisingly, this paper does not describe the exact testing protocol. Based on the Ashworth scale guidelines, Lee et al. (1989) investigated the inter- and intra-rater reliability of spasticity measurement using a recorded and summated spasticity score. While it was not possible to draw any conclusions on the reliability of the Ashworth scale as a measure of spasticity in individual joints, there are important data analysis issues that need to be highlighted. If it is accepted that the Ashworth scale is not an interval or ratio level measurement of spasticity, then the use of parametric measures of intra-rater reliability may be questioned. Similarly, the summing of individual joint scores to produce a summated Ashworth score is methodologically flawed.

Nuyens et al. (1994) investigated the inter-rater reliability of the Ashworth scale to measure spasticity in selected muscles of the lower limb, although it is not entirely clear how the authors differentiated between some muscle groups tested (e.g. M. soleus and M. gastrocnemius). Based on an initial assumption that it was an ordinal measure of spasticity, the authors supported the continued use of the Ashworth score as a clinical measure of spasticity. They also suggested that the inter-rater reliability of the scale when measuring spasticity in the lower limb may vary according to the muscle group being tested and concluded that the inter-rater reliability was better for the distal than the proximal muscle groups. In the same study, they summed the (non-parametric) Ashworth scores obtained from individual muscles to obtain a total score and showed that the median of these totals was similar for both assessors, even though the two raters often assessed spasticity differently. This latter finding highlights how the use of a summated score in intervention and reliability studies may mask any unreliability arising with the use of individual joint scores.

Modified Ashworth scale

Bohannon & Smith (1987), as well as being the originators, were the first to test the inter-rater reliability of the modified Ashworth scale. They concluded that the inter-rater reliability at the elbow was acceptable, but noted the possibility that the high degree of agreement may have been attributable to the interactions (mutual testing and discussions) between assessors. Bodin & Morris (1991) investigated the inter rater reliability of the scale for measuring wrist flexor spasticity and concluded that it was a reliable measure of wrist flexor spasticity when used by two trained testers. The authors were of the view that the good agreement was independent of interactions between assessors during the study period. Sloan et al. (1992) investigated the reliability of the scale in measuring spasticity of the elbow flexors and extensors and the knee flexors. Assuming an ordinal level of measurement, they concluded that the modified Ashworth scale was a reliable measure of spasticity at the elbow but not at the knee. The results from this study were similar in some respects to those of Bohannon & Smith (1987) and supported the conclusions that the modified Ashworth scale may have sufficient reliability to classify resistance to passive motion at the elbow.

Allison et al. (1996) investigated the intra- and inter-rater reliability of the modified Ashworth scale when measuring ankle plantar flexor spasticity and concluded, despite reservations, that it had sufficient reliability in measuring spasticity at the ankle in the clinical setting. The authors also highlighted some practical difficulties experienced when using the scale to classify spasticity in the ankle plantar flexors.

Comparison of the Ashworth and the modified Ashworth scales

Hass et al. (1996) compared the inter-rater reliability of the Ashworth and the modified Ashworth scales achieved by two assessors grading spasticity in the lower limbs of 30 subjects with spinal cord injury. Using the Cohen's κ to test for the inter-rater reliability, they concluded that both scales should be used with extreme caution since the inter-rater reliability in classifying spasticity in the lower limb was poor. They also showed that inter-rater reliability was better for the original Ashworth scale.

It could be argued that by adding an extra level of classification to increase the sensitivity, Bohannon & Smith (1987) also had increased the probability of errors occurring in the modified Ashworth scale. In addition as pointed out earlier there is a certain degree of ambiguity between the grades 1 and 1+ in the modified Ashworth scale. The lower reliability observed when using the modified Ashworth scale to grade spasticity could be explained by the above two factors.

Ashworth scales – conclusions and recommendations

Based on the published evidence, the Ashworth scale and the modified Ashworth scale can be regarded as ordinal and nominal level measures of resistance to passive movement, respectively. However, they may only be regarded as measures of spasticity if the velocity of passive joint movement is kept low, the joint range of movement is not compromised and in the absence of pathologies which may cause other forms of increased tone, such as rigidity. The use of parametric procedures such as a recoded and/or summated Ashworth score in the place of individual joint (or muscle) scores is not recommended, as two individuals who rate resistance to passive movement quite differently can produce similar summated scores.

Some further key points which arise are:

- Although the use of the frequency distributions, median and interquartile ranges (mean and standard deviation/confidence intervals) may be used in descriptive studies, it is appropriate only to use categorical/non-parametric data analysis techniques in reliability and intervention studies (Chatfield & Collins, 1980; Bland, 1995; Agresti, 1996).
- In any clinical trials, it is essential that the investigators apply the scales as described in the source publications (Ashworth, 1964; Bohannon & Smith, 1987) and are not tempted to introduce intermediate levels (e.g. spasticity grades of 2.5) (Agresti, 1996).
- Given the uncertainty surrounding the inter-rater reliability of these scales, it is advisable that a single assessor is used in all clinical trials. If this is not possible (e.g. multi-centre studies), then it is suggested that the consistency between assessors be tested before the actual trial.
- While an implicit assumption in the original scales is that the resistance to passive movement is tested through the full range of passive movement (except grade 4), this may not always be possible in clinical practice. Although many investigators provide information related to passive range of movement, few provide a measure of the starting position of the limb or an indication of whether the subject experienced pain during the assessment of spasticity. It should be remembered that reflex excitability may be influenced by the resting length of the limb and pain (Burke, 1988; Rothwell, 1994; Rymer & Katz, 1994). Thus, it is recommended that in future studies, information on the passive range of movement, the resting limb posture before stretch and pain during the stretch be recorded.
- Many authors use repeated cycles of passive stretching prior to grading spasticity (Hufschmidt & Mauritz, 1985). It is also important to realize that the visco-elastic contributions to the resistance to passive movement are likely to decrease with repeated cycles of stretching (Pandyan, 1997) while the changes in the tone-related components will need to be considered indeterministic (i.e. it could increase, reduce or remain unchanged and will depend on many extraneous factors). It is therefore essential that repeated movements are kept to a minimum and the guidelines described by Nuyens et al. (1994) would be recommended in future clinical trials.

- Environmental and postural considerations are also likely to be important. For instance measurements should always be carried out in a room of the same temperature on each occasion, and the posture of the subject should be kept the same at each measurement occasion.
- It would appear that the modified Ashworth scale, when compared with the original Ashworth scale, has lower reliability if used to classify resistance to passive movement at the lower limb. It is possible that the difference arises from the modified Ashworth scale having an additional level classification (Sloan et al., 1992; Nuyens et al., 1994; Hass et al., 1996). In addition, the loss of reliability in the lower limb may be attributable to difficulties in perceiving reflex mediated stiffness when moving the heavier shank and foot segments.

Further work is now required to examine both the validity and the reliability of both the Ashworth and modified Ashworth scales thoroughly, particularly as there may be an increase in their clinical use with the advent of more therapeutic interventions focused at reducing spasticity.

Biomechanical approaches

Since the usual definition of spasticity concerns the relationship between velocity of passive stretch and resistance to motion, it is logical to investigate biomechanical approaches to quantification. For instance, techniques have been developed to use a motor powered system to apply the motion and measure the resistance in a controlled manner.

Wartenberg test

The procedure that has received the most attention is the pendulum test, originally proposed by Wartenberg (1951), in which the knee is released from full extension and the leg allowed to swing until motion ceases. In his original paper, Wartenberg observed that in the normal healthy subject the leg would swing approximately six times after release and proposed a test for the assessment of spasticity involving counting the number of swings before the limb comes to rest. This procedure was further examined by Bajd & Vodovnik (1984) who attached a goniometer to the knee and recorded the movements at the joint after release. They then proposed a relaxation index, based on the rate of decay of oscillation, as a measure of spasticity. However, despite quite extensive technical development, they did not validate the technique in clinical practice. While, superficially, this test should provide a measure of spasticity according to the Lance definition, it must be remembered that the reflex system is complex with a number of important variables. In order to study this, He & Norling (1997) have performed a mathematical modelling study of the test taking into account both the thresholds and the gain in the reflex arc together with the non-linear force production properties of muscle. This study highlights the complex behaviour of reflexes during the experiment and the difficulties of making a simple interpretation. In particular, it demonstrates how this complexity can lead to patterns of movement that are distinctly different from those of a simple damped pendulum.

From the practical clinical viewpoint, Leslie and colleagues (1992) have examined the relationship between measurements of spasticity in patients with multiple sclerosis, made on the Ashworth scale and those obtained from the Wartenberg test. They established that the two methods appear to assess similar features of muscle function but that there were significant changes in the relaxation index within a single Ashworth grade, suggesting that the pendulum test is a rather more sensitive measure of spasticity. Katz and colleagues (1992) have reported the use of this test, and have suggested that it is an acceptable clinical measure which corresponds to the clinical perception of spasticity.

While the Wartenberg pendulum test can be used in cases of relatively mild spasticity, it is likely to be unsuitable for the commonly occurring clinical situations in which spasticity prevents true oscillation of the limb (in engineering terms, when the viscous damping attributable to spasticity is near to, or greater than, critical). In this situation there is a need for a technique which does not rely upon the measurement of damped oscillations, but which provides a soundly based physical measurement. Duckworth & Jordan (1995) performed a preliminary study in which they used a 'Myometer' (a single axis force transducer) to measure resistance to motion. While the technique probably does not conform with the definition of spasticity, early results were encouraging from the point of view of reliability. Lamontagne and colleagues (1998) used a similar technique and found it reliable for the measurement of non-reflex components of resistance to passive motion.

Powered systems

The need to study the relationship between joint motion and resistance has led to a number of projects using powered biomechanical systems for the measurement of spasticity. Before going on to describe these systems, it is useful to highlight the important biomechanical parameters which can, potentially, be studied. In biomechanical terms, a joint and muscle exhibiting spasticity can be regarded as a system exhibiting both elastic (recoverable) and viscous (energy absorbing) behaviour. These two aspects are illustrated in Figure 3.2 showing a *hysteresis loop*, which is the relationship between the displacement and moment measured at a joint being moved in cyclical flexion and extension. Essentially two quantities can be measured from this graph. While the average gradient is a measure of the elastic behaviour, the area within the curve represents the energy absorbed and therefore the viscous behaviour. Jones et al. (1992) have used a powered device to move the joint in a known manner and showed that it could provide useful measurement. However, while they demonstrated the ability to measure joint stiffness and hysteresis there are no further data on clinical validation of the system. Katz & Rymer (1989) have

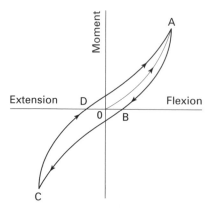

Fig. 3.2   An idealized hysteresis loop obtained from cyclical movement of a joint affected by spasticity. Two key variables may be measured from this graph – the mean slope which represents elastic stiffness, and the area within the loop which represents hysteresis effects associated with spasticity.

demonstrated a powered system for the measurement of stiffness at the wrist but concluded that this was probably not a useful measure of spasticity. They have suggested, in particular, that an increase in stiffness may be related more to contracture than spasticity, and have proposed, instead, that it may be more appropriate to measure joint torque at some specified joint angle. In later studies, Given et al. (1995) have demonstrated that while there are changes in the hysteresis elements of torque angle curves at the wrist, the elastic stiffness appears unchanged. Becher and colleagues (1998) have followed a similar approach and have used a powered system to investigate the resistance of lower limb muscles and the associated emg signals while applying sinusoidal motion at the ankle. In a preliminary study, they were able to detect differences in stiffness between the impaired and unimpaired sides of patients with hemiplegia and were able to demonstrate that muscle stiffness remained unchanged after local anaesthesia. Lehmann and colleagues (1989) have used a similar technique and demonstrated an analytical method to separate passive from reflex responses. However, the method has not been validated clinically. All of these studies demonstrate that, while powered systems highlight important changes in muscle function, the interpretation of the data is difficult and certainly not at a level for routine clinical use.

Interesting studies have been performed by Walsh (1996) who, using a low inertia electrical drive to apply powered oscillation at the wrist, was able to demonstrate some novel phenomena. In particular, he showed that, after the application of a number of cycles of movement, the resistance to motion would be reduced and that a larger amplitude oscillation could be sustained. This situation was maintained for as long as the movement was applied but the joint returned to its previous state after a resting period. This phenomenon is not fully explained but may be

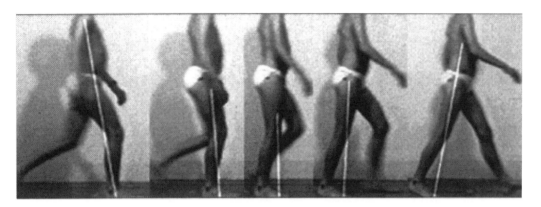

Fig. 3.3   An illustration of the relationship between the ground reaction force vector (seen as a white line) and the hip, knee and ankle during normal gait. Note how the vector passes close to the knee and hip signifying a low turning moment.

due to some change in muscle and, possibly, reflex behaviour. This interesting work has not been repeated by other workers nor has it led to any clinically useful method of measurement. However, this effect of reducing resistance after prolonged excitation may be of importance when designing research studies. In a related study (Lakie et al., 1988), the same research group have used this powered system to assess spasticity in patients with hemiplegia. While they established that both resonant frequency and damping were increased in these patients, they did not propose a measurement of spasticity as such.

Clearly, the application of powered systems allows detailed studies of the relationship between resistance to motion and kinematic variables. However, while such systems may be powerful research tools, the techniques are almost certainly too complex for regular clinical use.

Indirect biomechanical approaches – gait analysis

While, so far we have looked at the measurement of spasticity at the impairment level, there is also a need to consider measurements of disability such as gait analysis. There can be little doubt that gait disorders result from spasticity but the exact relationships would seem to be far from clear. Probably the best way to examine this link is to consider the changes in external loading of the hip, knee and ankle during gait and, in particular, to look at the moments at the joints. The moment at a joint, which may be considered as the turning effect of the ground reaction force, is determined by the magnitude of that force and the distance of the force vector from the joint in question. While such biomechanical measurements require relatively sophisticated measurement equipment, the video vector technique, pioneered by the Orthotics Research and Locomotor Assessment Unit (ORLAU) in Oswestry (UK), allows a rapid visualization of these joint moments. Figure 3.3

Ground reaction Force – Abnormal gait

(a)   (b)   (c)

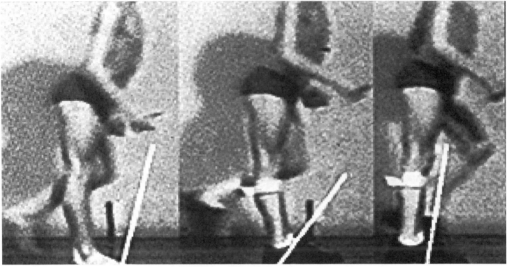

Fig. 3.4   In these illustrations, the relationship between the ground reaction force vector and the
hip and knee during pathological gait can be clearly seen. In (a) the large distance
between the vector and the knee is shown; in (b), although the vector now originates at
the heel, it is still at a large distance from the knee. In (c), the use of a 'tuned' orthosis
aligns the vector more closely with the knee and so reduces the effects of spasticity.

illustrates the visual output of the system in which the ground reaction force vector,
shown as a white line, can be seen superimposed upon the image of the subject. It
will be seen in this illustration of normal walking that the distance between the
vector and the centres of hip and knee is relatively small. This indicates that the
moment of the force and, therefore, the activity of the associated muscles, about
these joints is small. In contrast, Figure 3.4 shows the equivalent output for a child
with cerebral palsy in which the large distance between the vector and the hip and
knee is clearly visible (Butler et al., 1992). In this situation there must be greatly
increased muscle activity to resist these moments. It is also interesting to note how
the position of the vector is changed according to the orthotic treatment indicating that the effects of the spasticity within the gait cycle may be changed by provision of an orthosis. However, it must be stressed that, while this technique
demonstrates the excessive and poorly synchronized muscle activity that may be
associated with spasticity, this situation does not correspond directly with the
definition of spasticity. This last point is of particular importance and highlights
the need for further research investigating the exact relationships between spasticity and these phenomena.

Neurophysiological approaches to measurement

As spasticity results from altered conduction in the reflex pathways (see Chapter 2), there have been numerous attempts to quantify it by investigating the abnormalities in the reflex pathways – i.e. altered presynaptic inhibition and reciprocal inhibition, excitability in the 1a afferent pathway and increased alpha motor neurone excitability. The three common techniques that have been used for clinical quantification are spasticity tendon jerks, H-reflex studies and F-wave studies.

Tendon jerks

The most commonly used method to illustrate a spinal reflex is the tendon jerk, which is obtained by a rapid (but small) stretch of a muscle. The ensuing response is reported primarily to involve the monosynaptic pathway, although it has also been suggested that this action could be influenced by oligosynaptic pathways (Rothwell, 1994). It has been reported that tendon jerks are more readily elicited in people with spasticity – that is, they can be elicited with smaller levels of stimuli than normal, and the response to these stimuli has a higher amplitude and is more diffuse (i.e. can involve muscles that were not originally stimulated). Therefore it has been hypothesized that the tendon jerk can be a quantifiable measure of spasticity. However, it is important to note that increase in tendon jerk is not exclusive to spasticity. Furthermore, whether the increase in the tendon jerk response is related to increased gain, decreased threshold or a combination of both needs to be resolved.

H-reflexes

The H-reflex is a long latency reflex that is obtained by electrically stimulating a mixed nerve submaximally. The muscle response that follows results from conduction via the Ia afferent pathways. Although these reflexes are thought of as being primarily monosynaptic (Liveson & Ma, 1992), there is evidence that oligosynaptic reflex pathways could also be involved (Burke et al., 1983). (It should be noted that the H-reflex response is independent of the muscle spindle activity.) The H-reflex has to be used to study both excitability in the Ia afferent pathways and abnormalities in presynaptic and reciprocal inhibition, in spasticity (Panizza et al., 1990, 1995; Harburn et al., 1992; Katz et al., 1992; Rothwell, 1994). Despite the reported ease of conducting these tests, there can be a varied outcome. This is reported to result from variations in stimulus intensity, the resting posture of the limb, the ability of a subject to relax or the neck and vestibular reflexes, and would suggest that the results should be treated with caution (Katz & Rymer, 1989; Liveson & Ma, 1992; Katz, 1994). In order to normalize for this variability, the H-reflex response has been expressed as a percentage of the M-response – i.e. the stimulus of a muscle to supramaximal stimulation. It should be noted that when using this ratio there is an assumption that the presynaptic component in the reflex response is fixed. While there are reports that H/M ratios are increased in spasticity, it has also been demonstrated that the ratios do not decrease following treatment of spasticity (Matthews, 1966). It has also been reported that the correlation between H/M ratios and the severity of spastic hyperreflexia was poor (Matthews, 1966; Katz et al., 1992). There have been attempts to use the influence of vibration on the H-reflex. Since in normal subjects the vibration of muscle inhibits H-reflex activity, it has been hypothesized that, in spastic limbs, this inhibition should be reduced. However, more work is needed to develop this as a clinically usable technique to quantify spasticity (Rothwell, 1994).

F-waves

F-waves are obtained by the supramaximal stimulation of a mixed nerve and have been used as a measure of alpha motor neurone excitability. Unlike H-reflexes, the F-wave does not result from stimulation of a sensory nerve but from the antidromic stimulation of the alpha motor neurone. Furthermore, unlike the H-reflex that shows an inverse relationship with the M-wave, the F-wave, which follows the M-wave, shows no correlation with M-wave amplitudes. In addition, the amplitude of the F-wave is much smaller than that of the H-reflex (Liveson & Ma, 1992). Although the F-wave provides a more stable signal, which is less influenced by resting posture and the ability of a subject to relax, the average F-wave response from repeated tests is often used because of variations in latency and amplitude. In spastic patients it has been demonstrated that subjects show increased F-wave amplitudes suggesting increased motor neuronal excitability (Eisen & Odusote, 1979). However, more work is still required to develop this technique as a reliable clinical measure of spasticity.

The primary problem with existing electrophysiological methods to quantify spasticity appears to be the poor correlation with the other clinical techniques. The fact that the most commonly used clinical scales to quantify spasticity have been shown not to be an exclusive measure of spasticity adds further to this confusion. In conclusion, although there are a number of tests available to measure spasticity, the clinical usefulness of many of these techniques still remain unproven and further work will be required to prove their validity, reliability and clinical applicability.

Overall conclusions

The measurement of any variable depends upon an adequate definition. In the case of spasticity, it appears that the complexity of any comprehensive definition makes direct clinical measurement very difficult. While the Lance definition provides a useful basis for measurement and appears to have a biomechanical interpretation, the complex behaviour of the reflex arcs and the wide variations in pathology probably make a single universal definition impossible. As a direct result, a universal measurement system may also be impossible to achieve. It is almost certainly this background that has confounded attempts to produce reliable instruments.

Despite all of the more recent studies, the original Ashworth scale would still appear to be the most reliable measure of spasticity. It has been shown, however, that the possible contradictions within the modified version of this scale may lead to problems of interpretation. Although biomechanical approaches to measurement are attractive, there are real problems in producing systems which are universally applicable and which can be used in the clinical setting. However, the simplest of these methods, the Wartenberg pendulum test is attractive in that it provides a simple method of measurement based on relatively well-defined biomechanical principles. It is believed that this is worthy of further investigation. Finally, while gait analysis provides much useful data on the disability of patients with spasticity it cannot be regarded as a measure of the actual impairment.

It is believed, therefore, that the Ashworth scale (and possibly the modified Ashworth scale) will continue to be used in the clinic. If this is the case, then it is essential that the limitations highlighted in this chapter are recognized and that the appropriate statistical procedures are used.

Acknowledgements

I would like to express my thanks to Dr David Pandyan for many hours of stimulating discussion on this topic and for the provision of material on neurophysiological approaches to measurement. Acknowledgement is also due to Orthotics Research and Locomotor Assessment Unit (ORLAU), Oswestry, for providing Figures 3.3 and 3.4.

REFERENCES

Agresti, A. (1996). *An Introduction to Categorical Data Analysis.* New York: John Wiley & Sons Inc.

Allison, S. C., Abraham, L. D. & Petersen, C. L. (1996). Reliability of the modified Ashworth scale in the assessment of plantar flexor muscle spasticity in patients with traumatic brain injury. *Int J Rehabil Res,* **19**: 67–78.

Ashworth, B. (1964). Preliminary trial of carisoprodal in multiple sclerosis. *Practitioner,* **192**: 540–2.

Bajd, T. & Vodovnik, L. (1984). Pendulum testing of spasticity. *J Biomed Eng,* **6**: 9–16.

Becher, J., Harlaar, J., Lankhorst, G. J. & Vogelaar, T. W. (1998). Measurement of impaired muscle function of the gastrocnemius, soleus, and tibialis anterior muscle in spastic hemiplegia: a preliminary study. *J Rehabil Res Develop,* **35**: 314–26.

Bland, M. (1995). *An Introduction to Medical Statistics.* 2nd edn. Oxford: Oxford Medical Publications.

Bodin, P. G. & Morris, M. E. (1991). Inter rater reliability of the modified Ashworth scale for wrist flexors spasticity following stroke. *World Confederation of Physiotherapy, 11th Congress, 1991.* Pp. 505–7.

Bohannon, R. W. & Smith, M. B. (1987). Inter rater reliability of a modified Ashworth scale of muscle spasticity. *Phys Ther,* **67**: 206–7.

Burke, D. (1988). Spasticity as an adaptation to pyramidal tract injury. *Adv Neurol,* **47**: 401–22.

Burke, D., Gandevia, S. C. & McKeon, B. (1983). The afferent volleys responsible for spinal proprioceptive reflexes in man. *J Physiol,* **339**: 535–52.

Butler, P. B., Thompson, N. & Major, R. E. (1992). Improvements in walking performance of children with cerebral palsy: preliminary results. *Dev Med Child Neurol,* **34**: 567–76.

Chatfield, C. & Collins, A. J. (1980). *Introduction to Multivariate Analysis.* London: Chapman & Hall.

Duckworth, S. & Jordan, N. (1995). Peripheral nerve blockade with phenol in spasticity – a myometric and functional assessment. Proc. of British Association of Neurologists. *Abstract J Neurol Neurosurg Psychiatry,* **59**: 214.

Eisen, A. & Odusote, K. (1979). Amplitude of F-wave: potential means of documenting spasticity. *Neurology,* **29**: 1306–9.

Given, J. D., Dewald, J. P. A. & Rymer, W. Z. (1995). Joint dependent passive stiffness in paretic and contralateral limbs of spastic patients with hemiparetic stroke. *J Neurol Neurosurg Psychiatry,* **59**: 271–9.

Harburn, K. L., Hill, K. M., Vandervoort, C. H., Kertesz, A. & Teasell, R. W. (1992). Spasticity measurement in stroke: a pilot study. *Can J Public Health,* **83** (Suppl. 2): S41–S45.

Hass, B. M., Bergstrom, E., Jamous, A. & Bennie, A. (1996). The inter rater reliability of the original and of the modified Ashworth scale for the assessment of spasticity in patients with spinal cord injury. *Spinal Cord,* **34**: 560–4.

He, J. & Norling, W. R. (1997). A dynamic neuromuscular model for describing the pendulum test for spasticity. *IEEE Trans Biomed Eng,* **44**: 175–83.

Hufschmidt, A. & Mauritz, K. (1985). Chronic transformation of muscle in spasticity: a peripheral contribution to increased tone. *J Neurol Neurosurg Psychiatry,* **48**: 676–85.

Jones, E. W., Plant, G. R., Stuart, C. R., Mulley, G. P. & Johnson, F. (1992). Comments on the design of an instrument to measure spasticity in the arm – SAM. *Eng Med* **11**: 47–50.

Katz, R. T. (1994). Electrophysiologic assessment of spastic hypertonia. *Phys Med Rehabil: State Art Rev,* **8**: 465–71.

Katz, R. T., Rovai, G. P., Brait, C. & Rymer, W. Z. (1992). Objective quantification of spastic hypertonia. Correlation with clinical findings. *Arch Phys Med Rehabil,* **73**: 339–47.

Katz, R. T. & Rymer, W. Z. (1989). Spastic hypertonia: mechanisms and measurement. *Arch Phys Med Rehabil,* **70**: 144–55.

Lakie, M., Walsh, E. G. & Wright, G. W. (1988). Assessment of human hemiplegic spasticity by a resonant frequency method. *Clin Biomech*, 3: 173–8.

Lamontagne, A., Malouin, F., Richards, C. L. & Dumas F. (1998). Evaluation of reflex and non-reflex induced muscle resistance to stretch in adults with spinal cord injury using hand held and isokinetic dynamometry. *Phys Ther*, 78: 964–77.

Lance, J. W. (1980). Pathophysiology of spasticity and clinical experience with Baclofen. In *Spasticity: Disordered Motor Control*, ed. J. W. Lance, R. G. Feldman, R. R. Young & W. P. Koella, pp. 185–204. Chicago: Year Book Medical Publishers.

Lehmann, J. F., Price, R., deLateur, B. J., Hinderer, S. & Traynor, C. (1989). Spasticity: quantitative measurement as a basis for assessing effectiveness of therapeutic intervention. *Arch Phys Med Rehabil*, 70: 6–15.

Lee, K., Carson, L., Kinnin, E. & Patterson, V. (1989). The Ashworth scale: a reliable and reproducible method of measuring spasticity. *J Neurol Rehabil*, 3: 205–9.

Leslie, G. C., Muir, C., Part, N. J. & Roberts, R. C. (1992). A comparison of the assessment of spasticity by the Wartenberg pendulum test and the Ashworth grading scale in patients with multiple sclerosis. *Clin Rehabil*, 6: 41–8.

Liveson, J. A. & Ma, M. D. (1992). Late responses. In *Laboratory Reference for Clinical Neurophysiology*, pp. 237–46. Philadelphia: F. A. Davis & Co.

Matthews, W. B. (1966). Ratio of maximum H-reflex to maximum M-response as measure of spasticity. *J Neurol Neurosurg Psychiatry*, 29: 201–4.

Nuyens, G., De Weerdt, W., Ketelaer, P., Feys, H., De Wolf, L., Hantson, L., Nieuboer, A., Spaepen, A. & Carton, H. (1994). Inter rater reliability of the Ashworth scale in multiple sclerosis. *Clin Rehabil*, 8: 286–92.

Pandyan, A. D. (1997). *Use of electrical stimulation to prevent wrist flexion contractures in post stroke hemiplegia*. PhD Thesis, University of Strathclyde; Glasgow.

Pandyan, A. D., Price, C. I. M., Curless, R. H., Johnson, G. R., Barnes, M. P. & Rodgers, H. (1999). A review of the properties and limitations of the Ashworth and modified Ashworth scales as measures of spasticity. *Clin Rehabil*, 13: 373–83.

Panizza, M., Lelli, S., Nilsson, J. & Hallett, M. (1990). H-reflex recovery curve and reciprocal inhibition in different kinds of dynstonia. *Neurology*, 40: 824–8.

Panizza, M., Balbi, P., Russo, G., Nilsson, J., Panizza, M., Balbi, P., Russo, G. & Nilsson, J. (1995). H-reflex recovery curve and reciprocal inhibition of H-reflex of the upper limbs in patients with spasticity secondary to stroke. *Am J Phys Med Rehabil*, 74: 357–63.

Rothwell, J. C. (1994). *Control of Human Voluntary Movement*. 2nd edn. London: Chapman & Hall.

Rymer, W. Z. & Katz, R. T. (1994). Mechanism of spastic hypertonia. *Phys Med Rehabil: State Art Rev*, 8: 441–54.

Sloan, R. L., Sinclair, E., Thompson, J., Taylor, S. & Pentland, B. (1992). Inter-rater reliability of the modified Ashworth scale for spasticity in hemiplegic patients. *Int J Rehabil Res*, 15: 158–61.

Walsh, E. G. (1996). Thixotropy: a time dependent stiffness. In *Muscle, Masses and Motion*, pp. 78–102. Oxford: MacKeith Press.

Wartenberg, R. (1951). Pendulousness of the legs as a diagnostic test. *Neurology*, 1: 18–24.

4

Physiotherapy management of spasticity

Roslyn N. Boyd and Louise Ada

Introduction

Much of the controversy about the management of spasticity stems from the lack of commonly accepted clear definitions of the disorder, the difficulty in measuring spasticity as well as the changing nature of the motor disability with growth and maturation of the patient. There is also a paucity of data to validate current clinical practice.

While many disciplines are involved in the management of spasticity, physiotherapists have a unique role in applying their understanding of the biomechanics of movement to the analysis of motor disability and their knowledge of motor learning principles to training of motor function. The theoretical basis for the physiotherapy management of spasticity needs to take account of current literature in the movement sciences (Shepherd, 1995).

In this chapter, the emphasis is on contemporary thinking and the intervention that follows from these current theories. We advocate, therefore, training to improve muscle activity in order that everyday actions may be readily undertaken (Carr & Shepherd 1987, 1998; Ada & Canning, 1990) rather than preparing the patient for function by affecting abnormal reflex activity which has been the focus in the past (Bobath, 1990; Mayston, 1992). In addition, we will discuss the physiotherapists' goals in using orthoses, and the role of pharmacological and surgical interventions. Clinical applications for children with cerebral palsy and adults after stroke will be highlighted because these individuals form the largest group of brain damaged people with spasticity.

What is spasticity?

Spasticity is one of the impairments that affects function following brain damage. It is typical to consider the impairments associated with the upper motor neuron syndrome as either positive or negative. Negative impairments are those features that have been lost, following brain damage (e.g. loss of strength and dexterity)

Table 4.1. Table of definitions of spasticity and other disorders

Term	Definition
Spasticity	A motor disorder characterized by a velocity-dependant increase in tonic stretch reflexes (muscle tone) with exaggerated tendon jerks, resulting from hyperexcitability of the stretch reflex as one component of the upper motor neurone syndrome (Lance, 1980, p. 485).
Hyper reflexia	A greater than normal reflex response, e.g. the presence of reflex responses during slow stretch of a relaxed muscle.
Muscle tone	The resistance felt when moving a limb passively through range, normally due to inertia and the compliance of the tissues.
Hypertonia	A greater than normal resistance felt when moving a limb passively through range.
Overactivity	Excessive muscle activity for the requirements of the task.
Passive stiffness	The force required to lengthen a muscle at rest, i.e. the slope of the force displacement curve.
Active stiffness	The force required to lengthen a muscle that is active, i.e. the slope of the active force displacement curve.
Viscosity	Force, velocity dependent lengthening.
Impairment*	Less or abnormality of physiological, psychological or anatomical structure.
Disability*	Restriction or lack of ability to perform an activity.
Activity limitation[†]	Limitation of societal involvement.
Handicapped*	Disadvantage suffered by individuals as a result of ill health due to inability to fulfill a role which is normal for someone of that age, sex and culture.

Notes:
* World Health Organization (1980).
[†] World Health Organization (1999).

whereas positive impairments are those features that are additional (e.g. spasticity and abnormal postures) (Jackson, 1958; Burke, 1988; Lance, 1990; Landau, 1990).

The most widely used definition of spasticity is that of Lance (1980, p. 485). This definition puts the problem clearly in the realm of an abnormality of the reflex system. It is common for clinicians to argue for a broader definition of spasticity, often inclusive of the whole upper motor neurone syndrome, rather than viewing spasticity as one feature of the syndrome. We argue that it is important to accept Lance's relatively narrow but clear physiological definition (Table 4.1).

Increasingly, the independence of the positive and negative features has been recognized (e.g. Burke, 1988). Viewing the positive and negative impairments as separate features of the syndrome will affect assessment and management procedures.

For example, it is important initially to differentiate the relative contributions of the impairments so that intervention specific to the problem can be instituted. Grouping all impairments seen following an upper motor neuron lesion under one category, as a spastic 'syndrome', does not help this process.

How important a determinant of disability is spasticity?

If spasticity is only one of several impairments following brain damage, physiotherapists need to clarify how spasticity affects the ability to move. Historically, spasticity was seen as the major determinant of disability. However, Landau (1974) questioned this assumption and a variety of experiments have since supported his position. First, experiments eliminating spasticity in specific muscles in adults after stroke (McLellan, 1977) and in children with cerebral palsy (Nathan, 1969; Neilson & McCaughey, 1982) did not result in improved performance of that particular muscle. Second, studies examining the relationship between spasticity and muscle performance found no correlation between them (Sahrmann & Norton, 1977; O'Dwyer et al., 1996). These experimental findings resulted in dexterity being viewed as a separate impairment rather than the result of spasticity. However, these findings are often misinterpreted as suggesting that spasticity either does not exist or is never a problem. Severe spasticity will obviously interfere with everyday functioning. Rather, the implication of these findings is that reducing spasticity will not automatically improve function and the abnormal negative features require specific training.

Experiments on the nature of the abnormality of the stretch reflex after brain damage may help us to understand how spasticity can contribute to disability. Clinically, the picture of spasticity is one of increased resistance to passive movement of a relaxed muscle caused by abnormal reflex activity. There is an assumption that this abnormal reflex activity will be exaggerated when the person attempts to move. However, there is growing evidence that, rather than the picture of a small reflex abnormality under relaxed conditions being exaggerated under active conditions, the reflex is not modulated. That is, the reflex responses do not get larger under active conditions. Lack of modulation of the reflex has been found when studying tonic stretch reflexes (Ibrahim et al., 1993a,b; Ada et al., 1998). This paints a picture, not of an abnormal 'out-of-control' reflex, but of a reflex that is not being modulated. Normally, the reflex is modulated up and down according to the requirements of the task. In the presence of spasticity, the reflex is 'on' all the time regardless of conditions. Perhaps the amount the reflex is 'on' is the determining factor as to whether spasticity interferes with movement control. A person with an abnormal stretch reflex that is 'on' a small amount will register as spastic when measured clinically but the reflex response may not increase with movement, thereby not interfering with function. This suggests that patients who are measured as mildly to moderately spastic under passive conditions are not necessarily hampered by this spasticity during function. On the other hand, if the reflex is always 'on' a large amount, even if the response does not increase with effort, it will interfere with movement. That is, moderate to severe spasticity may contribute to disability by causing excessive muscle contraction which resists lengthening of the affected muscle during everyday actions.

Confusion between spasticity and other impairments

The difficulty in assessing the contribution of different impairments to disability makes it possible for other impairments to be mislabelled as spasticity. One of the major confusions is between the neural and peripheral causes of hypertonia, a term often used interchangeably with spasticity. Hypertonia refers to the excessive resistance that may be felt when the limb of a brain-damaged person is moved passively. The resistance felt when a normal limb is moved slowly through range is the result of the inertia of the limb and the compliance of the soft tissues (Katz & Rymer, 1989). Normally, there is no contribution from reflex activity – i.e., the muscles are electrically silent (Burke, 1983). The increase in resistance often felt after brain damage is usually assumed to be the result of hyperreflexia – i.e., it is a neural problem, in line with Lance's definition. However, the increased resistance may be the result of a peripheral problem, specifically muscle contracture. Animal studies into the biology of muscle contracture have revealed that contracture is associated with an increase in muscle stiffness due to a remodelling of the connective tissue (e.g., Goldspink & Williams, 1990). Furthermore, in humans the ability of a muscle with contracture to produce an increase in the resistance to passive movement has been verified. O'Dwyer et al. (1996) found that muscle stiffness can be associated with muscle contracture, even in the absence of hyperreflexia. The confusion is further reinforced because the most common clinical measure of hypertonia – the Ashworth scale – does not differentiate between neural and peripheral causes of hypertonia. It is important, however, for physiotherapists to be able to differentiate between these two causes of hypertonia because the intervention for muscle contracture differs from that for spasticity. Figure 4.1 illustrates figuratively two possible mechanisms of hypertonia.

Another possible confusion between various types of motor impairment is that between spasticity and muscle overactivity. When the person with spasticity activates a muscle, thereby stretching the muscle spindle and exciting the hyperactive stretch reflex, this in turn causes the muscle to contract excessively relative to the original neural input. While spasticity is undoubtedly one cause of overactivity exhibited by people with brain damage, another may be lack of skill. Unskilled

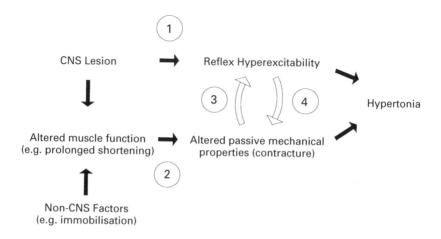

Fig. 4.1　　Two possible mechanisms of hypertonia following an upper motor neurone lesion. The solid arrows indicate well-established mechanisms, while the open arrows indicate more hypothetical mechanisms (with permission O'Dwyer & Ada, 1996).

performance is usually accompanied by excessive, unnecessary muscle activity (Basmajian, 1977; Basmajian & Blumenstein, 1980). Several studies have demonstrated that an increase in skill is accompanied by a decrease in muscle activity (Payton & Kelley, 1972; Payton et al., 1976; Hobart et al., 1995). It may be that some of the motor behaviour that clinicians have viewed as spastic is the result of lack of skill. For example, Figure 4.2 illustrates an attempt by a person after stroke to lift a glass off the table, but instead of the wrist radially deviating, the elbow flexes. Behaviour such as this is often attributed to biceps spasticity. However, overactivity in the biceps in this case is unlikely to be the result of spasticity since, following feedback about her performance, the patient successfully lifts her hand without any accompanying elbow flexion. Canning et al. (2000) examined adults following chronic stroke who demonstrated excessive, unnecessary activity during the performance of a task, which was correlated with poor performance but not with spasticity.

Effect of pathology and maturation on spasticity

The operational definitions and relative importance of spasticity are confounded by the issue of how spasticity affects growth and maturation in children with spastic-type celebral palsy. It is a common clinical observation that muscle growth does not keep pace with bone growth in young children with cerebral palsy (Rang, 1990). It is assumed that decreased longitudinal growth of the muscle is caused by

(a)

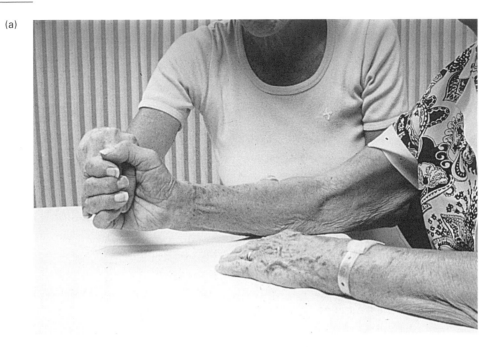

(b)

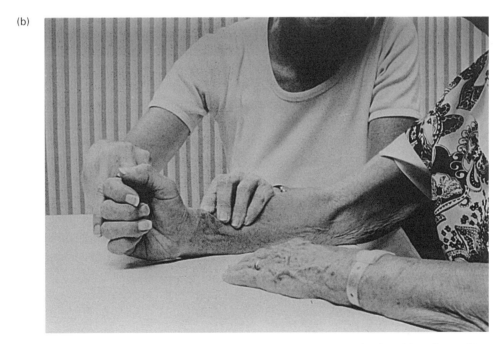

Fig. 4.2   (a): When this woman was asked to lift her hand off the table, she flexed her elbow. (b): However, when she understood that elbow flexion should not take place, with practise, she lifted her hand by bending at the wrist only (with permission, Carr et al., 1995).

overactivity due to spasticity. Animal models of spasticity have demonstrated the lack of longitudinal growth of the muscle relative to bone (Ziv et al., 1984). Furthermore, normal longitudinal muscle growth has been restored following intramuscular injections of botulinum toxin A (BTXA) to reduce spasticity thereby allowing full muscle excursion (Cosgrove & Graham, 1994). Human studies have supported the notion that the muscle normally grows in response to full muscle excursion (Koning et al., 1987).

In addition, how muscles respond to casting to lengthen muscles may vary with age. Animal studies have shown that the response of young muscle to immobilization in a lengthened position differs from that of older muscle (Tardieu et al., 1977). The young muscle initially responds in a similar way to adult muscle by the addition of sarcomeres. However, no further addition of sarcomeres but a relative lengthening of the muscle tendon in the young animal follows this. Although there should be some caution in extrapolating evidence from the animal literature to clinical practice, these findings may explain the tendency for an overlengthened calf muscle tendon and short gastrosoleus muscle belly frequently seen after growth periods in children with cerebral palsy. A similar response can be noted after extended periods of serial casting in these children.

There can be an appreciable difference in the peripheral components of hypertonia in a young child (1–4 years) with cerebral palsy compared with adolescents who have undergone their second growth spurt. Clinically, younger children tend to demonstrate overactivity, which leads to reduced muscle excursion, while adolescents are more likely to demonstrate contracture and weakness. In addition, the development of contracture in certain muscle groups may be faster according to the motor distribution. In children with hemiplegia due to cerebral palsy, it is often the calf muscles before the hamstring muscles that develop reduced excursion, whereas in children with diplegia it is often the hamstring and adductor muscles before the calf muscles (Boyd & Graham, 1997). The concept of the *biological clock* ticking faster in children with cerebral palsy in certain muscles according to motor type and aetiology has been proposed (Boyd & Graham, 1997). On the other hand, there may be a mechanical explanation. The child with cerebral palsy who spends most of his or her time sitting or crawling is likely to have shorter hamstring muscles. Prediction of which muscles are 'at risk' of shortening from observation of common patterns of overactivity and increased muscle stiffness will help in the prevention of muscle contracture.

The relative contribution of the positive and negative features in adults and children appears to differ due to pathology. In adult stroke patients, problems of weakness and dexterity are more apparent (Carr et al., 1995). In young children with cerebral palsy, the positive features of velocity-dependent hyperreflexia and inappropriate muscle overactivity lead to reduced muscle excursion and eventual contracture (Rang, 1990; Cosgrove et al., 1994). By adolescence, weakness and muscle contracture may become greater problems.

Measurement of spasticity

An important component of the clinical management of brain damage is careful assessment of the contribution of various impairments to disability. Unfortunately, this is not an easy task. Spasticity is most commonly measured clinically by either grading the response of the tendon jerk while the subject is relaxed (where an increased response is reported as hyperreflexia) and/or grading the resistance to passive movement while the subject is relaxed (where increased resistance is reported as hypertonia, e.g. Ashworth, 1964). Spasticity is most commonly measured in the laboratory by moving the joint (mechanically or manually), either by repeated oscillation (sinusoidal movement) or by a single ramp movement and quantifying the electromyographic activity in response to stretch (e.g. Neilson & Lance, 1978; O'Dwyer et al., 1996) and/or quantifying the resistance to movement (e.g. Gottlieb et al., 1978; Rack et al., 1984; Hufschmidt & Mauritz, 1985; Lehmann et al., 1989; Corry et al., 1997).

The difficulty is that both the clinical and laboratory measures of resistance to movement do not differentiate whether the cause of the hypertonia is neural or peripheral. The most valid measure of spasticity is the use of electromyography (EMG) during passive stretch of a muscle because the presence of stretch-evoked muscle activity is the only way of ascertaining a neural component. However, this is not a feasible technique for clinical use. In a recent study, no relation was found between clinically measured phasic stretch reflexes (tendon jerks) and laboratory measured tonic stretch reflexes (Vattanasilp & Ada, 1999). The lack of relationship between these two tests of reflex activity can be explained by the fact that they are measuring different components of the stretch reflex response. The tendon jerk excites a phasic, monosynaptic component of the stretch reflex in response to a rapid stimulus. In contrast, sinusoidal stretch in which the input is ongoing excites a tonic, polysynaptic component of the stretch reflex. Fellows et al. (1993) have previously pointed out that the tendon jerk has limitations in providing a complete picture of the pathological changes in reflex responses following stroke.

This leaves physiotherapists in a dilemma. While the Ashworth scale has been shown to measure resistance adequately (Vattanasilp & Ada, 1999), it measures both the neural and peripheral contributions to resistance without differentiating their individual contributions. However, the Tardieu scale (Tardieu et al., 1954; Boyd et al., 1998a,b; Boyd & Graham, 1999) appears to be better at identifying a neural component. By moving the limb at different velocities, the response to stretch can be more easily gauged since the stretch reflex responds differentially to

Table 4.2. Tardieu scale (adapted for stroke)

- Grading is always done at the same time of day.
- Constant position of the body for a given limb.
- Other joints particularly the neck must remain in a constant position throughout the assessment and from one test to another.
- For each muscle group, reaction to stretch is rated at a specified stretch velocity with two parameters X, Y.

Velocity of stretch

V1: As slow as possible (slower than the rate of the natural drop of the limb segment under gravity).

V2: Speed of the limb segment falling under gravity.

V3: As fast as possible (faster than the rate of the natural drop of the limb segment under gravity). Once V is chosen for a muscle it remains the same from one test to another.

Quality of muscle reaction (X):

0: no resistance throughout the course of the passive movement.

1: slight resistance throughout the course of the passive movement with no clear catch at a precise angle.

2: clear catch at a precise angle, interrupting the passive movement, followed by release.

3: fatiguable clonus (less than 10 seconds when maintaining the pressure) appearing at a precise angle.

4: unfatiguable clonus (more than 10 seconds when maintaining the pressure) at a precise angle.

Angle of muscle reaction (Y):

Measured relative to the position of minimal stretch of the muscle (corresponding to angle zero) for all joints except hip where it is relative to the resting anatomical position.

Lower limb:

To be tested in a supine position, at the recommended joint positions and velocities:

	X	Y (degrees)

Hip

Extensors (knee extended, V3)

Adductors (knee extended, V3)

External rotators (knee flexed by 90, V3)

Internal rotators (knee flexed by 90, V3)

Knee

Extensors (hip flexed by 30, V2)

Flexors (hip flexed, V3)

Ankle

Plantarflexors (knee flexed by 90, V3)

Plantarflexors (knee fully extended, V3)

Upper limb is to be tested in a sitting position, elbow flexed by 90 degrees (except when testing it), at the recommended joint positions and velocities:

Table 4.2 (*cont.*)

Shoulder
Horizontal adductors (V3)
Vertical adductors (V3)
Internal rotators (V3)

Elbow
Flexors (shoulder adducted, V2)
Extensors (shoulder abducted, V3)
Pronators (shoulder adducted, V3)
Supinators (shoulder adducted, V3)

Wrist
Flexors (V3)
Extensors (V2)

Fingers (angle PII of digit III – MCP)
Palmar interossei + FDS (wrist resting position, V3)

Source: (Tardieu et al., 1954; Held & Pierrot-Deseilligny, 1969; Boyd & Graham, 1999; personal communication from Jean Michael Gracies.

velocity (see Table 4.2). The modified Tardieu scale (Boyd & Graham, 1999) uses standardized conditions and measures the quality of muscle reaction as well as the angle at which it occurs. In children the point of resistance to a maximum velocity stretch (V3) is synonymous with the 'overactive stretch reflex' defined by Boyd as 'R1'. This is compared to the amount of muscle contracture or muscle length 'R2' obtained when a standardized velocity (V1) and force is applied. Compared with the modified Ashworth scale (Bohannon & Smith, 1987), the modified Tardieu scale has been shown to discriminate better between children with cerebral palsy who received intramuscular injections of BTXA and those who did not, when used by a 'blinded' assessor (Boyd et al., 1998a; Boyd & Graham, 1999).

Contracture can be measured under conditions in which hyperreflexia will be minimized. For example, by moving the limb slowly so as not to excite hyperexcitable reflexes and holding the muscle in a lengthened position for a while so as to dampen the reflex response, an accurate picture of muscle length can be gained. If a contracture is minor in extent, it may still be possible to achieve a normal range of motion by the application of sufficient force. For example, Halar et al. (1978) applied a force of 40 lbs and achieved similar magnitudes of ankle dorsiflexion in the affected and unaffected sides of hemiplegic patients, even in the presence of clinical contracture. Consequently, in order to assess the magnitude of joint

(a) (b)

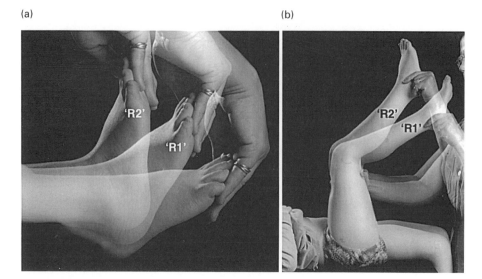

Fig. 4.3   Assessment if the range of motion at the (a) ankle and (b) knee using the modified version of the Tardieu scale (Boyd et al., 1998). 'R2' is the slow passive range of motion (conducted at Tardieu velocity 'V1'). 'R1' is the fast velocity movement of the ankle through full available range of motion to determine the point of 'catch' in the range of motion (Tardieu velocity 'V3'). The angle at which the muscle reaction ('catch' or 'R1') occurs is measured by goniometry. (a) the measure is performed at the ankle to test the gastrocnemius with the knee extended. (b) the measure is performed for the hamstring muscles with the hip flexed to 90° and the opposite hip extended.

motion, it is important not only to standardize the force applied but also not to exceed the magnitude of force that is normally sufficient to stretch the muscles through range (the 'R2'). It is more relevant to apply the magnitude of the force that reflects the normal forces applied at a joint during everyday use (e.g. forces applied to the ankle during walking are much larger than forces applied at the wrist during reaching). In addition, if a multi-joint muscle is being assessed, it is important to standardize the position of the joint not being measured. It is not easy to apply these controls in the clinical assessment of muscle contracture, yet without them contracture may be missed and therefore not treated.

The original Tardieu scale (see Table 4.2) has been modified by Boyd & Graham (1999) to assess specific muscles in the lower limb by standardizing conditions for limb placement and alignment (for the gastrosoleus, hamstrings and adductors) (see Figure 4.3). The 'dynamic component' or angle of the overactive stretch reflex is defined by Boyd at Tardieu velocity of stretch 'V3' and the slow passive range of motion or degree of muscle contracture 'R2' is graded as the angle at 'V1'. More important than the individual measures of 'R1' and 'R2' is the relationship between 'R2' minus 'R1'. A large difference between the two measures characterizes a large 'reflexive' component which is likely to respond to BTXA injections (Boyd et al., 1998a) whereas a small difference between 'R2' minus 'R1' means that there is predominantly fixed muscle contracture present. The expected outcome of treatment with BTXA will be influenced by the baseline value of 'R2' (amount of contracture) and the amount of 'R1' beyond that range (Boyd & Graham, 1999). The relative changes in 'R2' and 'R1' of the gastrosoleus determined clinically have been found to correlate with range of motion in gait as determined by sagittal plane kinematics (Boyd et al., 1998b).

Clinically, the most important measurement for physiotherapists is the level of disability – i.e., the level at which impairments affect the everyday life of the person who has suffered brain damage. Spasticity is just one of the impairments which affect function. The clinician needs carefully to assess the relative contribution of the individual impairments and how they impact on disability. In summary, in the clinic, muscle contracture and function can be measured, and it is possible to gain some insight into the contribution of spasticity to increased muscle stiffness.

Intervention

The current emphasis of physiotherapy for spasticity in adults is on training geared to addressing the more prevalent negative features of weakness and incoordination. In children with motor impairment, the emphasis is on management of emerging motor behaviours against the background of growth and maturation (Shepherd, 1995). In children with cerebral palsy, the impairments of overactivity, inappropriate muscle force, adaptive soft tissue changes due to overactivity and imbalances with growth are most evident in younger children whereas weakness and adaptive soft tissue changes due to non-use may become increasingly evident in the adolescent years.

Clinicians need to identify the contribution of spasticity to disability in order to plan effective management. Intervention needs to include training the patient to control muscles for specific tasks while eliminating unnecessary muscle activity during motor performance as well as maintaining soft tissue extensibility. It may be necessary to apply pharmacological treatment to dampen overactivity and reduce muscle stiffness or, if contracture already exists, to lengthen muscles by serial casting followed by training in these lengthened ranges (Boyd & Graham, 1997). If the lack of soft tissue extensibility is mostly contracture and/or bony deformity it may be appropriate to collaborate in surgical programmes that will restore biomechanical alignment and balance the soft tissue contractures (Gage, 1991). Where appropriate, orthoses may enhance carry over and provide the appropriate biomechanical alignment for practice. All these options must be accompanied by motor training to control muscles for specific tasks while eliminating unnecessary muscle activity during motor performance.

Elimination of unnecessary activity

In the past, it was common for therapists to avoid instructing the patient to contract any potentially spastic muscles (Bobath, 1990). One of the difficulties with this strategy is that all muscle activity not appropriate to an action is considered spastic. Avoiding encouraging muscle activity due to apprehension that it will cause spasticity has been challenged by studies showing that, after a strength-training programme, spasticity was not increased and in some cases was decreased (Butefisch et al., 1995; Sharp & Brouwer, 1997). Not only have spastic muscles been found to be weak in cerebral palsy (Wiley & Damiano, 1998) but strength training has also shown improvements in function with no mention of an increase in spasticity (MacPhail & Kramer, 1995; Damiano et al., 1995). In fact, strength training in children with cerebral palsy has been shown to be as effective in improving function as a selective dorsal rhizotomy plus strength training (McLaughlin et al., 1998). It is important to train aggressively those muscles which are important for everyday function, for example the calf muscles, even if they are considered to be a common site of spasticity. Learning to control muscles eccentrically during task performance may be particularly useful as it involves the patient learning to decrease muscle activity. For example, the calf muscles work eccentrically during stance phase to control the movement of the shank forward over the fixed foot as the hip extends and then concentrically at push-off (Sutherland et al., 1980). Eccentric contractions can be practised by placing the forefoot on a wedge and lowering the bodyweight (Figure 4.4a). For push-off, the patient practises plantarflexion in step stance with the hip and knee extended and the ankle initially dorsiflexed (Figure 4.4b). By learning to control calf muscle activity in these positions, the risk of developing overactivity and/or muscle contracture is reduced.

In young children, such training is often more difficult to perform and tasks need to be adapted to account for the lack of motivation and poor concentration. The use of a suitable reward system can be effective. In training calf muscles in their lengthened range, the emphasis may be on walking up slopes, stair climbing and reaching in inclined standing with the hips and knees extended and the feet dorsiflexed under the body to ensure maximal lengthening. Carry over of training can be reinforced by the appropriate use of a fixed ankle foot orthosis (Butler et al., 1992) tuned with a wedge to correctly align the ground reaction force with the knee joint and ensure appropriate control of the calf muscle in gait. This training can progress to less constrained conditions by the use of high-topped boots which encourage dorsiflexion,

(a)

(b)

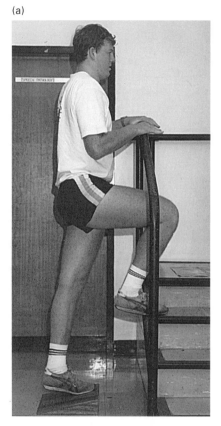
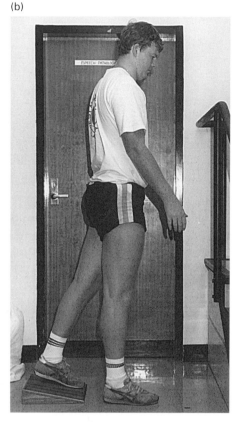

Fig. 4.4   (a): By standing with the ball of one foot on a wedge and raising and lowering himself, this patient practises controlling his plantarflexors eccentrically and concentrically in a lengthened range. (b): He practises plantarflexing during the last part of push-off by shifting his weight forward with his hip and knee in extension. (From Ada & Canning, 1990.)

thereby enabling achievement of heel strike at initial contact, whilst still allowing control of forward progression of the tibia during midstance.

Training of appropriate muscle force

Excessive, inappropriate muscle force can be a manifestation of spasticity or lack of skill. Either way, it is important to emphasize the correct application of muscle force during the performance of tasks. Practise may, therefore, need to be modified to allow the patient to participate without using unnecessary muscle activity. For example, during standing up from a seated position, the greatest extensor torque is required at thighs off and this is larger the lower the chair (Burdett et al., 1985). When standing up from a normal height chair (i.e. 44 cm) is outside the realms of possibility for a patient, the attempt may produce excessive weight shift to the intact side so that the knee extensor effort in the affected side causes the foot to move forward (often labelled as spasticity) rather than the trunk moving forward over a fixed foot. If the task is modified so that the patient practises standing up from a higher than normal chair, the extensor torque requirements are reduced and may enable more optimal practice. The patient will be able to keep more weight on the affected foot, thereby avoiding the adaptive responses seen when standing up from a normal height chair (Carr & Shepherd, 1989).

In children, it is more difficult for the physiotherapist to train the appropriate use of force in a motor task. There needs to be a greater emphasis on adaptation of the environment as well as use of auditory and visual cues to modify emerging motor behaviours. In grasping an object, children frequently use too much force, so it may be appropriate to train drinking from a cup by grasping a 'squashy' plastic cup. Using plasticine to make animal shapes also helps because the correct forces are needed to create the relevant shapes. Different textures may be needed to reduce excessive force such as with the task of holding a soft tomato without deformation and then progressing by using the other impaired hand to cut the tomato with a knife.

Forcing activation of the appropriate muscles

In young children and adults with hemiplegia, there can be a strong tendency for non-use of the affected limb, or more frequently, the lack of skill in that limb means it is rarely used except in bimanual tasks. Forced use of the affected limb, first suggested by Taub (1980), may be very effective in training underutilized muscles by careful restraint of the unaffected limb (Shepherd, 1995). Manual restraint of the unaffected limb can be unacceptable to children, so placing the arm inside the clothing, placing objects out of reach of the unaffected arm or use of that arm for support of the body can all be effective (Figure 4.5). Training tasks for young children need to be motivating, so that successful completion of the task will give positive feedback and knowledge of results.

Prevention of adaptive soft tissue changes

Diligent prevention of muscle contracture is important, not only because full muscle length is necessary for optimal function but because of the possible causal relation between spasticity and contracture. Both the immobility that is a major consequence of adult brain damage and the overactivity that is prevalent in children with brain damage may lead to increased muscle stiffness and contracture. Muscle length should be maintained, preferably through active training but where necessary by passive methods.

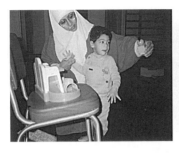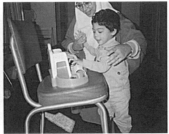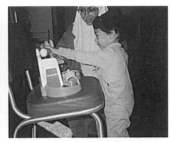

Fig. 4.5   A young boy with left hemiplegia has his unaffected arm restrained by his mother during training of reaching and manipulation. The task is designed so that attainment of the goal (dropping the toy through the slot) is only achieved by appropriate manipulation of the toy.

Muscles at risk of shortening should be trained in a lengthened part of the range so that the voluntary contraction of the muscle and its antagonist can be practised. For example, in adults following stroke, muscles around the shoulder that are particularly at risk of shortening when muscle activity is poor are the internal rotators and horizontal adductors. By side lying with the shoulder in 90° abduction and the arm rotated to face the wall while moving the arm in small excursions from this position, these muscles are being lengthened and are required to contract eccentrically (Figure 4.6). Once some control has been regained over agonist and antagonist muscle groups in different ranges around the joint, the risk of developing contracture is diminished.

In young children with cerebral palsy, the greater issue is overactivity leading to increased muscle stiffness and reduced muscle excursion rather than inactivity leading to soft tissue adaptations. However, in adolescence, this relative contribution of overactivity and adaptive changes in inactive or weak muscle is altered. It is important for the clinician to predict in which muscles overactivity will lead to increased muscle stiffness (such as the adductor and medial hamstring muscles which result in scissoring postures in standing and stepping in children with spastic diplegia). If reduced muscle excursion continues, lateral displacement of the hip may occur. It will be useful to encourage abducted postures and training of reciprocal leg movements in an abducted position (e.g. riding a bike with adapted footplates). Frequently overactivity of the adductor muscles occurs during a large portion of the day, so it may be appropriate to utilize functional bracing which still allows sitting, stepping, sit to stand and crawling in an abducted range (Figure 4.7).

It is necessary to determine the relative contribution of muscle overactivity and length to alignment. For example, it is common for children with cerebral palsy to stand up on their toes (in equinus) with their knees flexed due to hamstring

(a)

(b)

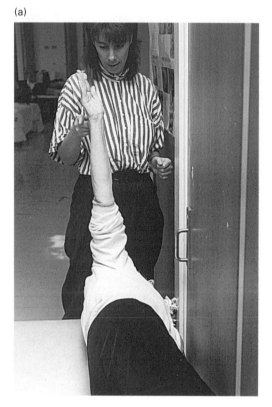
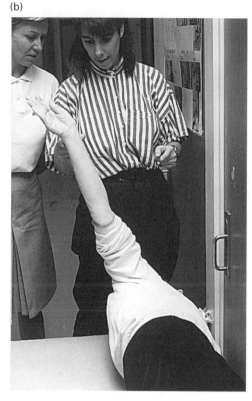

Fig. 4.6   (a): By lying on her side with her arm facing the wall, the muscles at risk of developing contracture (such as the horizontal adductors and internal rotators) are in a lengthened range. (b): The patient can then practise using her weak shoulder muscles in a relatively gravity eliminated position by making small excursions from this position. (Ada & Canning, 1998).

contracture and/or quadriceps weakness. A biomechanical analysis needs to differentiate whether the plantarflexed posture of the ankles is 'true equinus' (predominantly due to an overactive calf muscle) or whether it is 'apparent' equinus with the flexed knee position (predominantly due to hamstring overactivity). In apparent equinus, management needs to focus on training the hamstrings in the lengthened position as well as training the weak quadriceps using squat to stand manoeuvres. For example, Damiano et al. (1995) demonstrated the effectiveness of a quadriceps strengthening programme in improving crouch gait. If calf muscle length is adequate then techniques to lengthen the calf muscles alone would be ineffective.

Where patients are immobilized due to paralysis following stroke, severe overactivity due to cerebral palsy and/or unconsciousness following head injury, muscle length may have to be maintained using passive methods. The most important principle is to keep the muscle at risk of shortening in a lengthened position for

(a)

(b)

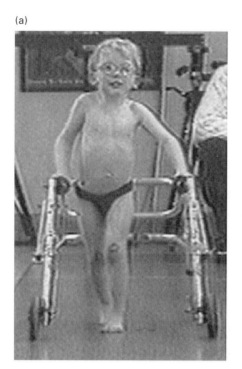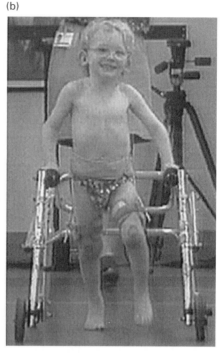

Fig. 4.7   (a): A young boy with spastic type diplegia usually walks with a scissoring posture of the lower limbs. (b): Use of a variable hip abduction orthosis puts the adductors in a lengthened position during walking.

some time. Evidence from the animal literature gives indications of the proportion of time the muscle needs to be in a lengthened position (Tardieu et al., 1988; Williams, 1988). Sustained periods of lengthening may be achieved by using sandbags to weight a limb and keep it in one position, as well as gaiters or splints to control limb position. Positioning to lengthen multiarticular muscles needs to take into account the position of all the joints that the muscle crosses, for example, lengthening the hamstrings requires hip flexion as well as knee extension.

In severe cases of four-limbed cerebral palsy or traumatic brain injury, maintaining muscle length will require sustained positioning using special seating and standing frames in positions that will allow functional training of the upper limbs for eating, play and communication (Finnie, 1974). It may be necessary to focus on training motor behaviours such as standing and stepping, and by-passing others such as crawling, as certain important muscles which tend to shorten with growth may not be utilized in their lengthened range in crawling. This is the case when the hamstring muscles shorten in children with cerebral palsy who predominantly crawl, sit between their heels and who therefore find full knee extension for standing and stepping more difficult.

There is ample evidence that serial casting, the most extreme form of positioning available to the physiotherapist, is effective in lengthening muscles which have already shortened (e.g. Booth et al., 1983; Copley et al., 1996; Moseley, 1997; Brouwer et al., 1998). It can also be a preventative measure to avoid muscle shortening in muscles known to be overactive in severe head injured patients (Conine et al., 1990). The emphasis should be for short periods of casting with frequent changes to serially lengthen the muscle because extended periods of casting may lead to weakness, and stiffness can remain. While there may be a shift in the muscle's length tension relationship (Herbert, 1988), this may revert quickly when casting ceases if the muscle is weak after sustained immobilization and active training in the lengthened range has not been undertaken.

Pharmacological and surgical options

There are many pharmacological and surgical options available in the management of spasticity, which may be focal or general, reversible or permanent in action (Boyd & Graham, 1997). Several other chapters in this book will address these options in detail, so our emphasis here is upon the physiotherapist's role in patient selection, evaluation of outcome and most importantly, motor training to achieve maximum benefit.

In pharmacological management, the physiotherapist's role is to identify the relative contribution of the positive impairments such as spasticity, muscle stiffness, muscle contracture, and the negative impairments such as weakness and poor selective control so that a total programme can be planned which is aimed at the individual impairments. A combination of options may be adopted. For example, an initial intramuscular injection with BTXA to address overactive or stiff muscles may need to be followed by short periods of serial casting to address any residual muscle contracture. A training programme is essential to address any negative features of incoordination and weakness, which may be evident. Management may require suitable orthoses that are geared to providing the appropriate biomechanical alignment outside training sessions. For example, improvement in gait is not always seen following BTXA injection alone. Active training and use of orthoses for carry-over has been shown to be essential in achieving improved motor performance (Boyd & Graham, 1997). In some cases, these interventions have enabled carry-over of effects of BTXA injections well beyond the estimated six months' pharmacological response (Boyd & Graham, 1997; Boyd et al., 2000) (Figure 4.8).

In assessing suitability of patients for pharmacological agents, it is important to recognize the expected action of the agent on the motor impairments, and choose appropriate tools to evaluate functional outcome. For example, studies of intrathecal baclofen (ITB) in children with generalized spasticity have shown a decrease

(a)   (b)   (c)

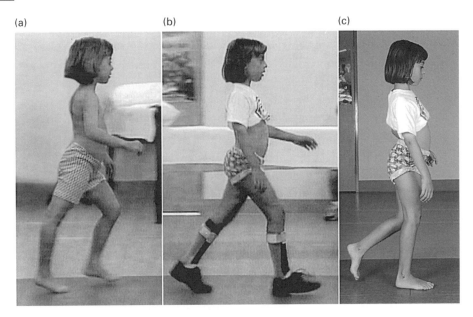

Fig. 4.8   (a): A girl with spastic type diplegia walks with an overactive plantarflexion-knee
extension couple due to overactivity of the calf muscles. (b): Following intramuscular
injection of botulinum toxin A to the gastrocsoleus, a fixed ankle–foot orthosis is used to
provide the appropriate biomechanical conditions to train knee control during gait. (c):
Thirteen months later, adequate length of the calf muscles has been maintained and
improved knee and ankle position without the orthosis has been achieved.

in hypertonia (according to the Ashworth scale) and improved joint range of
motion (Albright et al., 1991). However, unlike other pharmacological agents, an
improvement in function has not been demonstrated with ITB in a randomized or
controlled trial. In addition, it is important to establish whether efficacy in the
target muscle group has been established.

Where spasticity is generalized and persistent, surgical procedures such as selective dorsal rhizotomy (SDR) have been proposed. Results from three randomized
controlled trials appear variable (Lin, 1998). McLaughlin et al. (1998) compared a
strengthening programme with SDR plus strengthening and showed no difference
between the groups in terms of function. SDR aimed at managing spasticity may
have been inappropriate, as weakness rather than hyperreflexia may have been the
main problem (Guiliani, 1991). These findings illustrate the importance of training the negative features of brain damage as well as attending to the positive features.

In children with cerebral palsy where muscle contracture and poor biomechanical alignment have become severe, a programme of single event multilevel surgery

(SEMLS; Boyd & Graham, 1997) may be appropriate as opposed to multiple surgical events at single levels ('the birthday syndrome'; Rang, 1990; Gage, 1991). SEMLS should only be undertaken after the initial growth period and when gait performance has plateaued, around seven to ten years of age. An effective programme of management of muscle overactivity (with BTXA) and motor training is used to delay SEMLS until gait maturation (Boyd & Graham, 1997). The outcome from SEMLS will not be optimal if overactivity continues to cause reduced muscle excursion and interfere with motor function. This surgical approach of restoring bony lever arm alignment and balancing soft tissues in one occasion of treatment needs to be followed by an active training and strengthening programme. Children may be taller and straighter following SEMLS but not necessarily more effective in motor performance. The physiotherapist must train control of lengthened and transferred muscles in the context of motor tasks (e.g. stepping up and down, sit to stand), using objective assessment of gait to prescribe appropriate ankle foot orthoses and gait aids. They should continue to suggest training programmes to build confidence, stamina, gait independence and participation in activities of daily living and sport.

Conclusion

Effective intervention for disability associated with adult stroke and children with cerebral palsy requires careful assessment of the contributing impairments, specific motor training for function and avoidance of the development of adaptive soft tissue changes. Recent findings have identified the complexity of the contribution of both the negative and positive impairments to motor disability. In this chapter, we have used these findings to present a science-based model of clinical intervention for both adults and children following brain damage. Examples of strategies presented have taken into account the modifications necessary to cope with growth, maturation and motor learning in children. There is now a need to confirm efficacy of these interventions by clinical trials so that physiotherapy practice can become evidence-based (e.g. Fetters & Klusick, 1996; Dean & Shepherd, 1997).

Acknowledgements

The authors would like to thank Professor Meg Morris, Janice Collier and Professor H. Kerr Graham for their helpful comments during the preparation of this manuscript. Roslyn Boyd is a doctoral student in the School of Human Biosciences, an adjunct senior lecturer in the School of Physiotherapy, La Trobe University, Melbourne and Senior Research Physiotherapist, Hugh Williamson Gait Laboratory. Dr. Louise Ada is a senior lecturer at the School of Physiotherapy, University of Sydney.

REFERENCES

Ada, L. & Canning, C. (1990). Anticipating and avoiding muscle shortening. In *Key Issues in Neurological Physiotherapy*, eds. L. Ada & C. Canning, pp. 219–36. Oxford: Butterworth Heinemann.

Ada, L., Vattanasilip, W., O'Dwyer, N. & Crosbie, J. (1998). Does spasticity contribute to walking dysfunction after stroke? *J Neurol Neurosurg Psychiatry*, **64**: 628–35.

Albright, A. L., Ceervi, A. & Singeltary, J. (1991). Intrathecal baclofen for spasticity in cerebral palsy. *JAMA*, **265**: 1418–22.

Ashworth, B. (1964). Preliminary trial of carisoprodal in multiple sclerosis. *Practitioner*, **192**: 540–2.

Basmajian, J. V. (1977). Motor learning and control: a working hypothesis. *Arch Phys Med Rehabil*, **58**: 38–40.

Basmajian, J. V. & Blumenstein, R. (1980). *Electrode Placement in EMG Biofeedback*. Baltimore: Williams and Wilkins.

Bobath, B. (1990). *Adult Hemiplegia, Evaluation and Treatment*, 3rd edn. London: Butterworth Heinemann.

Bohannon, R. W. & Smith, M. B. (1987). Interrater reliability of a modified Ashworth scale of muscle spasticity. *Phys Ther*, **67**: 206–7.

Booth, B. J., Doyle, M. & Montgomery, J. (1983). Serial casting for the management of spasticity in the head-injured adult. *Phys Ther*, **63**: 1960–6.

Boyd, R. N., Barwood, S. A., Ballieu, C. & Graham, H. K. (1998a). Validity of a clinical measure of spasticity in children with cerebral palsy in a randomised clinical trial. (Abstract.) *Dev Med Child Neurol*, **40**: 7.

Boyd, R. N. & Graham, H. K. (1997). Botulinum toxin A in the management of children with cerebral palsy: indications and outcome. *Eur J Neurol*, **4** (Suppl. 2): 15–22.

Boyd, R. N. & Graham (1999). Objective measurement of clinical findings in the use of botulinum toxin A in the management of children with cerebral palsy. *Eur J Neurol*, **6** (Suppl. 4): S23–S35.

Boyd, R. N., Pliatsios, V. & Graham, H. Kerr (1998b). Use of objective measures in predicting response to botulinum toxin A in children with cerebral palsy. (Abstract.) *Dev Med Child Neurol*, (Suppl.). (Full paper in press: *Dev Med Child Neurol*.)

Boyd, R. N., Pliatsios, V., Starr, R., Nattrass, G. & Graham, H. K. (2000). Biomechanical transformation of the gastrocsoleus muscle by injection of botulinum toxin A in children with cerebral palsy. *Dev Med Child Neurol*, **42**: 32–41.

Brouwer, B., Wheeldon, R. K., Stradiotto-Parker, N. & Allum, J. (1998). Reflex excitability and isometric force production in cerebral palsy: the effect of serial casting. *Dev Med Child Neurol*, **40**: 168–75.

Burdett, R. G., Hasasevich, R., Pisciotta, J. et al. (1985). Biomechanical comparison of rising from two types of chairs. *Phys Ther*, **65**, 1177–83.

Burke, D. (1983). Critical examination of the case for or against fusimotor involvement in disorders of muscle tone. In *Motor Control Mechanisms in Health and Disease. Advances in Neurology*, ed. J. E. Desmedt, vol. 39, pp. 133–50. New York: Raven Press.

Burke, D. (1988). Spasticity as an adaptation to pyramidal tract injury. In *Functional Recovery in Neurological Disease. Advances in Neurology*, ed. S. G. Waxman, vol. 47, pp. 401–3. New York: Raven Press.

Butefisch, C., Hummelsheim, H. & Mauritz, K.-H. (1995). Repetitive training of isolated movements improves the outcome of motor rehabilitation of the centrally paretic hand. *J Neurol Sci*, **130**: 59–68.

Butler, P. B., Thompson, N. & Major, R. E. (1992). Improvement in Walking performance of children with cerebral palsy: preliminary results. *Dev Med Child Neurol*, **34**: 567–76.

Canning, C., Ada, L. & O'Dwyer, N. J. (2000). Muscle activation patterns associated with low dexterity following stroke. *J Neurol Sci*. (In press.)

Carr, J. H. & Shepherd, R. B. (1987). *A Motor Relearning Programme for Stroke*, 2nd edn. Oxford: Butterworth Heinemann.

Carr, J. H. & Shepherd, R. B. (1989). A motor learning model for stroke rehabilitation. *Physiotherapy*, **75**: 372–80.

Carr, J. H. & Shepherd, R. B. (1998). *Neurological Rehabilitation: Optimizing Motor Performance*. Oxford: Butterworth Heinemann.

Carr, J. H., Shepherd, R. & Ada, L. (1995). Spasticity: research findings and implications for intervention. *Physiotherapy*, **81**: 421–9.

Conine, T. A., Sullivan, T., Mackie, T. & Goodman, M. (1990). Effect of serial casting for the prevention of equinus in patients with acute head injury. *Arch Phys Med Rehabil*, **71**: 310–12.

Copley, J., Watson-Will, A. & Dent, K. (1996). Upper limb casting for clients with cerebral palsy: a clinical report. *Aust Occup Ther J*, **43**: 39–50.

Corry, I. S., Cosgrove, A. P., Walsh, E. G., McClean, D. & Graham, H. K. (1997). Botulinum toxin A in the hemiplegic upper limb: a double blind trial. *Dev Med Child Neurol*, **39**: 185–93.

Cosgrove, A. P., Corry, I. S. & Graham, H. K. (1994). Botulinum toxin in the management of the lower limb in cerebral palsy. *Dev Med Child Neurol*, **36**: 386–96.

Cosgrove, A. P. & Graham, H. K. (1994). Botulinum toxin prevents development of contracture in the heriditary spastic mouse. *Dev Med Child Neurol*, **36**: 379.

Damiano, D. L., Vaughan, C. L. & Abel, M. F. (1995). Muscle response to heavy resistance exercise in children with spastic cerebral palsy. *Dev Med Child Neurol*, **37**: 731–9.

Dean, C. M. & Shepherd, R. (1997). Task related training improves performance of seated reaching tasks: a randomised controlled trial. *Stroke*, **28**: 722–8.

Fellows, S. J., Ross, H. F. & Thilmann, A. F. (1993). The limitations of the tendon jerk as a marker of pathological stretch reflex activity in human spasticity. *J Neurol Neurosurg Psychiatry*, **56**: 513–17.

Fetters, L. & Klusick, J. (1996). The effects of neurodevelopmental treatment versus practise on the reaching of children with spastic cerebral palsy. *Phys Ther*, **76**: 346–58.

Finnie, N. (1974). *Handling the Cerebral Palsy Child at Home*, 2nd edn. London: William Heinemann Medical Books.

Gage, J. R. (1991). *Gait Analysis in Cerebral Palsy. Clinics in Developmental Medicine*, No 121. Oxford: MacKeith Press.

Goldspink, G. & Williams, P. E. (1990). Muscle fibre and connective tissue changes associated with use and disuse. In *Foundations for Practice. Topics in Neurological Physiotherapy*, ed. A. Ada & C. Canning, pp. 197–218. London: Heinemann.

Gottlieb, G. L., Agarwal, G. C. & Penn, R. (1978). Sinusoidal oscillation of the ankle as a means of evaluating the spastic patient. *J Neurol Neurosurg Psychiatry*, **41**: 32–9.

Guiliani, C. A. (1991). Dorsal rhizotomy for children with cerebral palsy: support for concepts of motor control. *Phys Ther*, **71**: 248–59.

Halar, E. M., Stolov, W. C., Venkatesh, B., Brozovich, F. V. & Harley, J. D. (1978). Gastrocnemius muscle belly and tendon length in stroke patients and able-bodied persons. *Arch Phys Med Rehabil*, **59**: 476–84.

Held, J. P. & Pierrot-Deseilligny, E. (1969). *Reeducation Motrice des Affections Neurologiques'*, pp. 31–42. Paris: J. B. Baillere.

Herbert, R. (1988). The passive mechanical properties of muscle and their adaptations to altered patterns of use. *Aus J Physiother*, **34**: 141–9.

Hobart, D. J., Kelley, D. L. & Bradley, L. S., (1995). Modifications occurring during acquisition of a novel throwing task. *Am J Phys Med*, **51**: 1–24.

Hufschmidt, A. & Mauritz, K.-H. (1985). Chronic transformation of muscle in spasticity: a peripheral contribution to increased tone. *J Neurol Neurosurg Psychiatry*, **48**: 676–85.

Ibrahim, I. K., el-Abid, M. A. et al. (1993a). Patients with spastic hemiplegia at different recovery stages: evidence of reciprocal modulation of early/late reflex responses. *J Neurol Neurosurg Psychiatry*, **56**: 386–92.

Ibrahim, I. K., Verger, W. & Trippel, M. (1993b). Stretch-induced electromyographic activity and torque in spastic elbow muscles. *Brain*, **116**: 971–89.

Jackson, J. H. (1958). Selected writings. In *John Hughlings Jackson*, ed. J. Taylor. New York: Basic Books.

Katz, R. T. & Rymer, W. Z. (1989). Spastic hypertonia: mechanisms and management. *Arch Phys Med Rehabil*, **70**: 144–55.

Koning, J. T. de, Milan, H. F., Wsither, R. D. & Huijing, P. A. (1987). Functional characteristics of rat gastrocnemius and tibialis anterior muscles during growth. *J Morphol*, **194**: 75–84.

Lance, J. W. (1980). Symposium synopsis. In *Spasticity: disorder of motor control*, ed. R. G. Feldman, R. R. Young & W. P. Koella, pp. 485–94. Chicago: Year Book Medical Publishers.

Lance, J. W. (1990). What is spasticity? *Lancet*, **335**: 606.

Landau, W. M. (1974). Spasticity: the fable of a neurological demon and the emperors of a new therapy. *Arch Neurol*, **31**: 217.

Landau, W. M. (1990). Spasticity: what is it? What is it not? In *Spasticity: Disordered Motor Control*, eds. R. G. Feldman, R. R. Young & W. P. Koella, pp. 17–24. Chicago: Year Book Medical Publishers.

Lehmann, J. F., Price, R., de Lateur, B. J., Hinderer, S. & Traynor, C. (1989). Spasticity: quantitative measurements as a basis for assessing effectiveness of therapeutic intervention. *Arch Phys Med Rehabil*, **70**: 6–15.

Lin, J. P. (1998). Dorsal rhizotomy and physical therapy. (Editorial.) *Dev Med Child Neurol*, **40**: 219.

McLaughlin, J. F., Bjornson, K. F., Astley, S. J., Graubert, C., Hays, R. M., Roberts, T. S., Price, R. & Temkin, N. (1998). Selective dorsal rhizotomy: efficacy and safety in an investigator – masked randomised clinical trial. *Dev Med Child Neurol*, **40**: 220–32.

McLellan, D. L. (1977). Co-contraction and stretch reflexes in spasticity during treatment with baclofen. *J Neurol Neurosurg Psychiatry*, **40**: 30–8.

MacPhail, H. E. & Kramer, J. F. (1995). Effect of isokinetic strength-training on functional ability and walking efficiency in adolescents with cerebral palsy. *Dev Med Child Neurol*, **37**: 763–75.

Mayston, M. J. (1992). The Bobath concept – evolution and application. In *Movement Disorders in Children*, eds. H. Forssberg & H. Hirschfeld, pp. 1–6. Basel: Karger.

Moseley, A. M. (1997). The effect of casting combined with stretching on passive ankle dorsiflexion in adults with traumatic head injuries. *Phys Ther*, **77**: 240–58.

Nathan, P. W. (1969). Treatment of spasticity with perineural injections of phenol. *Dev Med Child Neurol*, **11**: 384.

Neilson, P. D. & Lance, J. W. (1978). Reflex transmission characteristics during voluntary activity in normal man and patients with movement disorders. In *Cerebral Motor Control in Man: Long Loop Mechanisms. Progress in Clinical Neurophysiology*, ed. J. E. Desmedt, vol. 4, pp. 263–9. Basel: Karger.

Neilson, P. D. & McCaughey, J. (1982). Self-regulation of spasm and spasticity in cerebral palsy. *J Neurol Neurosurg Psychiatry*, **45**: 320–30.

O'Dwyer, N. J., Ada, L. & Neilson, P. D. (1996). Spasticity and muscle contracture following stroke. *Brain*, **119**: 1737–49.

O'Dwyer, N. J. & Ada, L. (1996). Reflex hyperexcitability and muscle contracture in relation to spastic hypertonia, *Curr Opin Neurol*, **9**: 451–5.

Payton, O. R., Payton, O. D., Su, S., et al. (1976). Abductor digiti quinti shuffle board: a study in motor learning. *Arch Phys Med Rehabil*, **57**: 169–74.

Payton, O. D. & Kelley (1972). Electromyographic evidence of the acquisition of a motor skill. A pilot study. *Phys Ther*, **52**: 261–6.

Rack, P. M. H., Ross, H. F. & Thilmann, A. F. (1984). The ankle stretch reflexes in normal and spastic subjects. *Brain*, **107**: 637–54.

Rang, M. (1990). Cerebral palsy. In *Paediatric Orthopaedics*, ed. R. T. Morrissey, 3rd edn., pp. 465–506. Philadelphia: J. B. Lippincott & Co.

Sahrmann, S. & Norton (1977). The relationship of voluntary movement to spasticity in the upper motor neurone. *Ann Neurol*, **2**: 460–5.

Sharp, S. A. & Brouwer, B. J. (1997). Isokinetic strength training of the hemiparetic knee: effects on function and spasticity. *Arch Phys Med Rehabil*, **78**: 1231–6.

Shepherd, R. B. (1995). *Physiotherapy in Paediatrics*, 3rd edn. Oxford: Butterworth Heinemann.

Sutherland, H. D., Cooper, B. A. & Daniel, D. (1980). The role of the plantarflexors in normal walking. *Journal of Bone and Joint Surgery*, 62-A, 3, 354–63.

Tardieu, G., Lepargot, A., Tabary, C. & Brett, M. D. (1988). For how long must the soleus muscle be stretched each day to prevent contracture? *Dev Med Child Neurol*, **30**: 310.

Tardieu, G., Shentoub, S. & Delarue, R. (1954). A la recherche d'une technique de mesure de la spasticite imprime avec le periodique. *Rev Neurol*, **91**: 143–4.

Tardieu, C., Tabary, J. C., Tabary, C. & Huet de la Tours E. (1977). Comparison of the sarcomere number adaptations in young and adult animals influence of tendon adaptation. *J Physiol*, **73**: 1045–55.

Taub, E. (1980). Motor research with monkeys: implications for rehabilitation medicine and behavioural psychology. In *Rehabilitation Medicine: Clinical Applications*, ed. L. P. Ince, pp. 371–401. Baltimore: Williams & Wilkins.

Vattanasilp, W. & Ada, L. (1999). Relationship between clinical and laboratory measures of spasticity. *Aus J Physiother*, **45**: 135–9.

Wiley, M. E. & Damiano, D. L. (1998). Lower extremity strength profiles in spastic cerebral palsy. *Dev Med Child Neurol*, **40**: 100–7.

Williams, P. E. (1988). Use of intermittent stretch in the prevention of connective tissue accumulation in muscle. *J Anat*, **158**: 109.

World Health Organization (1980). *International Classification of Impairments, Disabilities and Handicaps*. Switzerland: Geneva.

World Health Organization (1999). *International Classification of Impairments, Disabilities and Handicaps* (ICIDH-2 Beta draft).

Ziv, I., Blackbum, N., Rang, M. & Koresta, J. (1984). Muscle growth in normal and spastic muscle. *Dev Med Child Neurol*, **26**: 94–9.

5

Seating and positioning in spasticity

Craig A. Kirkwood and Geoff I. Bardsley

Introduction

Spasticity can create complex seating requirements for a wide variety of people with disabilities – from children with cerebral palsy, young adults with head injuries, people in middle life with multiple sclerosis to older users who have suffered cerebrovascular accidents. The nature of spasticity is complex and controversial, as is discussed elsewhere in this volume. Clinical characteristics which are described as constituting spasticity and which influence seating include increased muscle tone, changes in muscle structure and function, hyperactive stretch reflexes, and abnormal activity caused by posture, for example tonic neck and labyrinthine reflexes (Ford, 1986; Shepherd, 1995).

Spasticity, in itself, is not necessarily a problem and may assist in maintaining a seated posture. This is in contrast to individuals with hypotonia where providing seated support in a functional position is often inherently very difficult. There are, however, three key problems that spasticity can create for a person in a seated position:

- postural instability;
- reduced upper limb function;
- joint contractures.

Correct positioning of the person can assist in reducing these problems (Zollars, 1993). Addressing one of these problems usually has a largely beneficial effect on the others, so there is little trade-off in applying strategies to tackle these problems. Barnes (1993) states: 'positioning of the individual is the most important element in the management of spasticity' (see also Vaughan & Bhakta, 1995).

Appropriate seating should be seen as an adjunct to other approaches discussed in this volume which may have greater precedence with increasing severity of spasticity (e.g. pharmacological, surgical (Richardson & Thompson, 1999)). This is important to note as there are often expectations that correct seating will tackle all problems an individual has resulting from spasticity, when other methods have been unsuccessful.

As Barnes (1993) notes, the management of spasticity requires a team approach with the involvement of 'nurses, physiotherapists, physicians, occupational therapists, orthotists and wheelchair specialists' in addition to the patient and their carers. This multidisciplinary approach should be regarded as 'best practice' as often the various health professionals seek to tackle spasticity with little knowledge of other, sometimes conflicting, involvement.

This chapter is concerned mainly with the seated aspect of positioning, particularly for those who spend long periods in a wheelchair. People, however, also spend many hours lying down and correct positioning during this period is equally important (Scrutton, 1971, 1978; Todd, 1974; Bell & Watson, 1985; Nelham et al., 1992). Whilst the same principles in terms of positioning and design considerations apply, a variety of positions over a 24-hour period are required to move joints through their range of motion (ROM) and prevent soft tissues becoming contracted in a 'seated' position.

Clinical assessment

Detailed assessment is essential to draw up a full picture of the patient's seating requirements and their problems relating to spasticity in order that clear, specific and realistic objectives can be agreed by all those involved with the patient's care. A detailed prescription can then be produced to achieve the objectives.

Assessing the patient with spasticity for seating may involve four procedures to assist in determining the effect of the spasticity:

(1) *History taking* – soliciting information of the particular problems that occur with increased tone and factors which are found to exacerbate tone and produce associated reactions. This background information is very significant as the clinical situation itself can have a significant effect on the patient's presentation (Harburn & Potter, 1993). They may also recently have had medication to control spasticity, particularly if travelling a distance to an appointment. It may be useful for video to be used to monitor the patient unobtrusively in particular situations where there is a problem, such as during feeding.

(2) *Examination on plinth in supine* – whilst determining range of joint motion, account can be taken of resistance to motion and variation according to speed of movement. Care needs to be taken in interpreting this information as overall tone may be different to the seated position.

(3) *Support in seated posture* – whilst the patient is well supported in a seated posture (by one or more staff), account can be taken of tone in body (by those supporting) and changes to apparent range of motion in lower limbs. As sitting balance is affected by the level of spasticity (Yang et al., 1996), it may be useful to grade this using, for example, the Chailey scale (Green & Nelham, 1991).

(4)   *Support in a seating simulator* – a seating simulator allows the patient to be supported in a variety of configurations by altering the relative position of the support surfaces and their orientation in space. Account can therefore be taken of functional ability – e.g. trying to lift a cup and drink – and the simulator can be adjusted to check for variations in function and level of spasticity (Bardsley & Taylor, 1982).

Principles of seating and positioning

The basic philosophy of seating is the same for all patients: 'that the body should be maintained in a balanced, symmetrical and stable posture that is both comfortable and maximizes function' (Barnes, 1993). It is the nature of spasticity to produce postures that are unbalanced, non-symmetrical and unstable, with the result that the patient is uncomfortable and there is impairment of functional ability.

The following are 10 principles that should be considered when seeking to achieve an 'optimum' seated position for those with spasticity. The diverse range of factors which relate positioning and spasticity and which may affect postural stability, function and the development of contractures are explored.

Sustained muscle stretch

The key principle in reducing spastic contraction is the same as that applied in physiotherapy. That is, sustained muscle stretch working against the spastic muscle (Bobath, 1977). Stretching reduces spasticity directly in the muscle being stretched by depressing muscle spindle activity (Kaplan, 1962). It also reduces the possibility of contractures (Harburn & Potter, 1993; Bakheit, 1996). Such a reduction of spasticity may reduce overall tone in the body and hence may also permit greater use of the upper limbs (Nwaobi, 1987a).

As such, correct positioning in seating is consistent with a physiotherapy programme which emphasizes the importance of daily ROM exercises and static muscle stretch to prevent contractures and reduce spasticity (Little & Massagli, 1993). Odeen (1981) reported increased ROM and decreased activation of the antagonist in voluntary abduction by using a mechanical leg abductor for thirty minute treatment sessions.

The prevention or reduction of contractures by muscle stretching is particularly significant because of the pain contractures can produce and the difficulties they can create in treatment regimes. The muscle contracture itself may potentiate the stretch reflex (O'Dwyer et al., 1996) causing further problems with spasticity.

When applying a muscle stretch using seating support elements, the same principle as serial casting (Brouwer et al., 1996) can be utilized whereby gains in com-

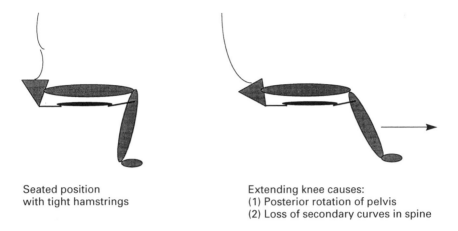

Seated position
with tight hamstrings

Extending knee causes:
(1) Posterior rotation of pelvis
(2) Loss of secondary curves in spine

Fig. 5.1   Effect of hamstring stretch on seated posture.

fortable ROM at a joint can be consolidated and increased by providing progressively greater stretch. This implies that the seating requires to be monitored and frequently adjusted to build on gains and address failures. One possible exception to this principle, when applied to the seated posture, is stretching of the hamstrings to extend knee joints to 90° or more. The hamstrings extend over two joints with the result that extending the knee also acts to rotate the pelvis posteriorly (Zollars, 1996) which in turn pulls the person out of the wheelchair and produces a kyphotic spinal posture (Figure 5.1). In order for a hamstring stretch to be effective the pelvis must be firmly secured both anteriorly and posteriorly to prevent movement but in practice this is difficult to achieve.

The link between hip flexion and hand function is controversial. No relationship was reported by Seeger et al. (1984) but Nwaobi et al. (1986) reported that 90° hip flexion gave better function compared to 50°, 70° and 110°. Using supported standing for load bearing (Odeen & Knutsson, 1981; Tremblay et al., 1990) has been successful in producing a muscle stretch which reduced spasticity. This position has other benefits, such as bladder drainage and increasing bone density, for those who spend long periods sitting.

Maintenance of hip integrity

A common problem encountered in seating children with cerebral palsy is hip subluxation and dislocation. Kalen & Bleck (1985) identified the primary aetiology and therefore the primary focus of treatment to be adductor and iliopsoas spasticity and contractures. X-rays have shown that the acetabulum of the adducted hip does not develop normally, with increasing subluxation and eventual dislocation of the hip (Fulford & Brown, 1976). Howard et al. (1985) found from examining the X-rays of hips of patients with cerebral palsy that 79% of bilateral hemiplegics had abnormal hips; the majority of these were non-walkers, the others required a frame or rollator. Young et al. (1998) found that in patients with spastic quadriplegia, 25% had hip dislocation and 63% subluxation. This reinforces the need to address hip status particularly among children with more involved cerebral palsy.

In addition to the pain that can be caused to the patient by compromised hips (Bagg et al., 1993), there is an asymmetry in the interface between the patient's pelvis and hips and the seated surface thus producing an asymmetric pelvis and consequent postural scoliosis. This may become less flexible with time and there is an increased risk of pressure sores on the more heavily loaded side of the pelvis.

Helping to maintain hip joint integrity is therefore an important role of seating in wheelchairs. Problems are particularly likely in patients with adductor spasticity. The distal end of the femur is pulled to the midline and tends to pull the femoral head away from the socket therefore compounding the lack of normal weight bearing in promoting acetabulum development. Scrutton (1991) emphasized the need for correct positioning and the experience of standing for those under four years of age as this is when such problems begin to develop.

A common, related problem is 'windsweeping' where there is an abduction contracture of one hip and an adduction contracture of the contralateral hip with subluxation or dislocation (Lonstein & Beck, 1986). This is often related to pelvic obliquity and scoliosis thus presenting a significant seating problem. Young et al. (1998) state: 'those with asymmetry of tone and severe spasticity seem to be at the greatest risk for dislocation, with a windswept hip deformity toward the opposite side.'

Tight, and eventually contracted adductors, with consequent dislocated hips causes serious toileting problems (Cornell, 1995). This represents a common indication for surgery, taking account of the impossibility of relocating the hip joint by soft-tissue operations alone (Samilson et al., 1967). Spencer (1999) emphasizes the complexity of surgery, the problem of post-operative pain for the child and great difficulty in treating painful dislocated hips in young adults. These are strong indicators for prevention through the close monitoring and conservative management of hips in children with cerebral palsy.

This problem needs to be addressed primarily by abducting the hips. In seating it is important that sufficient abduction is used to produce the required muscle stretch and maintain the integrity of the interface of the femoral head to the acetabulum. Many pommels that are commonly used in cushions are relatively narrow in width and therefore serve mainly to simply prevent contact between the thighs, thus limiting adduction without producing abduction. This may be general practice because a pommel wide enough to produce an abducted hip position would have poor cosmesis and may be impractical when skirts are worn.

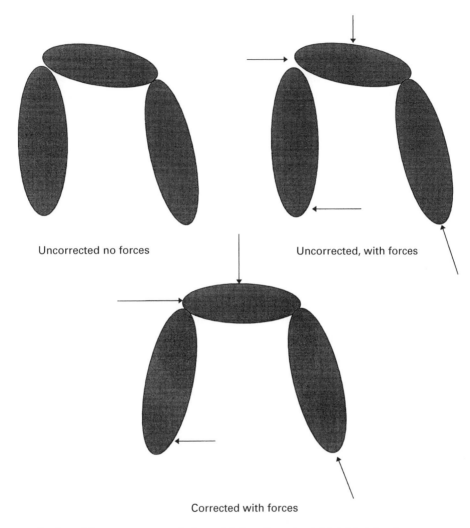

Uncorrected no forces   Uncorrected, with forces

Corrected with forces

Fig. 5.2   Application of forces to correct windswept deformity and establish hip integrity.

An alternative option is the use of a hip abduction orthosis (Bower, 1990) to maintain the relationship between the femurs and pelvis combined with use of a seating system. Another approach is to use a seating orthosis combining a spinal jacket and abduction orthosis (Carlson & Winter, 1978) which gives better control of hip position.

An approach commonly used in seating which addresses the problem of windsweeping is the application of a knee block (Scrutton, 1978; Green & Nelham, 1991). Figure 5.2 illustrates the application of forces to produce a corrected position. The knee block works by applying a derotational force along the femur of the abducted hip and an abducting force to the adducting hip together with stabilization of the pelvis. It is critical that a knee block is adjusted and used correctly for it to be effective. Before this approach is adopted, however, a thorough examination of hip integrity on the abducted side is required to ensure it is able to withstand the de-rotational forces.

Proper positioning following hip surgery is also required in order to maximize its benefits (Scrutton, 1989). It is vital therefore, particularly when casts are removed, that the hips are positioned correctly when seated in the wheelchair to consolidate gains made by surgery.

Trunk orientation

Appropriate orientation of the trunk in space is an important consideration in any seating system. As a number of patients present with anterior trunk postural stability problems, it is often tempting to use a seated orientation that is tilted back. This utilizes the effects of gravity to locate the patient against the backrest, therefore reducing the need for activation of postural support muscles.

Research with able-bodied people has shown that sitting against a more reclined backrest reduces activation of the back extensors (Andersson et al., 1974, 1975). This finding, however, cannot be transferred to those with spasticity where factors such as labyrinthine responses and a feeling of disorientation and falling (Green et al., 1992) can have a significant effect.

It has been shown that muscle activity and movement time of upper limbs increased in children with cerebral palsy when a backrest reclined from the upright was used (Nwaobi & Trefler, 1985; Nwaobi, 1987a).

Nwaobi (1986) studied 12 children with mild to moderate spastic diplegia. They were tested in an upright and 30° tilted back position. There was a marked and statistically significant ($P<0.05$) increase in activity of back extensors when tilted back. The activity levels of the hip adductors and ankle plantar flexors showed small increases in mean value but were not statistically significant.

The variability of such studies was shown when Nwaobi et al. (1983) investigated 11 children with cerebral palsy in seven combinations of seat and backrest inclination. This study showed a trend for mean electromyography (EMG) to increase with a rearward inclined backrest ($P<0.05$). There was, however, a marked and significant change with the backrest inclined forward by 15°.

Rearward tilting has a further detrimental effect on the ability to interact with the environment and decreases social stimulation and visual awareness. Compromises may be achieved in a device with variable tilt which can be readily adjusted to suit the different functional requirements of the individual. Care is required to ensure that such devices are used appropriately and not simply left tilted backwards for the convenience of the carer. The use of such devices requires careful discussion with the patient's carers to ensure that it is tilted back only when appropriate – e.g. if the user falls asleep.

Restraint of arm movement

Any form of restraint used with individuals is a sensitive issue and may require specific authorization. However, it may be appropriate in certain situations, that unwanted arm movement is restrained to help reduce tone and associated reactions and produce functional gains.

Restraint of non-dominant arm

Patients presenting with athetosis often request that the non-dominant arm be restrained in order to gain better control of the dominant arm, for example to facilitate the use of a joystick on a powered wheelchair. Sometimes this effect has been achieved by patients themselves wedging their non-dominant arm within the wheelchair/seating system to restrict its movement.

A single case study by Nwaobi (1987b) showed a marked reduction in deltoid activity in the restrained arm and some reduction in the non-restrained arm. It was also found that quadriceps activity in both legs reduced notably, showing that there was no overflow to distal segments caused by the restraint and in fact that there is a generalized reduction in tone.

Restraint of both arms

Where both arms are non-functional and athetosis is a problem, then it may be appropriate to restrain both arms to achieve functional gains with, for example, chin control of an electric wheelchair.

Trefler (1986) found in a study of 14 children with athetoid cerebral palsy using arm-restraint trays, that they were perceived by all parents and teachers as providing more function and comfort and that they were generally well received by the children.

Restraining movement – safety aspects

Some patients combine strong muscle contractions with osteoporosis. Consideration has to be given in these cases, to the safety of restricting motion of some body segments. This is of particular clinical relevance where a patient has strong extensor thrust at hips and knees and will therefore be seated with a belt restricting the motion of the pelvis. With these elements restrained, the remaining body part that moves is the lower leg as the knee extends. Restricting the motion by foot straps can result in sufficient force to fracture the leg.

Postural stabilization

A detailed biomechanical analysis of maintaining a seated posture and its facilitation by seating is a highly complex subject and has yet to be reported. An empirical summary with clinical application is provided by Bardsley (1993).

The importance of an integrated approach to postural stabilization has been examined by Myhr & von Wendt (1990, 1991, 1993) and Myhr (1994). These studies have explored a 'functional sitting position' which has as key elements:

(1)   symmetrical fixation of pelvis with firm posterior support and hip belt anchored under seat;

(2)   abduction orthosis, which also externally rotates the thighs;

(3)   placement of the line of gravity of the upper body anterior to the axis of rotation of the ischial tuberosities.

The seated position also incorporates a tray to assist upper body support as a result of (3) and free positioning of the feet (which tend to move backward).

The authors found that stabilization of position utilizing the combination of the above elements had the greatest effect in improving postural control and upper limb function by reducing pathological movements and spasticity than any single element.

Reduction of unnecessary upper limb activity

In past years it was standard practice to prescribe occupant propelled wheelchairs, often one-arm drive, to patients with hemiparesis during their rehabilitation to encourage physical activity and promote independence. However, it was often noted that the effort involved in propelling the wheelchair increased tone and associated reactions in such patients (Ashburn & Lynch, 1988). This follows the general principle that associated reactions are caused by forceful movements in other parts of the body (De Wald, 1987). This was considered, therefore, to undermine the efforts of physiotherapists to reduce spasticity.

Cornell (1991) looked at 10 subjects with hemiparesis undergoing rehabilitation. Both attendant and occupant propulsion were used on a test track with photographs being taken before, during and after the test run. The photographs were independently assessed to indicate the level of spasticity by body position. In general, the level of spasticity increased, often markedly, with occupant propulsion whereas in general there was little difference with attendant propulsion.

Dvir et al. (1996) after examining the relationship between graded effort and associated reactions, concluded that 'this study indicates that there is a direct relationship between levels of effort induced in the nonplegic forearm and the associated reactions elicited in the plegic forearm of post-stroke patients.' For this reason, it may often be more appropriate to use a powered wheelchair, at least initially so that independence can be gained without producing associated reactions and an increase in spasticity. Although, as Ashburn & Lynch (1988) comment, there is a danger in becoming dependent on the wheelchair with resulting disuse of motor skills, pain, stiffness and difficulties in extending lower limbs together with the difficulty of taking a wheelchair away from a patient once issued. In addition it should be noted that Blower et al. (1995) found that wheelchair propulsion ability at three weeks post-stroke was 'the most accurate guide to walking potential that has been reported to date'.

The same rationale means that any unnecessary activity involving significant exertion whether in the upper limbs or lower limbs (e.g. propelling by foot paddling) should be avoided (Bobath, 1977) and therefore activities should be constructed to minimize exertion and thereby avoid increasing spasticity.

Although there are those such as Blower (1988) who feel that the benefits of independent manual wheelchair use outweigh any disadvantages accruing from an increase in spasticity, the benefits of independence and morale are equally true of using a powered chair and perhaps more so as they give a greater range of travel and leave the users less fatigued to perform activities on arrival at their destination.

The use of manual and powered chairs and encouraging walking therefore requires careful judgement to balance the relative advantages and disadvantages in the early rehabilitation of stroke patients. All patients with spasticity using manual chairs should therefore be monitored for adverse effects.

Reduction of noxious stimuli

The provision of seated postural support must also take account of the fact that it is not only external, physical factors altering position that influence the level of spasticity but also the patient's mental state and perceptions which can have an important mediating effect. For example, biofeedback can be utilized to control the stretch reflex gain. O'Dwyer et al. (1994) found that after a training programme involving feedback of the gain of the tonic stretch reflex, the stretch reflex gain was significantly reduced in all subjects.

Katz (1988), Barnes (1993) and Bakheit (1996) have highlighted the importance of avoiding noxious stimuli, including prompt treatment of urinary tract complications, preventing pressure sores and contractures and proper management of the bowels and bladder. In the context of providing seated support, noxious stimuli can arise from factors such as discomfort from long periods of sitting (insufficient pressure relief), excessive pressure being applied to maintain seated posture and inappropriate seating causing pain (e.g. pressure from wheelchair backrest tubes).

An important aim, therefore, is that the seating system should be comfortable, in all aspects, for a reasonable sitting duration. Implicit in this is the recognition that changes in seated position are important throughout the day. Therefore an armchair for relaxation should receive the same consideration for selection as the wheelchair.

The variability of the patient's physical status during the day needs to be considered. For example, tiredness, excitement or tone reduction immediately after medication may lead to dramatic variations in sitting ability. A seat which gives the required support for these states needs to be provided.

The patient may sit well in a clinic when highly stimulated to maintain posture and when no upper limb activities are being performed. However, in everyday situations, they may find their activities limited by, for example, fear of imbalance when using upper limbs giving rise to an increase in tone because of the perceived problem. This is similar to the fear of falling which increases spasticity in ambulant hemiplegic patients (Bobath, 1977). The effect of a clinic event resulting in patients sitting unrealistically well should not be underestimated (Bishop, 1977). Conversely, a clinic event may give rise to anxiety and worsening of spasticity. The user's perception of postural security and comfort may be as important as the 'actual' support and pressure distribution provided.

Factors such as the importance of outdoor clothing to maintain temperature also deserve consideration (Shirado et al., 1995).

Alternative postures

Variation in posture is important to maintain joint mobility, to reduce the effects of sustained application of pressure and to facilitate different types of activity. The imaginative use of alternative postural support systems can help greatly to provide this variability. Examples are provided below:

Horseback riding

In addition to the static aspects of sitting, the dynamics of sitting are emphasized in horseback riding (Bertoti, 1988; Heine, 1997) where a combination of sitting posture with legs held in flexion, abduction and external rotation together with the movement of the horse are believed to help reduce spasticity. Quint & Toomey (1998) used a horse riding simulator and reported increased pelvic mobility after use, indicating that hip abduction and rhythmical movement may reduce spasticity.

Seating and mobility (SAM) system

The SAM system developed by Pope et al. (1988) includes the use of a saddle type of seat to promote hip abduction whilst allowing hip extension. The authors conclude that 'indications exist which suggest that the control of spasm is more a function of trunk posture relative to the supporting base than of the degree of hip flexion'.

Standing

Noronha et al. (1989) reported no difference in upper limb function between sitting and prone standing. However, Odeen & Knutsson (1981) found significant reductions in spasticity with paraplegic patients' weight-bearing using a tilt table to weight bear and stretch calf muscles. Similarly, Tremblay et al. (1990) reported significant reductions in spasticity in 22 children with spastic cerebral palsy standing with feet dorsiflexed on a tilt table.

Positioning in the seat

A well-designed seating system is only as good as the accuracy within which the person is positioned. A particular difficulty frequently encountered is that an appropriately prescribed seating system is not used correctly and therefore has reduced effectiveness.

Typically, when a patient is hoisted to transfer into a seat, there is an increase in tone, often producing hip extension or knee flexion. This results in the patient assuming an inappropriate posture when lowered into the seat (Scrutton, 1966). Time needs to be taken to allow the tone to reduce and to move affected joints slowly to allow repositioning in the seat. Similarly, adjustable or removable components require to be used and positioned appropriately. Misuse can not only negate the effectiveness of the seat but also be detrimental through the adverse positions and forces it can generate. This is particularly the case for components such as straps, belts and knee-blocks where adjustment can be critical.

The abilities of patients and carers for accurate positioning in the seat and to use removable/adjustable components can have an overriding influence on prescription. There is little point providing a device that will not be used effectively by the patients and their carers.

Position of tasks

Whilst it is important to reduce upper limb effort (as already discussed), it is of equal importance to consider the placement of even minimal effort tasks relative to the wheelchair user. The task should be orientated to minimize the need for the patient to move out of the supported position. In the field of ergonomics, a sloping work surface has been found to have a significant impact on upper body posture (Bridger, 1988). Bendix (1987) states 'The influence on posture from [angle of desk surface] is greater than that of optimizing the chair'.

Seat design and spasticity

Implementation of the preceding principles in a seating system requires careful consideration of the seat design as illustrated in the following sections.

Strength and durability

Support surfaces providing resistance to muscle contraction or providing muscle stretch require to be relatively non-compressible so that they will not yield under the often very high forces produced during extensor thrust. Forces in these surfaces can be very high, for example when patients go into body extension. To be effective, the surfaces require not to yield in these conditions. Not only must they be able to resist the highest force produced, but also the materials must be fatigue resistant and so withstand repeated extensor thrusts over a long period. The effects of such fatigue problems should not be underestimated. In clinical practice in Dundee (Scotland), one patient has been able to fracture specifically reinforced seating systems. In this regard it is important to note that strengthening one part of a seating system may transfer forces to other components which consequently may need strengthening. For example, reinforcing the seat section to resist strong hip extension may result in forces being transferred to the backrest.

Pressure reduction

Whilst structures require strength and fatigue endurance to resist the applied muscle forces, the surfaces through which the forces are applied should not produce excessively high pressures. Therefore the area of contact between these surfaces and the relevant body segment should be maximized. This could involve either contouring the support system or incorporating a layer of more compliant surface material to increase the area of support.

Complexities in cushion design arise for patients who have pressure sore susceptibilities combined with the need for postural support. A firm base is required, contoured to give the required posture, whilst the minimum surface padding is used. Areas of high vulnerability may incorporate extra pressure relief such as a gel pad leaving the rest of the cushion made from firmer material to give the required postural support. As discomfort can itself increase spasticity, as a noxious stimulus, good pressure distribution is a prerequisite of the seating system.

Shear force reduction

Unstable postures and movements produced by spasticity also tend to produce high shear forces at the body/seat interface. These can contribute significantly to pressure sores to the extent that they may be their prime cause. Hence, equal importance may be attached to inhibiting movement as well as distributing loads. Secure location of the person in the seat is a significant step towards reducing the potential for skin breakdown.

Adjustability

Many pathologies involving spasticity are of a changing nature resulting in continual improvements or deterioration of their condition. These can be rapidly changing such as in multiple sclerosis children and acute stroke patients. Many designs of seating systems are adjustable to permit easy variation of seat to match the changing needs of the patient.

Despite this major advantage, adjustable systems suffer drawbacks such as:
- increased size, cost, weight and complexity;
- may readily go 'out-of-adjustment';
- may be put 'out-of-adjustment' by untrained staff/parents carers, etc.;
- can be difficult to record settings for later re-manufacturing.

Hence care is necessary during prescription to ensure adjustable systems are appropriate for the environments and people with whom they will be used.

Evaluating success of seating systems

Many seating systems are claimed to reduce spasticity and thereby promote good seated posture, reduce joint contractures and improve upper limb function. Ideally the choice of a seating system should be based on scientific evidence of its applications. Most claims of effectiveness are largely qualitative and hence difficult to substantiate. Nevertheless some authors have reported attempts to address this issue.

Nwaobi (1983) cautions against using upper limb function as a measure of the success of interventions to reduce spasticity. After reviewing the literature, he concludes that 'basic neural deficits, such as prolonged EMG summation time required for voluntary movement and decreased firing frequency of motor units, may be significant factors in limiting voluntary movement in patients with upper motor neurone (UMN) lesions'.

Measuring spasticity is difficult (Katz & Roger, 1989) not least in view of the debate of the nature of spasticity. Pierson (1997) proposes that a battery of tools may be the best approach to take including measurement of technical and functional outcomes, patient satisfaction and cost-effectiveness of treatment.

Much of the research in the area of positioning and spasticity, cited in this chapter, is based on very small samples, with few using over 12 subjects. The difficulty in research is compounded by the non-homogeneous nature of the subject's presentation and the wide variations that occur within an individual. As Harburn & Potter (1993) note: 'Until the time arrives when spasticity can be sensitively, validly, and reliably measured, it will be difficult to measure the efficacy of treatment approaches designed to reduce spasticity . . . Rather, use of the treatment or treatment approaches that the clinician believes to be efficacious is appropriate.'

From clinical experience it is certainly apparent that the deformities seen in patients from former generations who were not adequately seated and were largely nursed in bed, are now seen much less frequently. It is hoped that this is a result of improved health care, including the provision of better seating.

Such observations are difficult to substantiate but Medhat et al. (1986) reported for 111 patients who were prescribed custom seating systems by an interdisciplinary seating clinic team: 32% had improvement in spasticity; 86% felt more comfortable; 82% indicated better positioning; and 35% improved in learning abilities.

Choosing seating systems

Having considered the relevant principles of seating for associated design considerations, there remains the question of how to select the most appropriate seating system. There is a wide range of commercial seating systems potentially applicable to people with spasticity. This range is continuously expanding and improving, making discussion of specific examples inappropriate. However, the above discussion principles should provide guidance in evaluating the usefulness of a particular commercial system. A variety of types of systems is summarized by Bardsley (1993).

Braus & Mainka (1993) highlight the importance of correctly setting up an adjustable wheelchair. Albeit based on a small sample, they report a correctly adjusted wheelchair resulting in a decrease in spasticity compared with a standard, non-adjustable wheelchair.

Anderson & Anderson (1986) describe the construction of a seat for neonates and infants to help promote normal posture whilst reducing extensor tone. The seat positions the child 'with hips flexed to a greater than 90° angle, hips abducted to a greater than 20° angle, body and head well supported, and shoulders well protracted'. The position is designed to reduce extensor tone. The seat consists of a rigid plastic exterior with positioning pieces of firm foam and is covered with lambs' wool. The seat thus combines the design features of firm support to resist movement whilst giving a soft and warm interface. The authors report that 'agitated behaviour and irritability decrease when the infant is in the seat, probably because the discomfort of the extensor pattern, which leaves the infant out of control, is decreased'.

Custom moulded plastic seating (Trefler et al., 1978; Nelham, 1975; Ring et al., 1978; Bardsley, 1984; Medhat & Redford, 1985) has been used extensively, particularly for those with severe cerebral palsy who often have joint contractures and spinal deformity. This type of seating provides intimately contoured support to maintain position and is firm and strong thus resisting spastic muscle contraction. Many users of this type of system would in former years have been regarded as 'unseatable' and therefore left in postures where further contractures often developed.

An alternative to individually contoured seating, which often has a relatively fixed configuration, is to provide a highly adjustable system which can be tailored to suit the user's needs. Barnes (1993) highlights the need for seats to have a variety of adjustments and supports including 'foot straps, knee blocks, adductor pommels, lumbar supports, lateral trunk supports, and head and neck support systems' It is important that such seats are configured correctly and that the configuration is not adjusted except following clinical review of needs.

One approach which seeks to maximize the adjustability and provide all the relevant components for positioning young children utilizes a car-seat style plastic shell into which firm foam pads can be attached by Velcro® in the desired configuration (Bardsley, 1993). It also includes a foot support with straps and an adjustable pommel.

Consideration should also be given to the need for transportation in a vehicle, especially if it requires to be folded and/or dismantled. Whilst there are a growing number of wheelchair accessible vehicles, a large number of wheelchairs are still transported in the boot of a car. As seating systems and their chassis increase in support offered and adjustability, so inevitably the weight rises and the ability to store in a small space decreases. Alternatively, the system may be used within the vehicle as one of its seats and therefore requires to be designed and tested to resist crash forces.

Conclusion

Carefully designed, correctly used seating is indispensable in managing the spasticity of the seated individual. Appropriate seating not only produces immediate functional benefits but serves to limit the development of contractures and subsequent deformities.

This review has highlighted the wide extent of work in this area, although much of it is either subjective or based on small sample studies. It is important that research, although difficult to carry out, continues in this field in order that the findings described may be fully validated and the relative effectiveness of each be compared. In this regard the choice of appropriate outcome measures in measuring the benefit obtained for an intervention is an area of current activity (Pierson, 1997; Nielson & Bardsley, 1998; Richardson & Thompson, 1999).

REFERENCES

Anderson, L. J. & Anderson, J. M. (1986). A positioning seat for the neonate and infant with high tone. *Am J Occ Ther*, **40**: 186–90.

Andersson, B. J. G., Ortengren, R., Nachemson, A. & Elfstrom, G. (1974). Lumbar disc pressure and myoelectric back muscle activity during sitting. *Scand J Rehabil Med*, **6**: 104–14.

Andersson, B. J. G., Ortengren, R., Nachemson, A. L., Elfstrom, G. & Broman, H. (1975). The sitting posture: an electromyographic and discometric study. *Orthop Clin N Am*, 6: 105–19.

Ashburn, A. & Lynch, M. (1988). Disadvantages of the early use of wheelchairs in the treatment of hemiplegia. *Clin Rehabil*, 2: 327–31.

Bagg, M. R., Farber, J. & Freeman, M. (1993). Long-term follow-up of hip subluxation in cerebral palsy patients. *J Pediatr Orthop*, 13: 32–6.

Bakheit, A. M. O. (1996). Management of muscle spasticity. *Crit Rev Phys Rehabil Med*, 8: 235–52.

Bardsley, G. (1984). The Dundee seating programme. *Physiotherapy*, 70: 59–63.

Bardsley, G. (1993). Seating. In *Bimechanical Basis of Orthotic Management*, ed. P. Bowker, D. N. Condie, D. L. Bader & D. J. Pratt, pp. 253–80. Oxford: Butterworth-Heinemann.

Bardsley, G. & Taylor, P. M. (1982). The development of an assessment chair. *Prosthet Orthot Int*, 6: 75–8.

Barnes, M. P. (1993). Local treatment of spasticity. *Baillieres Clin Neurol*, 2: 55–71.

Bell, E. & Watson, A. (1985). The prevention of positional deformity in cerebral palsy. *Physiother Prac*, 1: 86–92.

Bendix, T. (1987). Adjustment of the seated workplace – with special reference to heights and inclinations of seat and table. *Dan Med Bull*, 34: 125–39.

Bertoti, B. (1988). Effect of therapeutic horseback riding on posture in children with cerebral palsy. *Phys Ther*, 68: 1505–12.

Bishop, B. (1977). Spasticity: its physiology and measurement. *Phys Ther*, 57: 371–401.

Blower, P. (1988). The advantages of the early use of wheelchairs in the treatment of hemiplegia. *Clin Rehabil*, 2: 323–5.

Blower, P. W., Carter, L. C. & Sulch, D. A. (1995). Relationship between wheelchair propulsion and independent walking in hemiplegic stroke. *Stroke*, 26: 606–8.

Bobath, B. (1977). Treatment of adult hemiplegia. *Physiotherapy*, 63: 310–13.

Bower, E. (1990). Hip abduction and spinal orthosis in cerebral palsy. *Physiotherapy*, 76: 658–9.

Braus, D. F. & Mainka, R. (1993). Current trends of wheelchair provision after stroke. *J Rehabil Sci*, 6: 124–7.

Bridger, R. S. (1988). Postural adaptations to a sloping chair and work surface. *Hum Fact*, 30: 237–47.

Brouwer, B., Wheeldon, R. & Allum, J. (1996). The effects of serial casting on spasticity and muscle strength. *Dev Med Child Neurol*, 38 (Suppl. 74), 43.

Carlson, J. M. & Winter, R. (1978). The 'Gillette' sitting support orthosis for non-ambulatory children with severe palsy or advanced muscular dystrophy. *Minn Med*, 61: 469–73.

Cornell, C. (1991). Self-propelling wheelchairs: the effects on spasticity in hemiplegic patients. *Physiother Theor Prac*, 7: 13–21.

Cornell, M. S. (1995). The hip in cerebral palsy. *Dev Med Child Neurol*, 37: 3–18.

De Wald, J. P. A. (1987). Sensorimotor neurophysiology and the basis of neurofacilitation therapeutic techniques. In *Stroke Rehabilitation*, ed. E. M. Brandstater & J. V. Basmajin. Baltimore: Williams & Wilkins.

Dvir, Z., Penturin, E. & Prop, I. (1996). The effect of graded effort on the severity of associated reactions in hemiplegic patients. *Clin Rehabil*, 10: 155–8.

Ford, F. (1986). Neuro-motor dysfunction as it relates to therapeutic seating. In *Seating for Children with Cerebral Palsy: a Resource Manual*, ed. E. Trefler, pp. 10–23. Memphis: University of Tennessee Center for the Health Sciences.

Fulford, G. E. & Brown, J. K. (1976). Position as a cause of deformity in children with cerebral palsy. *Dev Med Child Neurol*, **18**: 305–14.

Green, E. M. & Nelham, R. L. (1991). Development of sitting ability, assessment of children with a motor handicap and prescription of appropriate seating systems. *Prosthet Orthot Int*, **15**: 203–16.

Green, E. M., Mulcahy, C. M. & Pountney, T. E. (1992). *Postural Management, Theory and Practice*. Birmingham: Active Design.

Harburn, K. L. & Potter, P. J. (1993). Spasticity and contractures. *Phys Med Rehabil State Art Rev*, **7**: 113–32.

Heine, B. (1997). Hippotherapy – a multisystem approach to the treatment of neuromuscular disorders. *Aus J Physiother*, **43**: 145–9.

Howard, C. B., McKibbin, B., Williams, L. A. & Mackie, I. (1985). Factors affecting the incidence of hip dislocation in cerebral palsy. *J Bone Joint Surg*, **67B**: 530–2.

Kalen, V. & Bleck, E. E. (1985). Prevention of spastic paralytic dislocation of the hip. *Dev Med Child Neurol*, **27**: 17–24.

Kaplan, N. (1962). Effect of splinting on reflex inhibition of sensorimotor stimulation in the treatment of spasticity. *Arch Phys Med Rehabil*, **43**: 565–9.

Katz, T. (1988). Management of spasticity. *Am J Phys Med Rehabil*, 108–16.

Katz, R. T. & Roger, W. Z. (1989). Spastic hypertonia: mechanisms and measurement. *Arch Phys Med Rehabil*, **70**: 144–55.

Little, J. W. & Massagli, T. L. (1993). Spasticity and associated abnormalities of muscle tone. In *Rehabilitation Medicine: Principles and Practice*, ed. J. A. DeLisa, 2nd edn., p. 673. Philadelphia: J. B. Lippincott Company.

Lonstein, J. E. & Beck, K. (1986). Hip dislocation and subluxation in cerebral palsy. *J Pediatr Orthop*, **6**: 521–6.

Medhat, M. A. & Redford, J. B. (1985). Experience of a seating clinic. *Int Orthop*, **9**: 279–85.

Medhat, M. A., Trautman, P., Haig, K. & Flanigan, J. (1986). Effect of seating on learning, feeding habits, spasticity, comfort, and positioning. *Arch Phys Med Rehabil*, **67**: 669.

Myhr, U. (1994). Influence of different seat and backrest inclinations on the spontaneous positioning of the extremities in non-disabled children. *Physiother Theor Prac*, **10**: 191–200.

Myhr, U. & von Wendt, L. (1990). Reducing spasticity and enhancing postural control for the creation of a functional sitting position in children with cerebral palsy: a pilot study. *Physiother Theor Prac*, **6**: 65–76.

Myhr, U. & von Wendt, L. (1991). Improvement of functional sitting position for children with cerebral palsy. *Dev Med Child Neurol*, **33**: 246–56.

Myhr, U. & von Wendt, L. (1993). Influence of different sitting positions and abduction orthoses on leg muscle activity in children with cerebral palsy. *Dev Med Child Neurol*, **35**: 870–80.

Nelham, R. L. (1975). The manufacture of moulded supportive seating for the handicapped. *Biomed Eng*, **10**: 379–81.

Nelham, R. L., Green, E. & Mulcahy C. (1992). 24 Hr postural management of children and young adults with cerebral palsy to improve ability and prevent deformity, *ISPO Newslett*, Summer, p. 24.

Nielson, A. & Bardsley, G. (1998). Outcomes of orthotic and seating interventions on people with disabilities. *Curr Opin Orthop*, **9**: 96–9.

Noronha, J., Bundy, A. & Groll, J. (1989). The effect of positioning on the hand function of boys with cerebral palsy. *Am J Occ Ther*, **43**: 507–12.

Nwaobi, O. M. (1983). Voluntary movement impairment in upper motor neuron lesions: is spasticity the main cause? *Occ Ther J Res*, **3**: 131–40.

Nwaobi, O. M. (1986). Effects of body orientation in space on tonic muscle activity of patients with cerebral palsy. *Dev Med Child Neurol*, **28**: 41–4.

Nwaobi, O. M. (1987a). Seating orientations and upper extremity function in children with cerebral palsy. *Phys Ther*, **67**: 1209–12.

Nwaobi, O. M. (1987b). Nondominant arm restraint and dominant arm function in a child with athetoid cerebral palsy: electromyographic and functional evaluation. *Arch Phys Med Rehabil*, **68**: 837–9.

Nwaobi, O. M., Brubaker, C. E., Cusick, B. & Sussman, M. D. (1983). Electromyographic investigation activity in cerebral-palsied children in different seating positions. *Dev Med Child Neurol*, **25**: 175–83.

Nwaobi, O. M., Hobson, D. A. & Trefler, E. (1986). Hip angle and upper extremity movement time in children with cerebral palsy. *Phys Ther*, **66**: 801.

Nwaobi, O. M. & Trefler, E. (1985). Body orientation in space and tonic muscle activity in patients with cerebral palsy. *Orthop Trans*, **9**: 84.

Odeen, I. (1981). Reduction of muscular hypertonus by long-term muscle stretch. *Scand J Rehabil Med*, **13**: 93–9.

Odeen, I. & Knutsson, E. (1981). Evaluation of the effects of muscle stretch and weight load in patients with spastic paraplegia. *Scand J Rehabil Med*, **13**: 117–21.

O'Dwyer, N. J., Ada, L. & Neilson, P. D. (1996). Spasticity and muscle contracture following stroke. *Brain*, **119**: 1737–49.

O'Dwyer, N., Neilson, P. & Nash, J. (1994). Reduction of spasticity in cerebral palsy using feedback of the tonic stretch reflex: a controlled study. *Dev Med Child Neurol*, **36**: 770–86.

Pierson, S. H. (1997). Outcome measures in spasticity management. *Muscle Nerve* Suppl, **6**: S36–S60.

Pope, P. M., Booth, E. & Goshing, G. (1988). The development of alternative seating and mobility systems. *Physiother Prac*, **4**: 78–93.

Quint, C. & Toomey, M. (1998). Powered saddle and pelvic mobility: an investigation into the effects on pelvic mobility of children with cerebral palsy of a powered saddle which imitates the movements of a walking horse. *Physiotherapy*, **84**: 376–84.

Richardson, D. & Thompson, A. J. (1999). Management of spasticity in hereditary spastic paraplegia, *Physiother Res Int*, **4**: 68–76.

Ring, N. D., Nelham, R. L. & Pearson, F. A. (1978). Moulded supportive seating for the disabled. *Prosthet Orthot Int*, **2**: 30–4.

Samilson, R. L., Carson, J. J., Preston, J. & Raney, F. L. (1967). Results and complications of adductor tenotomy and obturator neurectomy in cerebral palsy. *Clin Orthop Rel Res*, **54**: 61–73.

Scrutton, D. (1966). Prevention and management of incorrect spinal posture in cerebral palsy. *Dev Med Child Neurol*, **8**: 322–6.

Scrutton, D. (1971). A ramp-shaped cushion for prone lying. *Dev Med Child Neurol*, **13**: 228–30.

Scrutton, D. (1978). Developmental deformity and the profoundly retarded child. In *Care of the Handicapped Child*, ed. J. Apley. London: William Heinemann.

Scrutton, D. (1989). The early management of hips in cerebral palsy. *Dev Med Child Neurol*, **31**: 108–16.

Scrutton, D. (1991). The causes of developmental deformity and their implication for seating. *Prosthet Orthot Int*, **15**: 199–202.

Seeger, B. R., Caudrey, D. J. & O'Mara, N. A. (1984). Hand function in cerebral palsy: the effect of hip-flexion angle. *Dev Med Child Neurol*, **26**: 601–6.

Shepherd, R. B. (1995). *Physiotherapy in Paediatrics*, 3rd edn. Oxford: Butterworth Heinemann.

Shirado, O., Shundo, M., Kaneda, K. & Strax, T. E. (1995). Outdoor winter activities of spinal cord-injured patients: with special reference to outdoor mobility. *Am J Phys Med Rehabil*, **74**: 408–14.

Spencer, J. D. (1999). Reconstruction of dislocated hips in children with cerebral palsy. *BMJ*, **318**: 1021–2.

Todd, J. M. (1974). Physiotherapy in the early stages of hemiplegia. *Physiotherapy*, **60**: 336–42.

Trefler, E. (1986). Functional arm restraint for children with athetoid cerebral palsy. *Dev Med Child Neurol*, **28** (Suppl. 53), 56.

Trefler, E., Toom, R. E. & Hobson, D. A. (1978). Seating for cerebral-palsied children. *Inter Clin Info Bull*, **17**: 1–8.

Tremblay, F., Malouin, F. & Richards, C. L. (1990). Effects of prolonged muscle stretch on reflex and voluntary muscle activations in children with spastic cerebral palsy. *Scand J Rehabil Med*, **22**: 171–80.

Vaughan, C. & Bhakta, B. (1995). Recent advances in rehabilitation medicine. *J Roy Coll Phys (London)*, **29**: 534–9.

Yang, T. F., Chan, R. C., Wong, T. T., Bair, W. N., Kao, C. C., Chuang, T. Y. & Hsu, T. C. (1996). Quantitative measurement of improvement in sitting balance in children with spastic cerebral palsy after selective posterior rhizotomy. *Am J Phys Med Rehabil*, **75**: 348–52.

Young, N. L., Wright, J. G., Lam, T. P., Rajaratnum, K., Stephens, D. & Wedge, J. H. (1998). Windswept hip deformity in spastic quadriplegic cerebral palsy. *Pediatr Phys Ther*, **10**: 94–100.

Zollars, J. A. (1993). *Seating and Moving Through the Decades: A Literature Review on Seating and Mobility Through 1992*. Santa Cruz: PAX Press.

Zollars, J. A. (1996). *Special Seating: An Illustration Guide*. Minneapolis: Otto Bok.

6

Orthoses, splinting and casting in spasticity

Paul T. Charlton and Duncan W. N. Ferguson

Introduction

'An orthosis is an external device used to modify the structural or functional characteristics of the neuromuscular system' as defined by the International Standards Organisation. This definition encompasses all other devices referred to as splints, braces and casts. Although not so well defined, it is common practice for clinicians to refer to orthoses as those external devices provided by an orthotist whereas splints are commonly recognized as orthoses made of low temperature plastics or fabric by therapists other than orthotists. Non-removable orthoses made of plaster or casting tape are referred to as casts.

The use of orthoses (in all their forms) for adults presenting with spasticity has been controversial (Edwards & Charlton, 1996) and use varies from centre to centre depending on the treatment regime adopted by the therapist. However, in paediatrics, their use is more widely accepted partially due to the work of Meadows (1984) and those therapists using conductive education techniques promoted by the Peto Institute.

In adult neurology, treatment is often based on the Bobath concept of normal movement (Bobath, 1980), which for many years frowned on the use of splinting because of the obvious impingement on the ability to perform normal movement. Normal movement is the ultimate goal in neuro-rehabilitation. However, to expect all patients with a neurological deficit to make a full recovery is not realistic. It must be accepted that, despite our best efforts, at some stage recovery will plateau and the remaining deficit may require mechanical management to allow the person optimum function. This factor must be a consideration when the need for an orthosis is assessed and highlights the need for regular review, at which time thought can be given as to the true aim of intervention, rehabilitation or management. It is now generally accepted that there is a place for orthoses, when provided following proper assessment and selection.

The aim of orthotic intervention should be, where it is achievable, to realign the limb segments as near as possible to the normal position in the hope that normal posture will occur through recruitment of the appropriate muscle groups. It is this understanding which is crucial to correct orthotic assessment and provision.

Orthotic aims

The fundamental aim of providing an orthosis is to improve recovery and ultimately the quality of life of the patient. Where provision of an orthosis is part of the treatment regime, it should be recognized that one device may not provide for the patient's requirements throughout their rehabilitation and, as with other interventions, its use will require monitoring and adjusting as changes occur.

The aim of any orthosis should be clearly identified at the assessment stage. The most common aims are as follows.

Reduce or inhibit an abnormal pattern by positioning

Holding an ankle in slight dorsiflexion can inhibit the onset of an extensor pattern and is often achieved by the use of an ankle foot orthosis (AFO). Gross trunk extension can be managed by holding the hip in flexion and inducing a lumbar lordosis, as with special seating or a sitting brace often used in children. These devices must be sufficiently rigid to prevent movement beyond the desired position. Another example is the use of dynamic insoles and AFOs to reduce tone as described by Hylton (Hylton & Allan, 1997).

Prevent abnormal movement

By splinting in a position of maximum function with a rigid device even if the spasticity can not be inhibited, the abnormal movement caused by it may be prevented. This should be undertaken with care, as the forces generated can be considerable.

Promote normal alignment and movement

In many patients it is possible to fine tune the positioning in either sitting or standing such that the alignment of the body segments are as close as possible to the recognized normal. In standing this can be achieved with some accuracy with the use of gait analysis, which allows alignment with reference to the ground reaction force (Stallard, 1987). The effect of this is to place the body in optimum position to recruit normal movement and prevent compensatory movements. The most common example of this is the hemiplegic patient with an extensor pattern who typically presents with a plantar flexed ankle, hyperextended knee and flexed hip and trunk. By fixing the ankle in slight dorsiflexion, it is possible to push the knee

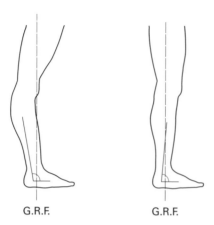

Fig. 6.1   Line of ground reaction force and ankle in normal subject compared to one with a hyperextended knee.

anteriorly, which then encourages the patient to extend the hip and trunk to maintain balance. Ideally a force platform with ground reaction force visualization is used and the ankle angle is altered until the ground reaction force is just posterior to the knee centre (Stallard, 1987; Figure 6.1).

This is a well-documented technique with cerebral palsy children but is equally effective with hemiplegic adults (Farmer et al., 1999).

Preventing contractures and maintaining or increasing joint ranges

There is now evidence that contractures are a common sequel to neurological damage and the importance of prevention is recognized. A greater understanding of the response of muscle to changes in length and position has led to improved orthotic management. However, there is much to understand about the role of orthoses for the prevention or alleviation of contractures. For example, we do not know how long the device needs to be in place during a 24-hour period in order to be effective.

Targeted motor learning

Butler & Major (1992) have strong evidence to suggest that an effective method of learning is to immobilize joints distally until sufficient control is gained proximally and then removing support at the next level until control is gained there. This is mainly geared towards the cerebral palsy child and starts with head control and works down each spinal level (Butler, 1998). The same logic is applicable to the lower limbs. It is difficult to work on improving hip control if there is little control of the knee supporting it.

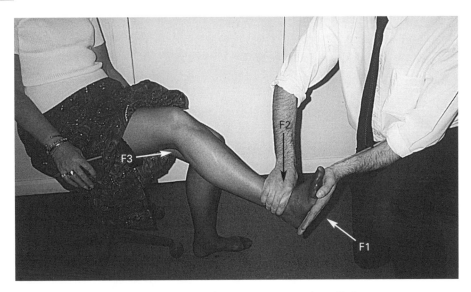

Fig. 6.2   Correction of a plantarflexed ankle and the forces (F1, F2, F3) applied.

Biomechanics and materials

A good understanding of this subject is essential to appreciate fully the forces involved and their influence on the design of orthoses. Those interested may find further reading (Bowker et al., 1993) useful.

Any external device must provide a force to have an effect and an important consideration of applying an orthosis is how and where to apply these forces and make them as tolerable and effective as possible. One of the main skills of the orthotist is to identify, minimize and optimize the forces and pressures generated at the patient orthosis interface. To do this, knowledge of basic mechanics is important. In particular, it is useful to note that most orthoses use the application of a set of three forces to produce the required effect. This is usefully illustrated by considering the correction of a plantar-flexed ankle.

To correct a flaccid foot (Figure 6.2) would merely require a force under the fore-foot (Force 1). However, if the ankle is tight or demonstrating clonus then the hands can be placed one over the top of the ankle (Force 2) and hand (Force 1) would be positioned to provide a better push on the base. If the foot is very tight or there is a strong extensor pattern then there is a danger that you push so hard as to tip the whole patient backwards. This is because it is possible to overcome the frictional force of the patient on the chair as indicated by force (Force 3).

An indication of how mechanics can influence orthotic design is shown in the diagrams depicting the forces involved in correcting a hyperextended knee. It can

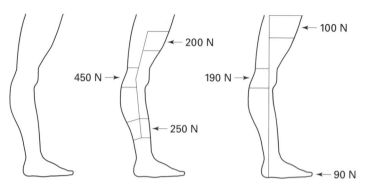

Fig. 6.3   Forces applied to control a hyperextending knee and the effect of increasing lever length.

be clearly seen how an increase in the overall length of the orthosis can lead to reductions in the applied forces, since the turning effect (moment) applied at the knee is determined by both the magnitude of the forces and the distance between them (Figure 6.3).

It is for this reason that a Swedish knee brace is likely to be uncomfortable and a long leg device may be the only practical orthotic solution for quadriceps spasticity.

The ability of an orthosis to manage spasticity will depend on how the spasticity presents. There is a need to be aware of any counter forces, which may have pressure, and skin care repercussions. The ability of the patient to tolerate the required forces necessary to achieve the aim of the device is of ultimate importance. It may be that, at review, a decision is made that the forces required are intolerable. In such a case the patient may be considered for other forms of spasticity management such as injection, pharmaceutical or surgical intervention as well as or instead of the orthosis.

Plastic orthosis or metal orthosis?

While it is not within the remit of this chapter to explore the varieties and limitations of available materials, it is worth explaining the most commonly asked question. It is often assumed that because metal is a stronger material, therefore metal orthosis are stronger and more effective than plastic orthoses at withstanding high forces. In fact often the opposite is true because of the method by which the orthosis acts upon the limb. The benefit of the plastic orthosis is that it can be moulded to the patient and so apply loads in precisely determined positions and frequently over a large area. The metal orthosis on the other hand usually depends on the patient's shoe being an integral part of the orthosis. This may lead to failures both in the fixing of the orthosis to the shoe (the socket) and the shoe itself deforming. It may also depend on some of the forces being applied by leather straps under the

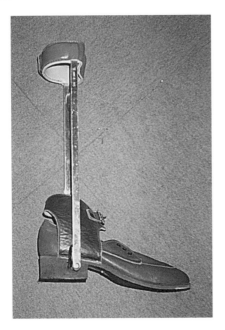

Fig. 6.4   Distortion of a shoe with metal ankle foot orthosis and T-strap by plantar flexion.

influence of the patient or carer. Metal orthoses are undoubtedly heavier than plastic orthoses but often the weight is as much due to the shoe socket as the calliper itself. In addition, the shoe may require reinforcing to prevent distortion from the forces applied, which may further increase weight (Figure 6.4).

Obviously any increase in weight is a disadvantage especially where there is a combination of weakness and spasticity as, for example, in multiple sclerosis.

Assessment

An orthotic assessment should ideally be performed by an orthotist and the treating therapist preferably with experience in orthotics. The team should then explore the history, current treatment and likely prognosis in order to define the aims of the orthosis.

Consideration of the prognosis is important and will help determine the practicality of an aggressive approach. For example, a young patient six weeks post-stroke presenting with a hemiplegia would hopefully recover sufficient motor control to attain a reasonable gait. The orthotic aim in such a case may well be to provide realignment to a degree that may challenge stability to ensure that compensatory positions are not recruited in favour of 'normal' activity, as it becomes available. In practice this may be a rigid AFO set in dorsiflexion to prevent knee hyperextension, even if tone in the quadriceps is not quite sufficient to maintain stability for any length of time. In an older patient, several years post-stroke, then the orthotic aim may well be purely to maintain stability or prevent pain.

It is worth noting that, depending on resources and the patient and therapist commitment, it is sometimes possible to change and improve quite established gait patterns (Butler et al., 1997). It is in these instances that the simulation of the effect of an orthosis before proceeding to a definitive one is extremely useful and gives some indication as to the possible outcome.

When examining the patient, consideration should be given to: joint range; muscle tone in rest and during activity; force required holding a position; skin condition; sensory loss; and oedema. If the use of a device seems a possibility, consideration should be given to the effect on other joints, the patient's function and the need for other intervention such as spasticity management, stretching regime or physiotherapy for gait re-education prior to or after supply.

To assist in making these decisions, it is extremely useful to simulate the effect of the orthosis either by bandaging the limb in the desired position or by adapting an existing orthosis. Even a brief glimpse as to how the patient may perform in a definitive orthosis will avoid unnecessary work. Prediction of functional effect is difficult without such a trial. Assessment tools may be stock orthoses or discarded bespoke orthoses. In particular, it is useful to have an assessment set of knee–ankle–foot orthoses, rigid leg gaiters or backslabs in plastic or plaster, which may allow the patient to experience full knee extension. The opportunity to apply a firm dorsiflexion bandage is also useful to simulate the effect of a rigid AFO. Common findings during assessment include:

- Weak hip flexors when the initial assumption was that lack of ankle dorsiflexion was the cause of poor foot clearance.
- Quiet zones – it is not uncommon with diplegic cerebral palsy children and some post-stroke hemiplegic people with extensor tone to find a range of ankle dorsiflexion where the spasticity can not be induced. In such patients the orthosis is made to limit movement to within that quiet zone (Meadows, 1984).
- Rigidity – the force can be so strong that it cannot be opposed tolerably and orthotic management may be limited to accommodation and stability.
- Positive support is a term commonly used by physiotherapists to describe the onset of spasticity in response to loading the foot. In such cases a dynamic insole can be used to accommodate the contours and dynamic arches of the foot to help this settle, this can be incorporated into an AFO (Small, 1995).
- It is our experience that a mechanism exists whereby a patient will tend towards an abnormal pattern of either flexion or extension in anticipation of having to weight bear on the side over which they do not have full control. This confidence factor we believe is demonstrated by patients who present with an abnormal

pattern yet can improve considerably by the provision of a relatively simple device such as an ankle stirrup. We know that the ankle stirrup does not apply the appropriate forces to control the limb but believe that because it gives the wearer greater confidence, they do not then recruit the abnormal activity in trying to improve stability themselves.

- Shunting has been described as the situation where the control of spasticity at one joint leads to its increase at another, usually the next, joint (Edwards, 1998). This is commonly seen in patients with spastic diplegia where the control of ankle position may result in increased knee flexion or internal hip rotation. In such a case, orthotic intervention may be contra-indicated.
- Severe spasticity can often generate sufficient force either to overcome the orthosis or to endanger tissue breakdown at the patient orthosis interface. If orthoses are used, this can be in conjunction with botulinum toxin injections, which can reduce the force generated. Even with other management techniques it is often accepted that the orthosis will not fully correct the affected joint. For instance, with the inverting ankle the orthosis is used to minimize damage to the joint. Because of the dangers of pressure, it is common to use the more tolerable correction of a padded leather T-strap and metal AFO than the less forgiving correction of a close-fitting plastic orthosis. The added benefit of the metal AFO and T-strap is that the degree of correction can be controlled by the length and tension of the strap. There are those who would argue that with severe spasticity, the presence of an orthosis encourages the muscle to pull against it and therefore reinforce the pattern, although there appears to be little evidence to support this.
- Assessment can also give the orthotist an idea of the forces involved and thus help to determine the type of orthoses required.

Once a specific presentation has been identified then it is worth exploring the underlying cause. An example of this is knee hyperextension, a common presentation in hemiplegia. The underlying mechanical cause of this can be:

- inability to get the heel to the ground due to tightness of the Achilles tendon;
- hamstring weakness;
- quadriceps weakness;
- quadriceps spasticity;
- weak hip extensors.

The simplest method of preventing knee hyperextension is the Swedish knee brace, which although not an effective definitive orthosis, is a very effective assessment tool. Often when the knee is controlled, ankle control is lost and it becomes apparent that the knee is a secondary problem to lack of range or control at the ankle. There is also benefit in using this orthosis as a therapy tool, as by preventing knee hyperextension then a far more effective stretch of the Achilles tendon is achieved on weight bearing (Figure 6.5).

(a)

(b)

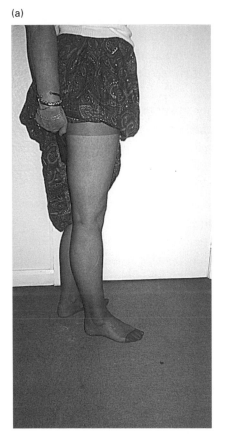 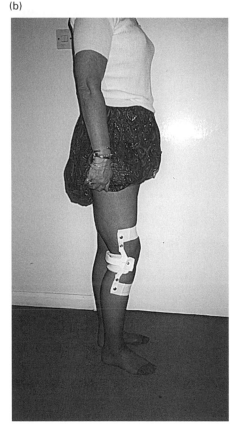

Fig. 6.5   Use of a Swedish knee brace to prevent hyperextension, and increase stretch on Achilles tendon.

A successful assessment does not necessarily result in the supply of an orthosis, although often the process of assessment will have other benefits such as highlighting and clarifying where problems lie and consequently, where treatment can be more specifically targeted.

Having identified deficits in motor control, joint range and other physical factors it is important to assess sensory and perceptual loss. We can now make a decision on the aims and objectives of the orthosis and identify which orthosis to provide. This decision may be influenced by a number of factors such as oedema, sensation, pressure tolerance or patient acceptance.

If the aim involves using the orthosis unsupervised on a daily basis, it is essential that individual acceptance is fully addressed. If the patient refuses to wear the orthosis, then supply is pointless. Acceptance is helped greatly if the patient or carer is made fully aware of the aims of the orthosis and shown any potential benefits and warned, at an early stage, of any practical implications, such as difficulty with footwear.

As with so many other forms of treatment, the final prescription may well be a compromise between the ideal, the practical and the acceptable. The most successful prescription is that which has been made with the full involvement of the patient and the carer.

Casting

There are several advantages of the use of casting over definitive orthoses, such as cost and availability. In addition, the freedom to change the position easily and accurately and the fact that the cast may not be removable, means that the limb has time to settle and accommodate to its new position. This will hopefully make the joint more amenable to a further stretch to a new position. By totally encasing the limb any corrective forces are spread over a maximum area, therefore reducing pressure. Consequently, serial casting has been found to be extremely effective in stretching out contractures (Zander & Healy, 1992), often with the final cast being bivalved and used as a removable splint to maintain the new range acquired. Having spent time enclosed in a cast it is often found that a spastic limb is less active to handle and therefore more likely to tolerate an orthosis. Full-length leg plaster back slabs are now commonly applied to the early neurological insult. This will minimize knee flexion and hamstring contraction but also allow for early weight bearing which will give effective stretch to the Achilles tendon.

Plasters are also a useful prelude to a definitive orthosis both for early application and assessment. The development of modern casting materials and the availability of casting courses for therapists have meant that the ability to apply good casting technique is accessible in most hospitals and centres. It is still essential that skill is used to ensure a smooth patient cast interface and the distally exposed limb is monitored for any signs of problems beneath the plaster such as swelling, discoloration or temperature changes which may indicate pressure problems and necessitate cast removal. Clear guidelines exist for the application of casts and it is important that these are adhered to (ACPIN, 1998).

Timing of orthotic intervention

In order to minimize contractures it is generally recognized that early aggressive intervention is essential. However, the timing of intervention for rehabilitation of normal movement is not quite so well defined. Common sense may dictate that the earlier the patient can experience 'normal' positioning and alignment the better, although evidence for early intervention is lacking. It is important that optimum foot position and alignment is achieved before attempts are made to achieve free standing and walking. It is undesirable to teach normal hip and knee movement when there is insufficient ankle dorsiflexion to attain heel strike. This is practically impossible for the patient as without adopting some form of compensatory strategy there is a risk of tripping over the slightest obstacle. Failure to use an orthosis in this situation will lead to a higher energy cost or an unsafe gait.

Orthotics in paediatric management

As one might expect there are special considerations when dealing with children with spasticity. The absence of normal muscle tone on an immature skeleton can lead to considerable complications. Around the hip joint, for example, it is believed that spasticity can lead to malformation of the acetabulum and recurrent or permanent dislocation. A dislocated hip, as well as causing pain can lead to problems with seating and secondary spinal scoliosis. It is not uncommon for major orthopaedic intervention to be required to resolve these problems. Orthotic intervention can help as positioning hips in maximum abduction ensures maximum containment of the femoral head and optimizes development of the acetabulum.

Types of orthoses

Classification

A system has been developed whereby orthoses are classified and named by reference to the parts of the body over which they pass (Harris, 1973). For example, an orthosis around the ankle is called an ankle–foot orthosis (AFO) and a full leg calliper is termed a knee–ankle–foot orthosis (KAFO). This classification is useful but does not describe the function, construction or aim of the orthosis.

Footwear and adaptations to shoes

An extensor pattern of the lower limb is often accompanied by spasticity in the toe flexors. This leads to clawing, causing pain on the tops of the toes from pressure from the shoe and on the tips of the toes from weight bearing on them. This or any pain tends to increase tone and further compound the problems. Fabrication of a silicone orthosis under the toes to lift the tips from the ground can relieve this pain and help reduce over-activity. Patients with mild spasticity may benefit from careful selection of footwear. A common occurrence is over-activity in the ankle inverters and long toe flexors, which presents as lateral instability of the ankle and clawing of the toes. Shoes with a strong heel stiffener but soft deep forepart are frequently sufficient to resolve or manage these problems. Preferably the shoe should have a broad heel to increase stability but if these are not available, conventional shoes can be modified to have a broader heel, and a light tilt can be added to provide further stability. Insoles may be added to conventional shoes to achieve increased stability, an improved base of support, stretch on the plantar fascia or redistribution of pressure. The height of heel may be altered to accommodate loss of range of the Achilles

(a)   (b)

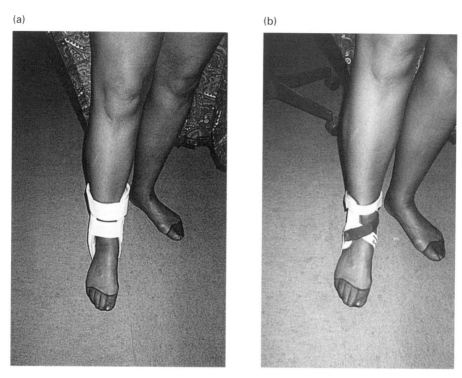

Fig. 6.6   Aircast ankle stirrup (a) and Malleolock ankle brace (b).

tendon and achieve a heel strike and knee alignment. It should be realized, however, that this is at the expense of stretching and that, once a heel raise has been used, there may be a loss of range which cannot be recovered. Tightness of the Achilles tendon can also lead to a compensatory collapse of the medial arch of the foot. It is common for the midfoot to evert and dorsiflex in order to achieve heel contact with the ground.

Ankle–foot orthoses (AFO)

The most commonly recognized AFO is probably that which gives some control to ankle plantar dorsiflexion. It should however be recognized that AFOs also include orthoses that control medio-lateral movement such as the 'Aircast' and 'Malleolock' (Figures 6.6a and 6.6b) as well as various soft orthoses that may offer compression or limitations of movement by strapping.

AFOs that assist the ankle into a dorsiflexed position are not useful in the management of spasticity, as the force of the spastic muscle can override it and render it ineffective. Static or limited motion orthoses include callipers with a range of movement adjustments of which there are many types. As mentioned earlier, it is important that the foot is well fixed into the shoe and the shoe does not distort.

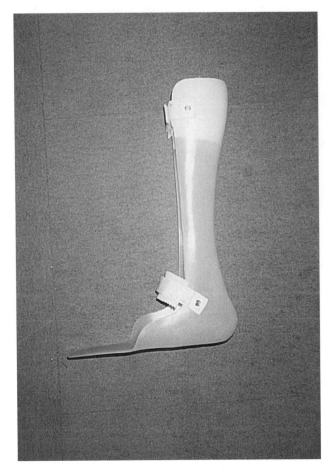

Fig. 6.7   Polypropylene ankle–foot orthosis with full foot piece and 45° ankle strap.

Although it is common to use the high-strength resilient material Ortholen for many AFOs, this is to be avoided with spasticity where rigidity is essential.

Yates (1968) examined the concept of the AFO made in polypropylene and some fundamental flaws were noted when applied to spasticity management. The AFOs were contoured to allow for the shoe pitch which placed the ankle in a plantar flexed position. As the spasticity increased the centre of gravity moved back and the heel elevated out of the orthosis because the shoe was unable to apply sufficient force to hold the foot. This, combined with plantar flexion for the pitch of the shoe, can lead to contracture of the calf muscles. The trim line behind the metatarsal head sometimes simulated a plantar grasp reaction thus increasing the level of spasticity.

Meadows (1984) endorsed the casting of AFOs at 90° with a stretch encouraged on the Achilles tendon from a fitted heel strap which bisected the foot and leg at 45° (Figure 6.7). This encourages better control of the hindfoot. The additional use of

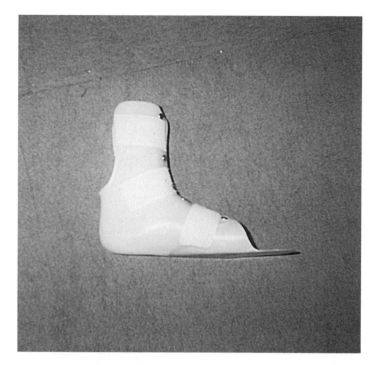

Fig. 6.8   Dynamic ankle–foot orthosis.

a sole wedge or rocker made the flow of mobility more fluent from heel strike to toe-off by maintaining a superior leg-over-foot position controlled by the proper application of forces around the knee through the walking cycle. The study went on to show there was a reduction in tone, the necessity for surgery was less, and long-term complications of scarring and a shortened spastic muscle were diminished.

Types of AFOs

Dynamic insoles and dynamic AFOs (DAFOs)

Much publicity was given to these by the work of Hylton (Hylton, 1989; Hylton & Allan, 1997) who advocated the use of a footplate or insole that was manufactured accurately to reinforce all of the dynamic arches of the foot, including the lateral arch (Figure 6.8). As well as aggressively supporting these arches, she also advocated building up and supporting the toes, other than the great toe. An insole made to this specification cradles the calcaneum and metatarsal heads providing an optimum weight-bearing surface, which is most likely to allow the foot to settle. This footplate was used as a basis for a DAFO, which unlike other AFOs extends only just proximal to the malleoli offering ankle alignment without addressing

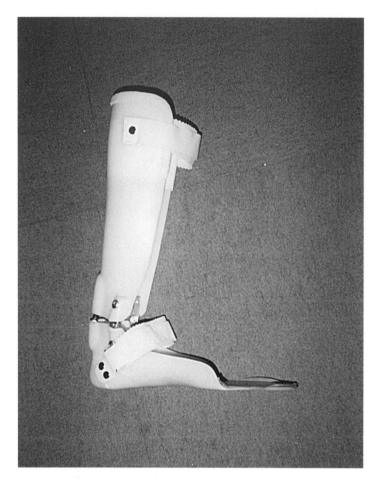

Fig. 6.9   Hinged ankle–foot orthosis with adjustable screw plantar flexion stop.

plantar dorsiflexion. The material used is thin malleable plastic and the aim of orthosis is to have a tone-reducing effect such that normal movement may be recruited. Often the ability of the patient to recruit dorsiflexion is absent. The foot-plate, however, is a useful adjunct to a conventional AFO in helping an overactive foot to settle.

Hinged AFO
A rigid polypropylene AFO may be cut at the ankle joint axis and a hinge introduced (Figure 6.9). A posterior stop may provide the desired resistance to plantar flexion while allowing a range of dorsiflexion. This is especially useful for those patients who have a quality of gait that allows walking over uneven ground and also makes simple tasks such as getting from sit to stand and negotiating stairs much easier. Care must be taken at the assessment stage as some patients have a deficit

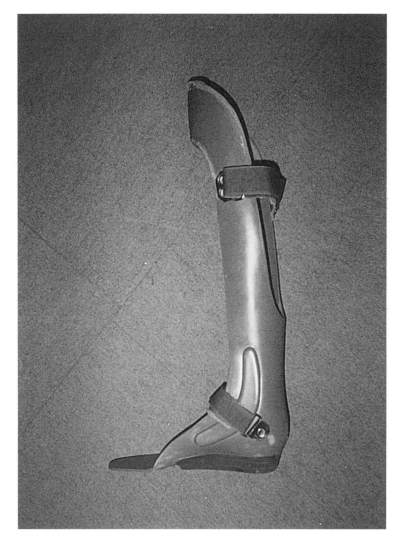

Fig. 6.10   Ground reaction ankle–foot orthosis.

that may benefit from some restriction to dorsiflexion (e.g. those prone to a flexed gait). By providing adjustable plantarflexion, then the position can be altered to fine-tune the orthosis for the patient.

Ground reaction AFO
This variation (Figure 6.10) of a rigid AFO is aimed at resisting dorsiflexion and therefore limits progression of the tibia over the foot during stance phase. This is sometimes useful in those patients presenting with a crouch gait. The anterior load bearing surface requiring a posterior opening ensures correct application of forces.

(a) (b)

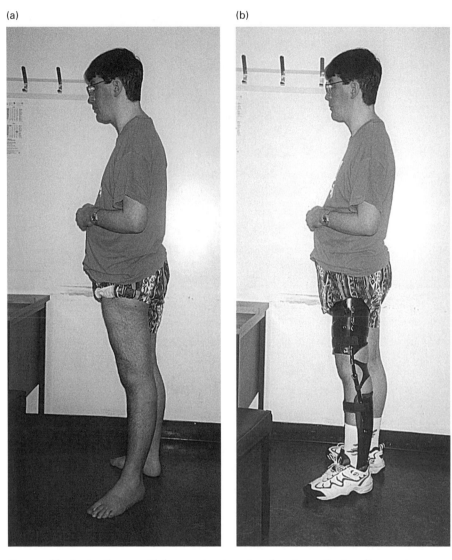

Fig. 6.11   Knee–ankle–foot orthoses with hyperextension stop showing patient realignment.

Knee orthoses and knee–ankle–foot orthoses
The principal aim of the knee orthosis is to prevent knee hyperextension in exten-sor tone and flexion in flexor tone. However, as previously mentioned, they are often too short to provide sufficient leverage to control the effect of spasticity about the joint. In either case, the joint should be realigned as near as possible to the normal standing position (Figures 6.11a and 6.11b). In the case of spasticity of the hamstrings, the forces involved are considerable and may make automatic knee

joints unreliable and, therefore, dangerous. The traditional manual knee locks are probably more appropriate to allow flexion for sitting.

Hip and hip–knee–ankle–foot orthoses

Hip orthoses, sometimes known as sitting braces can assist in postural control to help with windswept, scissoring and sacral sitting positions. This may be instead of or along with special seating. As mentioned earlier, hip position can play an important part in hip containment and development. The more complex orthoses such as the Parawalker (Butler & Major, 1987) and reciprocal gait orthosis (Douglas & Solomonow, 1987) developed for paraplegics both require relatively smooth symmetrical hip action and probably preclude all but the mildest of spasticity. 'Twisters' are functional hip orthoses that control internal rotation during gait and can be most effective and are most commonly used in children with diplegia.

Cervical orthoses and the cervical spine

Spasticity can affect the control of the head and neck. Some control may be provided by an intimately fitted collar (Figure 6.12) either moulded directly to the patient or made to a plaster cast. Care must be taken regarding pressure, as sometimes the forces generated are considerable. Sometimes the combination of a collar and the use of botulinum toxin injections may lead to the best success. Occasionally the extensors of the cervical spine are affected making fitting a collar extremely hazardous as the counter pressure is on the throat. This problem can be overcome by extending the orthosis down over the front of the clavicle and under the arm. By fastening around the back, this creates a three-point pressure with the back, the back of the head and the front of the clavicle. Although this is cumbersome, and some may feel impractical, it may have uses for helping with specific tasks such as eating.

The hemiplegic shoulder

Management of the hemiplegic shoulder is a source of frustration for patients and clinicians and the causes of the problems are not always clear. Sometimes it appears to be due mainly to subluxation whilst at other times tightness due to spasticity in the rotator cuff is the cause. The shoulder is often painful but, in addition, laxity and subluxation makes it prone to injury in handling. These problems can be exacerbated if the upper limb is oedematous and heavy, leading to misalignment of the whole trunk. The complexity of these interactions has been demonstrated by Price et al. (1999) when studying the variations in scapular motion in such patients.

Orthotic intervention, although common, is not usually satisfactory. The biomechanical aim is to reduce subluxation by unloading the shoulder joint by

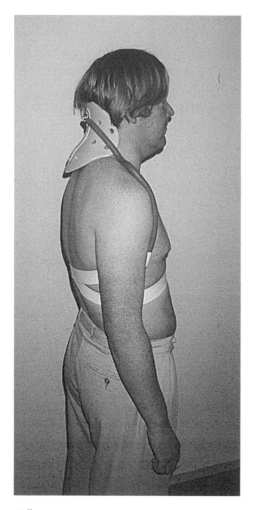

Fig. 6.12   Collar.

suspending the humerus in a cuff on a figure of eight bandage about the opposite shoulder. However, if subluxation is due to spasticity of downward acting muscles, as seems possible, then this strategy is unlikely to be successful.

In orthoses designed to prevent subluxation, a cylindrical cuff around the soft tissue of the upper arm is used to apply the necessary force. However, this is rarely successful since the humerus tends to slide through the cuff (Carus et al., 1993). Attempts to prevent this by increasing the cuff pressure can impede circulation, causing discomfort under the axilla. However, it is surprising how frequently the cuff is still used, despite its limitations. Among questioning users it is commonly accepted that its use can give confidence to the wearer and remind carers of the problem at the shoulder. A mechanically more effective device consists of a broad

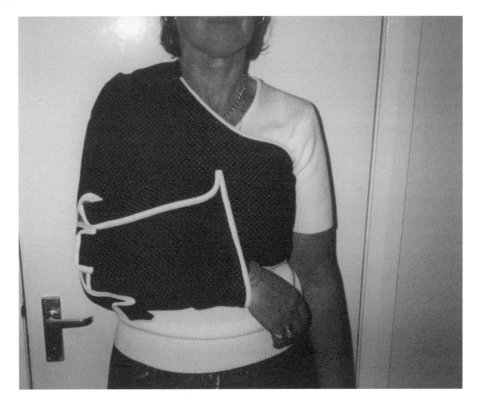

Fig. 6.13   Dr Berrhill jacket.

strap over the affected shoulder extending to a cuff just distal to the elbow. This provides a fulcrum about which the weight of the forearm and hand acting down produces an upward vertical force to the humerus that may reduce subluxation (Cool, 1989) However, this device does depend on some flexion of the elbow that is not always desirable as it may reinforce the typical flexor pattern which is often best avoided. Patients who present with reduced tone in the shoulder girdle and heavy arm, as described earlier, often benefit from strapping the arm to the body in a way as to distribute its weight evenly and minimize the effect of pulling down. An effective orthosis for this is similar to a half jacket spreading the load evenly. This is sometimes known as a Dr Berrhill jacket (Figure 6.13).

The hand and wrist

The fine movements of the hand and fingers make it difficult to apply any orthosis without interfering with function. Orthotic intervention for the spastic hand is therefore aimed at maintaining muscle length and trying to inhibit spasticity. This second claim is unclear and not defined well in the literature. It is possible that by applying a splint to the dorsal aspect of the wrist, tone is inhibited. Mechanically the most effective stretch can be applied by an orthosis applied to the volar aspect of the hand with straps over the wrist and metacarpo-phalangeal joints to stretch the spastic flexor groups. As with other orthoses this should be reviewed and alternatives tried if not successful. Often these orthoses are made of low temperature thermoplastics, which although easy to mould and adjust to achieve an accurate fit, have limited strength and durability. For patients using such orthoses long-term it can be beneficial to use a low temperature orthosis as a template for a high temperature more durable orthosis. An added benefit is the higher temperature (polypropylene) orthosis, which is more rigid and will give a more effective stretch, whereas the lower temperature orthoses often buckle under the force of the spastic muscle. An important consideration is hygiene. If the hand is allowed to stay flexed for a prolonged period then it may become impossible to open it sufficiently to clean it and trim fingernails. In such cases of neglect, it has been necessary to insert rods of gradually increasingly diameter to open the hand.

The list of available orthoses continues to grow. New designs are being developed and existing ones are always being customized to cater for the needs of individual patients. The important point is that the orthosis meets the function of the prescription that is derived from careful assessment and discussion with patients, carers and treating staff.

Future developments

In recent years the neoprene compression bracing used on arms, legs and trunk to give joint stability against gravity has been developed into elastic and lycra suits and segments. Systems in use in both North America and Australia have been reported to improve the functional ability of children with spasticity (Hylton & Allan, 1997).

The use of orthoses in conjunction with multilevel reconstruction surgery for cerebral palsy children (Gage, 1983) is probably the biggest advance in the use of orthoses. These techniques use gait analysis laboratories (Whittle, 1996) providing, amongst other things, visualization of the ground reaction force (Stallard, 1987). This facility is becoming more clinically accessible and will certainly lead to more accurate assessment and fine-tuning of orthoses. Advances are also being made in lighter stronger materials, which may make orthoses less obtrusive and more acceptable.

Conclusion

Orthoses can be highly effective tools in the management of spasticity. However, accurate and careful assessment, prescription and follow-up are required for the best results and thus a trained orthotist is an invaluable member of the spasticity team.

REFERENCES

Association of Chartered Physiotherapists with an Interest in Neurology (ACPIN) (1998). *Clinical Practice Guidelines on Splinting Adults with Neurological Dysfunction.* London: ACPIN.

Bobath, K. (1980). *A Neurological Basis for Treatment of Cerebral Palsy*, 2nd edn. London: Spastics International Medical Publications.

Bowker, P., Condie, D. N., Bader, D. L. & Pratt, D. J. (1993). *Biomechanical Basis of Orthotic Management.* London: Butterworth Heinemann.

Butler, P. B. (1998). A preliminary report on the effectiveness of trunk targeting in achieving independent sitting balance in children with cerebral palsy. *Clin Rehab*, **12**: 281–93.

Butler, P. B., Farmer, S. E. & Major, R. E. (1997). Improvement in gait parameters following late intervention in traumatic brain injury; a long term follow up of a single case. *Clin Rehab*, **11**: 220–6.

Butler, P. B. & Major, R. E. (1987). The parawalker: a rational approach to the provision of reciprocal ambulation for paraplegic patients. *Physiotherapy*, **73**: 393–7

Butler, P. B. & Major, R. E. (1992). The learning of motor control; biomechanical considerations. *Physiotherapy*, **78**: 1–6

Butler, P. B., Thompson, N. & Major, R. E. (1992). Improvement in walking performance of children with cerebral palsy: Preliminary results. *Dev Med Child Neurol*, **34**: 567–76.

Carus, D. A., Lamb, J. & Johnson, G. R. (1993). Upper limb orthoses. In *Biomechanical Basis of Orthotic Management*, ed. P. Bowker, D. L. Bader, D. Pratt et al., p. 206. Oxford: Butterworth Heinemann.

Cool, J. (1989). Biomechanics of orthoses for the subluxed shoulder. *Prosthet Orthot Int*, **13**: 90–6.

Douglas, R. & Solomonow, M. (1987). The LSU reciprocating gait orthosis. *J Rehabil Res Dev*, **25**: 57–8.

Edwards, S. (1998). Physiotherapy management of established spasticity. In *Spasticity Rehabilitation*, ed. G. Sheean, p. 85. London: Churchill Communications Europe Plc.

Edwards, S. & Charlton, P. T. (1996). Splinting and use of orthoses in the management of patients with neurological dysfunction. In *Neurological Physiotherapy: A Problem Solving Approach*, ed. S. Edwards, p. 161. London: Churchill Livingstone.

Farmer, S. E., Butler, P. B. & Major, R. E. (1999) Targeted training for crouch posture in cerebral palsy. *Physiotherapy*, **85**: 242–7.

Gage, J. R. (1983). Gait Analysis for decision-making in cerebral palsy. *Bull Hosp Joint Dis Orthop Inst*, **43**: 147–63

Harris, E. E. (1973). A new orthotic terminology: a guide to its use for prescription and fee schedule. *Orthot Prosthet*, **27**: 6–19.

Hylton, N. & Allan, C. (1997). The development and use SPIO Lycra compression bracing in children with neuromotor deficits. *Paediatr Rehabil*, **1**: 109–16.

Hylton, N. M. (1989). Postural and functional impact of dynamic AFOs and FOs in paediatric population. *J Prostheti Orthot*, **2**: 40–53.

Meadows, C. B. (1984). *The Influence of Polypropylene Ankle Foot Orthoses on the Gait of Cerebral Palsy Children.* PhD Thesis, University of Strathclyde, Glasgow.

Price, C. I. M., Franklin, P., Rodgers, H., Curless, R. H. & Johnson, G. R. (1999). A non-invasive method to evaluate shoulder problems post stroke. *Lancet*, **353**: 298.

Small, G. J. (1995). The orthotic management of the foot in cerebral palsy. In *Report of a Consensus Conference on the Lower Limb Management of Cerebral Palsy*, ed. D. N. Condie, pp. 123–6. Copenhagen: International Society for Prosthetics and Orthotics.

Stallard, J. (1987). Assessment of mechanical function of orthoses by force vector visualisation. *Physiotherapy*, **73**: 398–402.

Whittle, M. W. (1996). *Gait Analysis: An Introduction.* Oxford: Butterworth Heinemann.

Yates, G. (1968). A method for provision of lightweight aesthetic orthopaedic appliances. *Orthopaedics*, **1**: 153–62.

Zander, C. L. & Healy, N. L. (1992). Elbow flexion contractures treated with serial casts and conservative therapy. *J Hand Surgery(A)*, **17**: 694–7.

7

Pharmacological management of spasticity

Anthony B. Ward and Chit Ko Ko

Introduction

The management of spasticity requires a multiprofessional approach and is based on addressing the troublesome effects of the increased tone. Spasticity early on after a sudden loss of function often produces effects, which can be utilized in early rehabilitation. For example, a spastic leg may be a useful prop in mobilization after a stroke when there would otherwise be insufficient power to allow weight-bearing. Treatment should be within the context of goals set for rehabilitation and should be clearly set out (Ko Ko & Ward, 1997). Even in patients developing this impairment without much disability, treatment goals should be documented and agreed with the patient and significant others. Spasticity is not a condition that needs treatment in its own right and indeed medication may sometimes result in systemic side effects producing greater impairment. This chapter will discuss oral agents and their place in overall management strategies. Descriptions of other treatments are found elsewhere.

Primarily the treatment of spasticity is physical. Even when pharmacological agents are used, physical treatment should be carried on and pharmacological agents, in the main, should be regarded as additional rather than as substitutes for physical management (Ko Ko & Ward, 1997). The most important members of the management or rehabilitation team in this context are therefore the nursing staff with the assistance of physiotherapists, occupational therapists, speech and language therapists and doctors. Careful attention should be paid routinely to diminishing noxious and external stimuli, which require specific attention before pharmacological treatment for spasticity is considered (Katz, 1988). In order to achieve an optimal posture, whether the patient is in bed or in a chair, and to reduce noxious external and internal stimuli involves loosening of tight clothing, ensuring that tissue pressures are symmetrical through support of muscle weakness and attention to contractures, prevention of pain, incontinence, constipation and especially colonic faecal loading, infection and abscesses, pressure sores, etc. Limbs should be stretched as soon as practicable after the acute event and attention should be paid to reducing or dealing with cognitive or sensory deficits as soon as possible.

Table 7.1. Indications for pharmacological treatment of spasticity

Increasing tone despite physical stretching/casting limbs.
Pain due to spasticity.
Prevention and treatment of contracture formation.
Prevention of deformities.
Prevention and treatment of dysphagia.
Preservation of skin hygiene.
Preservation of sexual functioning.
Decrease carer burden to perform carer tasks.
Cosmetic effect.

Management strategy

Spasticity treatment is worthwhile if the patient's function or the carer's ability to care is impaired. Initially, treatment will be physical, as already discussed, and thereafter will be indicated through treatments shown in Table 7.1. Treatment choices are usually quite straightforward, but occasionally patients will seek correction of problems that have an impact on their self-esteem rather than purely their physical functioning. Over time, chronic spasticity leads to physiological and structural changes within the muscles, which leads in turn to shortening and eventually contracture of myocytes (Rack, 1966). This in turn leads to tendon shortening and contracture and eventually to limb deformity (Katz & Rymer, 1989) and is seen most commonly in anti-gravity muscles and is described elsewhere.

A management strategy is thus required. Treatment is initiated through oral anti-spastic agents. By and large, baclofen is the most commonly used agent, but is really only indicated for spasticity of spinal origin (Pedersen et al., 1974). Dantrolene sodium is regarded as more effective in cerebral spasticity although its cognitive side-effects do limit its desirability in traumatic brain injury (Monster, 1974). For patients with mild spasticity these drugs are quite effective, but success becomes more limited as the spasticity worsens. Because of the small therapeutic window between clinical effect and toxicity, patients frequently find that to get an effect from the drug involves intolerable side-effects. As a result, new treatments have been developed to compliment these more traditional therapies (Penn et al., 1984; Das & Park, 1989). These include botulinum toxin for the management of focal spasticity and intrathecal baclofen for generalized spasticity. Nerve and neuromuscular junction blockade with phenol or alcohol is still of value, particularly in combination with botulinum toxin and while it is more difficult to administer, it still has a place (Liversedge, 1960). Surgery is becoming less common and is mainly confined to tendon and soft tissue release in non-ambulant patients. All these other treatments are addressed in more detail elsewhere in this volume.

Patient types

Spasticity should be actively and effectively treated when it is causing harm. As stated above, it can sometimes be helpful, particularly in early rehabilitation, where it can support the patient in lieu of muscular strength. Oral agents are generally given to people with widespread spasticity rather than when it is a local problem. However, spasticity treatment is part of a rehabilitation process and its aims should fit into those of the overall rehabilitation objectives. Clear goals must therefore be communicated to the patient in order to ensure the right expectations (Wade, 1988). Their side-effects should be explained, particularly as they may cause drowsiness and there may thus be difficulties in patients with cognitive deficits. This impairment is one of the main reasons why their use has been limited in the rehabilitation of patients with severe disabilities. Generally speaking, these drugs are introduced at low doses and the dose increased to a point where there is an optimal clinical effect. The dose should therefore be titrated against the side-effect. If the latter is too troublesome, then the drug should be stopped or reduced. In this situation, combination treatment needs to be considered.

Different patient skills require different responses. The management of an ambulant-disabled person with spasticity will be quite different to that of a non-ambulant patient, whose cognitive abilities are quite impaired. If the aim is to get the patient to walk or to be dextrous, then a drug regimen that allows safety will be necessary, whereas drugs to achieve a better posture in a wheelchair may have different characteristics. Sometimes spasticity may require treatment not for the disabled person, but to assist the carer. Reducing spasticity to allow perineal hygiene, to ease dressing and to seat patients comfortably in chairs/wheelchairs decreases the burden on carers and this may be the primary treatment aim (Young & Delwaide, 1981).

Combination treatment

Most oral anti-spastic agents can be used in combination with each other. The only reason for this is to improve the clinical effect and lessen the incidence of side-effects, as it is ideally better to use one drug on its own. Combinations of baclofen with dantrolene sodium or with benzodiazepines are probably the commonest, but these are more likely to affect higher cerebral functioning. More importantly though, they can be used with newer treatments, such as botulinum toxin, phenol and intrathecal baclofen. Various studies are either underway, or are planned, to demonstrate this.

Outcome measures

Whenever any treatment is used for spasticity, it is important to measure the effect. Outcome measures have thus to be developed for easy use and to show the specific effect of the anti-spastic treatment. This applies to all forms of treatment, including physical therapy. These are discussed in more detail elsewhere, but measures should try to be as specific as possible in order to identify the individual patient's needs. They should thus be tied-in with goals of treatment, and goal attainment also should be included. Reducing the tone can be demonstrated through a change in the modified Ashworth score (Bohannon & Smith, 1986). This is now the most commonly used measure for this although it is not the most accurate, but it suffices as a clinical tool. Joint range of movement demonstrates a change in the impairment level and is easy to measure and identify. Because anti-spastic agents are used for generalized spasticity, there is a greater chance that it will be possible to measure a change in general physical functioning than with other agents. Sadly this is not the case, but there are occasions when specific changes are seen. This can be demonstrated by tests of impairments in limb functioning, such as, for example, the motricity index (Demeurisse et al., 1980), tests of disability and a timed walking test (Bradstater et al., 1983), the nine hole peg test (Mathiowetz et al., 1985) and stride length (Ward, 1999). Handicap and quality of life measures include the Nottingham Health Profile (Hunt et al., 1980) and Short Form 36 Questionnaire (Ware, 1993). For instance, many of these tests are quite sensitive for function in patients with progressive disability, such as multiple sclerosis, where they not only give an indication of patients' ability to ambulate, but also of their well-being.

Specific treatments

Physical measures are the mainstay of treatment in the early management of spasticity, with modification of muscle tone and maintenance of optimal muscle and joint condition. These measures are also beneficial in moderate to severe spasticity, particularly in optimizing the benefits of other treatment modalities such as pharmacological measures which are available as oral anti-spastic agents and as various forms of local pharmacological agents like intrathecal baclofen, phenol and botulinum toxin. Oral anti-spastic agents are usually indicated in patients with diffuse or regional muscle spasticity rather than localized muscle spasticity. Despite the large number of drugs, including cannabis, which were reported to influence the muscle tone, very few have been found useful in clinical practice. The commonly used anti-spastic drugs are baclofen, benzodiazepine, dantrolene sodium and tizanidine. These drugs could be used alone as monotherapy or in combination to reduce the spasticity effectively.

Baclofen

Baclofen is a structural analogue of gamma-aminobutyric acid (GABA) which is one of the main inhibitory neurotransmitters in the central nervous system. Chemically, baclofen has the structure of beta-4-chlorophenyl-gamma amino-butyric acid and is available as an approved drug only in its racemic mixture with about equal content of the two enantiomers, D-baclofen and L-baclofen. Laboratory studies have shown that L-baclofen is the active enantiomer (Olpe et al., 1978; Johnston et al., 1980) and D-baclofen antagonises the action of L-baclofen (Sawynok & Dickson, 1985; Fromm & Terrence, 1987).

Mechanism of action

Baclofen binds to the bicuculline-insensitive $GABA_B$ receptors (Price et al., 1984; Hwang & Wilcox, 1989) which are primarily located presynaptically at the Ia sensory afferent neurones or at the inter-neurones (Price et al., 1987) and some are also located post synaptically at the motor neurones (Wang & Dun, 1990). Upon binding at the $GABA_B$ receptor sites, the calcium influx through voltage-activated channels in the membrane of group Ia presynaptic terminals is inhibited and the release of endogenous excitatory neurotransmitters such as glutamate and aspartate are suppressed (Hill & Bowery, 1981; Davidoff, 1985; Noth, 1991; Curtis et al., 1997). The post-synaptic $GABA_B$ receptor-mediated inhibition is likely to occur by activating potassium channels through a membrane-delimited pathway and also through a second messenger pathway involving arachidonic acid (Misgeld et al., 1995). It also inhibits gamma motor neurone activity and reduces intrafusal spindle muscle sensitivity. The net result is inhibition of both monosynaptic and polysynaptic reflexes. In addition, animal studies have suggested that baclofen also has anti-nociceptive and analgesic properties possibly by reducing the release of substance P from nociceptive afferent nerve terminals (Henry, 1980).

Pharmacokinetics

Baclofen can be administered both by mouth and by intrathecal injection. After oral administration, it is rapidly and completely absorbed from the gastro-intestinal tract, with peak plasma levels occurring one to two hours after administration. Its plasma half-life is approximately 3.5 hours (range 2 to 6.8 hours). The serum protein binding rate is approximately 30%, and 70–80% of baclofen is excreted in unchanged form through the kidneys within 72 hours. A small proportion (about 10%) is metabolized in the liver (Faigle & Keberle, 1972). It can cross the placenta and only a small amount crosses the blood–brain barrier (Pedersen et al., 1974).

Clinical efficacy

Baclofen has been used as an anti-spastic drug for over 30 years. The majority of the clinical trials in several countries generally involve patients with multiple sclerosis and spinal cord lesions and have proved that baclofen is effective in reducing spasticity and sudden painful flexor spasms (Pinto et al., 1972; Duncan et al., 1976; Feldman et al., 1978). However, most of the studies failed to demonstrate improvement of mobility and activities of daily living (From & Heltberg, 1975).

In a double-blind, crossover trial of baclofen and placebo in 23 patients (18 with multiple sclerosis and 5 with spinal cord lesions), Hudgson & Weightman (1971) using the Ashworth scale confirmed that baclofen was significantly effective in reducing spasticity and was well tolerated. In 1976, Duncan et al. (1976) performed a double-blind, crossover study on 22 patients with spinal cord lesions and found that baclofen was effective in reducing spasticity and reflex spasms of legs and urinary bladder. The larger multicentre, double-blind, placebo-controlled trial in 106 patients with spasticity secondary to multiple sclerosis also confirmed that baclofen was effective in relieving symptoms of spasticity such as flexor spasms, clonus, pain, stiffness, resistance to passive movement of joints and tendon stretch reflexes (Sachais et al., 1977).

In three comparative studies (Ketelaer & Ketelaer, 1972; Cartlidge et al., 1974; From & Heltberg, 1975), baclofen was found to be significantly more effective than diazepam in reducing spasticity secondary to multiple sclerosis with considerably less daytime sedation. In a double-blind, crossover study (Roussan et al., 1987) of baclofen versus diazepam in 13 patients (7 with multiple sclerosis and 6 with spinal cord injury), both drugs produced similar improvement of spasticity but side-effects, especially excessive daytime sedation, were more common in those treated with diazepam. This study again showed the long-term efficacy and safety of baclofen therapy without evidence of drug tolerance, even after many years.

There have been few studies investigating the effect of baclofen in the treatment of spasticity of cerebral origin and the results described suggest a more limited benefit than that achieved among patients with multiple sclerosis and spinal cord lesions (Whyte & Robinson, 1990).

Dosage and administration

The recommended oral dosage ranges from 40 to 100 mg daily. In adults, the dosage begins with 5 mg orally, two to three times daily and is gradually titrated to achieve an optimal clinical response with minimal side-effects. If the dosage is too high or has been increased too rapidly, side-effects may occur, especially in patients who are immobile or elderly. Although the manufacturer's maximum recommended oral dosage is 100 mg daily, many patients with multiple sclerosis have received higher doses which were found to be well tolerated (Pinto et al., 1972; Smith et al., 1991). If the therapeutic effects are not evident in six weeks, it may not benefit the patient to continue with the therapy.

Elderly patients are more susceptible to side-effects and small initial doses with gradual increments under careful supervision are advised. In children, dosages in the range of 0.75 to 2.5 mg/kg body weight should be used and treatment usually initiates with 2.5 mg four times daily with gradual increments at approximately three-day intervals until a therapeutic response is achieved.

Side-effects

There is a low incidence of side-effects and these occur usually with initial treatment, with large doses or in the treatment of patients with spasticity of cerebral origin and of the elderly (Aisen et al., 1993). These adverse effects rarely require withdrawal of the medication and are frequently mild and transient. Modifying the dosage may lessen or eliminate the side-effects. Sometimes it may be difficult to distinguish between drug-induced undesirable effects and those caused by the underlying diseases being treated.

Mild gastro-intestinal disturbances such as dry mouth, nausea, vomiting, constipation or diarrhoea have been reported. Drowsiness and daytime sedation may occur especially at the initiation of treatment. Other reported neurological effects are lassitude, exhaustion, light-headedness, ataxia, confusion, dizziness, headache, insomnia, myalgia, muscle weakness, euphoria, hallucinations, nightmares, depression and dyskinesia (Hattab, 1980; Roy & Wakefield, 1986; Ryan & Blumenthal, 1993). Baclofen may interfere with attention and memory in elderly patients and in patients following acquired brain injury. In patients with epilepsy, seizure control may be lost during treatment with baclofen due to lower convulsion threshold. Sudden withdrawal of baclofen may lead to seizures, hallucinations, visual disturbances, anxiety, confusion, psychosis (Terrence & Fromm, 1981; Rivas et al., 1993) and, as a rebound phenomenon, temporary aggravation of spasticity. Baclofen might precipitate broncho-constriction in susceptible individuals. There was a report of baclofen-induced broncho-constriction in an asthmatic patient after taking baclofen on two separate occasions (Dicpinigaitis et al., 1993). Another asymptomatic patient with a history of exercise-induced dyspnoea and wheezing displayed bronchial hyper-responsiveness to inhaled methacholine only after taking a single dose of baclofen (Dicpinigaitis et al., 1993). Paradoxically, increased spasticity as a contradictory response to the medication has been reported in patients with spasticity of cerebral origin (Knutsson et al., 1974).

Benzodiazepines

The anti-spastic effect of benzodiazepines is mediated via the $GABA_A$ receptor, which consists of a GABA recognition site, a benzodiazepine binding site and a chloride ion channel (Davidoff, 1985). Among benzodiazepines, diazepam is the earliest anti-spastic medication used in widespread clinical practice and other benzodiazepine analogues such as clorazepate, clonazepam, ketazolam and tetrazepam have been shown to reduce muscle spasticity effectively.

Mechanism of action

The pharmacological and anti-spasticity effects of benzodiazepine are thought to be mediated by a functionally coupled benzodiazepine-$GABA_A$ receptor chloride ionophore complex (Costa & Guidotti, 1979; Olsen, 1987). Biochemical studies indicate that benzodiazepines enhance the affinity of GABA binding to $GABA_A$ receptors in rat brain (Guidotti et al., 1978; Skerritt et al., 1982; Skerritt & Johnston, 1983). Activation of the GABA recognition site initiates the opening of the chloride ion channel and the resulting increase in chloride conductance is responsible for the inhibitory post-synaptic effect of GABA. The benzodiazepines exert their anti-spastic action through facilitation of the post-synaptic effects of GABA, resulting in an increase in pre-synaptic inhibition at spinal and supraspinal sites and then a reduction of mono- and poly-synaptic reflexes at the spinal level (Schlosser, 1971; Polc et al., 1974; Schwartz et al., 1983).

Diazepam

Diazepam is a long-acting benzodiazepine and has been used widely as an anti-spastic drug for over 30 years.

Pharmacokinetics

Diazepam is well-absorbed after oral administration, with a peak blood level in one to two hours. It is metabolized in the liver to the active metabolites, N-desmethyl-diazepam and oxazepam. Excretion is through the kidneys in the form of conjugated oxazepam and temazepam. Diazepam is 98% protein-bound and its half-life varies from 20 to 50 hours whilst that of desmethyl-diazepam ranges up to 100 hours, depending on age and liver function. It crosses the placenta and is secreted into the breast milk. Diazepam is highly lipid soluble and readily crosses the blood–brain barrier.

Clinical efficacy

Diazepam has been used most extensively in patients with muscle spasticity resulting from spinal cord lesions, and its effectiveness has been demonstrated in these conditions in two double-blind, cross-over trials (Wilson & McKechnie, 1966; Corbett et al., 1972). It remains controversial as to whether it is more effective in patients with complete or incomplete spinal cord lesions (Cook & Nathan, 1967; Verrier et al., 1977). In children with cerebral palsy, diazepam has also been shown to be effective not only for spasticity but also for athetosis (March, 1965; Engle, 1966). Diazepam is generally unsuitable in patients with acquired brain injury because of its adverse effects on attention and memory (Kendall, 1964).

Although diazepam was marginally less efficacious than baclofen in reducing the symptoms of spasticity in the three comparative studies (Ketelaer & Ketelaer, 1972; Cartlidge et al., 1974; From & Heltberg, 1975), the double-blind, cross-over study (Roussau et al., 1987), however, showed both drugs to be equally effective in reducing spasticity in patients with multiple sclerosis and spinal cord injury. However, daytime sedation was much more common with diazepam, and clinicians and patients preferred baclofen in most of the studies.

Dosage and administration

Treatment with oral diazepam usually initiates with 2 mg twice daily and is then slowly titrated with 2 mg increments up to a maximum dose of 40–60 mg per day in divided doses. In children the dosage ranges from 0.12 to 0.8 mg/kg per day in divided doses.

Side-effects

Common adverse effects that are related to central nervous system depression, include drowsiness, sedation, unsteadiness and ataxia. The elderly are particularly sensitive to these centrally acting depressant effects and may experience confusion, especially if organic brain changes are present. Diazepam can suppress arousal, reduce motor co-ordination, and impair intellect, attention and memory (Kendall, 1964; Cocchiarella et al., 1967). Other rare adverse effects are headache, vertigo, visual disturbances, hypotension, gastro-intestinal upsets, urinary retention, changes in libido and skin rashes. The physiological dependence potential is low but this increases when high doses are used, especially when given over longer periods. This is seen particularly in patients with a history of alcoholism or drug abuse or in patients with marked personality disorders. Withdrawal symptoms such as depression, anxiety, nervousness, agitation, irritability, restlessness, tremor, muscle fasciculation and twitching, rebound insomnia, sweating, nausea and diarrhoea have been reported following abrupt cessation or rapid tapering of treatment with diazepam.

Other benzodiazepines

Clonazepam, which is commonly used in epilepsy, has been compared with baclofen as an anti-spastic efficacy in patients mostly of multiple sclerosis (Cendrowski et al., 1977), and was found to be as equally effective as diazepam, but was less well tolerated due to adverse effects such as sedation, confusion and fatigue, resulting in more frequent discontinuation of the drug. It is used mainly for suppression of nocturnal painful spasms. Clorazepate, a benzodiazepine analogue, has been shown in a double-blind study to be effective in reducing phasic stretch reflexes in stroke and multiple sclerosis patients (Lossius et al., 1985). Ketazolam, a benzodiazepine derivative, has been reported to be equally effective and slightly less sedating than diazepam in a double-blind, randomized, crossover study of 50 patients with spasticity of various causes (Basmajan et al., 1984, 1986). Tetrazepam, another benzodiazepine derivative, was reported to reduce the tonic stretch reflexes in patients with spasticity without effect on muscle strength (Milanov, 1992).

Dantrolene sodium

Dantrolene sodium, 1-([5-(p-nitrophenyl)furfurylidene]amino) hydantoin sodium hydrate, is a hydantoin derivative and is the only drug in clinical use for spasticity which produces relaxation of contracted skeletal muscle by affecting the contractile response at a site beyond the neuromuscular junction.

Mechanism of action

Dantrolene sodium acts peripherally on muscle fibres, where it is thought to suppress the release of calcium ions from the sarcoplasmic reticulum, thereby producing a dissociation of excitation–contraction coupling and diminishing the force of muscle contraction (Ellis & Carpenter, 1974; Putney & Bianchi, 1974; Hainaut & Desmedt, 1975; Pinder et al., 1977; Ward et al., 1986). In animal studies, the muscle relaxant effect is seen in both fast-contracting and slow-contracting muscle fibres but is more pronounced in the fast-contracting fibres (Bowman et al., 1979; Leslie & Part, 1981b; Jami et al., 1983). In addition, dantrolene exerts its greatest effect on contractile responses at the lower frequencies of nerve stimulation and at the shorter muscle length. These findings suggest that the clinical effects of dantrolene will depend on a balance between the frequency of motor unit firing in the particular muscle and the type of muscle fibre firing in that muscle. Dantrolene also affects both extrafusal and intrafusal muscle fibre contraction in the muscle spindles (Monster et al., 1974; Petite et al., 1980; Leslie & Part, 1981a), which indicates that its anti-spastic effect is partly contributed by alteration in muscle spindle sensitivity.

Pharmacokinetics

After oral administration, approximately 70% of dantrolene sodium is absorbed through the small intestine and the majority is metabolized into 5-hydroxydantrolene in the liver. It is then excreted in the urine and bile, with 15–25% in unchanged form in the urine. After an oral dose of 100 mg, the peak blood concentration of the free acid, dantrolene, occurs in three to six hours and its active metabolite occurs in four to eight hours. The half-life of dantrolene sodium is approximately 15 hours after an oral administration, and is about 12 hours after an intravenous administration (Herman et al., 1972; Ward et al., 1986). It is lipophilic and crosses the placenta and blood–brain barrier well.

Clinical efficacy

Most of the placebo-controlled trials have demonstrated that dantrolene is superior to placebo in adults and children with spasticity from various conditions, as evidenced by muscle and reflex responses to mechanical and electrical stimulation and by clinical assessment of disability and activities of daily living (Pinder et al., 1977). Although dantrolene is generally preferred for spasticity resulting from supraspinal lesions such as stroke, traumatic brain injury or cerebral palsy, this common belief remains controversial. Some workers have suggested that stroke patients are more likely to improve with dantrolene (Chyatte et al., 1971; Ketel & Kolb, 1984), whereas others have found that it did not clinically produce alteration in muscle tone or a change in functional outcome in patients with hemispheric stroke when dantrolene was commenced within eight weeks of onset of stroke (Katrak et al., 1992). It was reported that patients with spinal cord injury also responded well to dantrolene (Weiser et al., 1978). It is somewhat less effective in patients with multiple sclerosis (Gelenberg & Poskanzer, 1973; Tolosa et al., 1975). In four placebo-controlled clinical trials, dantrolene sodium was found to be an effective anti-spastic agent in children with cerebral palsy (Haslam et al., 1974). In three comparative studies (Glass & Hannah, 1974; Nogen, 1976; Schmidt et al., 1976), there was no significant difference between dantrolene and diazepam in terms of reduction in spasticity, clonus and hyper-reflexia, but dantrolene was significantly better in the side-effects profile.

Dosage and administration

The manufacturer's maximum recommended daily oral dosage in adults is 400 mg. The initial dosage is 25 mg per day and may be gradually increased up to 100 mg, four times per day. The dosage should be titrated against clinical improvement and the lowest dose compatible with optimal response is recommended. However, clinical responses are not clearly related to dose and may reach a plateau at a dosage of 100 mg per day (Meyler et al., 1981). If no clinical benefit is derived from administration of dantrolene after six weeks, it should be discontinued. In some of the clinical studies higher than the recommended dosage of 400 mg per day was used. In children, the dose begins at 0.5 mg/kg twice daily and the dosage and frequency are increased until the maximum clinical response is achieved (British National Formulary, March 2000). The maximum dosage in children is 3 mg/kg four times daily but not more than 100 mg four times daily.

Side-effects

Dantrolene commonly causes transient drowsiness, dizziness, weakness, general malaise, fatigue and diarrhoea at the start of therapy, but these are generally mild. Other side-effects include central nervous system disturbance, anorexia, nausea, vomiting and skin rash. Muscle weakness may be the principal limiting side-effect in ambulant patients, particularly in those with multiple sclerosis, and it could be hazardous in patients with pre-existing bulbar or respiratory muscle weakness (Pinder et al., 1977). Dantrolene has caused transient abnormalities in liver function, with symptomatic hepatitis in 0.35 to 0.5% and fatal, idiosyncratic hepatitis in 0.1 to 0.2 % (Utili et al., 1977; Wilkinson et al., 1979). The reactions occur at all doses, but are more frequent in patients taking over 400 mg per day. The risk of hepatic toxicity is greatest in women over 35 years, with concomitant medication such as oestrogen. Hence, liver function should be checked periodically during dantrolene therapy. Pleuro-pericardial reaction to treatment with dantrolene for two to three months has been reported and all the four patients developed peripheral blood eosinophilia (Petusevsky et al., 1979; Miller & Haas, 1984).

Central alpha-2 adrenergic receptor agonists

Clonidine and tizanidine are imidazoline derivatives that affect central alpha-2 adrenergic receptors and their anti-spastic effect may be related to restoration or enhancement of noradrenergic presynaptic inhibitory descending pathway. Clonidine has been used as an anti-hypertensive since early 1970s and tizanidine has only been licensed as an anti-spastic drug in the UK for two years, although it has been used in other European Union countries for some time.

Mechanism of action

The mechanism of action of clonidine is not fully understood, but probably acts at multiple levels as a selective alpha-2 adrenergic receptor agonist in the brain the brain stem and the substantia gelatinosa and intermediolateral cell columns of the dorsal spinal cord (Unnerstall et al., 1984). Other suggested mechanisms of action include suppression of alpha motor neurone excitability, enhancement of alpha-2 mediated presynaptic inhibition of sensory afferents and suppression of polysynaptic reflexes (Naftchi, 1982; Tremblay & Bedard, 1986; Schomburg & Steffens, 1988). Recent work suggests that clonidine's anti-nociceptive activity seems to be exerted either at the spinal and/or supraspinal level with the involvement of alpha-1 adrenergic, alpha-2 adrenergic and opioid receptors (Sierralta et al., 1996).

The precise mechanism of action of tizanidine is not clearly understood, but it has been postulated that its effects are mainly related to its central alpha-2 adrenergic agonist properties (Coward, 1994) and also its probable effect on imidazoline receptor sites (Sayers et al., 1980; Muramatsu & Kigoshi, 1992). Tizanidine acts presynaptically at the spinal level on the release of excitatory amino acids – i.e. glutamate and aspartate of interneurones – thus decreasing the excitability of alpha motor neurones (Davies, 1982; Davies et al., 1983). Another study has reported evidence for a possible depressant effect of tizanidine on the polysynaptic excitation of interneurones by postsynaptic reduction in the effectiveness of the release of excitatory amino acids (Curtis et al., 1983). In addition to the direct action at the spinal level, its supraspinal effect may also involve an alpha-2 adrenergic receptor-mediated influence on descending, facilitatory coeruleospinal pathways (Foote et al., 1983; Chen et al., 1987; Palmeri & Weisendanger, 1990). Recently Delwaide & Pennisi (1994) have postulated that tizanidine reinforces presynaptic inhibition as well as Ia reciprocal and Ib non-reciprocal postsynaptic inhibition and may reduce flexor reflexes.

Clonidine

Pharmacokinetics

Clonidine is well absorbed from the gastro-intestinal tract and its peak plasma concentrations are achieved three to five hours after oral administration. Its half-life is approximately 23 hours and is metabolized in the liver; about 20% is excreted in the faeces. About 65% is excreted in the urine, partly in an unchanged form.

Clinical efficacy

There are few clinical trials with clonidine as an anti-spastic agent and no double-blind placebo-controlled studies have been published. Two open-label trials have found the effectiveness of clonidine in reducing spasticity objectively and subjectively in patients with spinal cord lesion (Nance et al., 1985; Maynard, 1986). It has been shown to be an effective therapeutic agent in the management of spasticity in conjunction with baclofen in patients with spinal cord injury (Donovan et al., 1988). In a single-blind study of six spinal cord injury patients comparing clonidine with diazepam and placebo, clonidine has reduced spasticity, both subjectively and objectively, in terms of vibratory inhibition of the H reflex (Nance et al., 1989). In another comparative clinical trial, clonidine had a similar anti-spastic efficacy to baclofen and cyproheptadine in the spinal cord injured patients (Nance, 1994). In the single case report, a patient who developed spasticity after brain stem infarct, responded rapidly to clonidine (Sandford et al., 1988) and in a case series report, it was suggested that clonidine may also be useful in the management of spasticity associated with various forms of brain injury (Dall et al., 1996). One study suggested that it may be helpful in reducing spasticity in patients with multiple sclerosis who fail to respond to baclofen and diazepam (Khan & Olek, 1995). In addition to an oral form, the transdermal clonidine patch has also been reported to have an efficacy in the treatment of spinal spasticity with the advantage of fewer systemic side-effects (Weingarden & Belen, 1992; Yablon & Sipski, 1993). Clearly, double-blind placebo-controlled trials are needed to confirm and establish the efficacy and dosage of clonidine in the management of spasticity.

Tizanidine

Pharmacokinetics

Tizanidine is rapidly absorbed from the gastro-intestinal tract after a single oral dose, reaching peak plasma concentration in 0.75 to 2 hours. The half-life ranges from 2.1 to 4.2 hours. It is extensively metabolized in the liver via oxidation, and less than 3% of the administered dose is excreted in the urine in an unchanged form. About 20% of the administered dose is excreted in the faeces, and 53–66% in the urine as three main metabolites.

Clinical efficacy

A number of randomized, double-blind, placebo-controlled studies involving 544 patients have clearly demonstrated a beneficial effect of tizanidine in spasticity related to multiple sclerosis and in spinal cord injured patients, but no definite functional improvements were observed (Lapierre et al., 1987; Nance et al., 1994; Smith et al., 1994; United Kingdom Tizanidine Trial Group, 1994). Several double-blind, randomized, comparative trials have shown that tizanidine has a similar efficacy to baclofen in patients with multiple sclerosis or with spinal cord pathology (Hassan & McLellan, 1980; Smolenski et al., 1981; Newman et al., 1982; Stein et al., 1987; Bass et al., 1988; Eyssette et al., 1988; Hoogstraten et al., 1988; Pagano et al., 1988; Medici et al., 1989). It has also been compared to diazepam in a multi-centre, double-blind trial in patients with spasticity associated with hemiplegia resulting from stroke and traumatic brain injury (Bes et al., 1988). It had a similar clinical efficacy but showed a significantly better walking distance in the tizanidine treatment group. Most of these studies also showed objective improvement or preservation of muscle strength to a similar or greater extent in the tizanidine group compared with those receiving baclofen or diazepam. Tizanidine also had a favourable adverse effects profile although sedation was a prominent side-effect (Wagstaff & Bryson, 1997).

Dosage and administration

The most effective dose of tizanidine should be determined for each patient, and a titration period of two to four weeks appears adequate to ascertain the optimal therapeutic dosage. Tizanidine therapy is usually initiated with 2 mg twice daily, and is increased in 4 mg increments every four to seven days to a maximum of 36 mg per day, divided into three or four doses. At higher dosages, patients may experience sedation within an hour of administration which could be prevented by giving it in divided doses.

Side-effects

Common side-effects reported in clinical trials are dryness of mouth, drowsiness, somnolence, insomnia, dizziness, postural hypotension and muscle weakness. Side-effects are dose-related and often improve or resolve with a decrease in dosage. Other adverse effects are visual hallucinations and abnormalities of liver function (Wallace, 1994). Clinically significant increases in liver enzymes occurred in 5–7% of patients, resolving on withdrawal of tizanidine. An incident of fatal, acute fulminant hepatitis has been reported in a patient who was treated with tizanidine and oxazepam for about two months (Rustemovic et al., 1994). Another serious tizanidine induced hepatic injury was reported in a patient who received tizanidine for several months together with baclofen, diazepam, flurazepam and diclofenac (De Graaf et al., 1996). Measurement of liver function is recommended before initiation of tizanidine and then regularly after a month of treatment.

Cannabis

Cannabis has been widely used for several hundred years as an intoxicant or an herbal medicine. Delta-9tetrahydrocannabinol (THC) is the major active ingredient and is one of 66 cannabinoid constituents of the *Cannabis sativa* plant (Ross & Elsohly, 1995). Pure THC is now available as dronabinol (Marinol) or as the synthetic cannabinoid, nabilone (Cesamet). There have been anecdotal reports of muscle relaxant effect of smoking marijuana in spinal cord injured patients with spasticity (Dunn & Davis, 1974; Malec et al., 1982). In a double-blind trial of oral THC (either 5 mg or 10 mg of THC, or placebo) in nine patients with spasticity related to multiple sclerosis, both treatment groups were superior to placebo in reduction of spasticity scores (Petro & Ellenberger, 1981). In another double-blind, placebo-controlled, cross-over clinical trial of delta-9-THC in 13 patients with multiple sclerosis and spasticity, there was significant improvement in subjective ratings of spasticity at the dosage greater than 7.5 mg of THC (Ungerleider et al., 1987). Clifford (1983) reported that THC improved motor co-ordination in two out of eight multiple sclerosis patients who were severely disabled with tremor and ataxia, and a case report has suggested that THC has benefits for patients with the spasticity related to multiple sclerosis (Meinck et al., 1989). However, a double-blind, randomized, placebo-controlled study of the effect of smoking marijuana in patients with multiple sclerosis showed that posture and balance were deteriorated by the treatment (Greenberg et al., 1994) and similar findings were shown in normal volunteers (Kiplinger et al., 1971). In the literature there is no objective and conclusive evidence on the efficacy of THC or crude marijuana as anti-spastic agents.

Conclusion

Oral anti-spastic agents are first line treatment for the pharmacological management of generalized spasticity following physical therapy. There are now a number of useful agents, but their small therapeutic range make them ineffective in some patients before side-effects occur. However, they are essentially safe in most patients, and those with milder forms of spasticity generally tolerate them well. They are best used along with physical measures to reduce tone in the limbs and trunk, and can be employed in combination with other therapeutic agents. A good understanding of their uses, side-effects and limitations is essential in the rehabilitation of patients with neurological disorders producing significant spasticity and it is necessary for patients and their carers to take on realistic expectations of their place in the overall management of the condition. As more drugs become available and as more becomes known about spasticity, health professionals will become more skilled in utilizing different regimens. Spasticity management is a team-responsibility designed to address the needs of the disabled individual and the carer. The place of oral anti-spastic agents has been well established.

REFERENCES

Aisen, M. L., Dietz, M. A., Rossi, P., Cedarbaum, J. M. & Kutt, H. (1993). Clinical and pharmacokinetic aspects of high dose baclofen therapy. *J Am Paraplegia Soc*, **15**: 211–16.

Basmajan, J. V., Shandarkass, K., Russell, D. et al. (1984). Ketazolam treatment for spasticity: double-blind study of a new drug. *Arch Phys Med Rehabil*, **65**: 698–701.

Basmajan, J. V., Shandarkass, K. & Russell, D. (1986). Ketazolam once daily for spasticity: double-blind cross-over study. *Arch Phys Med Rehabil*, **67**: 556–7.

Bass, B., Weinshenker, B., Rice, G. P. A. et al. (1988). Tizanidine versus baclofen in the treatment of spasticity in patients with multiple sclerosis. *Can J Neurol Sci*, **15**: 15–19.

Bes, A., Eyssette, M., Pierrot-Deseilligny, E. et al. (1988). A multi-centre, double-blind trial of tizanidine, a new antispastic agent, in spasticity associated with hemiplegia. *Curr Med Res Opin*, **10**: 709–18.

Bohannon, R. W. & Smith, M. B. (1986). Interrater reliability of a modified Ashworth Scale of muscle spasticity. *Phys Ther*, **67**: 206–7.

Bowman, W. C., Houstan, J., Khan, H. H. et al. (1979). Effects of dantrolene sodium on respiratory and other muscles and on respiratory parameters in the anesthetized cat. *Eur J Pharmacol*, **5**: 293–303.

Bradstater, M. E., De Bruin, H., Gowland, C. & Clarke, B. M. (1983). Hemiplegic gait: analysis of temporal variables. *Arch Phys Med Rehabil*, **64**: 583–7.

Cartlidge, N. E. F., Hudgson, P. & Weightman, D. (1974). A comparison of baclofen and diazepam in the treatment of spasticity. *J Neurol Sci* , **23**: 17–24.

Cendrowski, W. & Sobczyk, W. (1977). Clonazepam, baclofen and placebo in the treatment of spasticity. *Eur Neurol*, **16**: 257–62.

Chen, D-F., Bianchetti, M. & Weisendanger, M. (1987). The adrenergic agonist tizanidine has differential effects on flexor reflexes of intact and spinalized rat. *Neuroscience*, **23**: 641–7.

Chyatte, S. B., Birdsong, J. H. & Bergman, B. A. (1971). The effects of dantrolene sodium on spasticity and motor performance in hemiplegia. *South Med J*, **64**: 180–5.

Clifford, D. B. (1983). Tetrahydrocannabinol for tremor in multiple sclerosis. *Ann Neurol*, **13**: 669–71.

Cocchiarella, A., Downey, J. A., Darling, R. C (1967). Evaluation of the effect of diazepam on spasticity. *Arch Phys Med Rehabil*, **49**: 393–6.

Cook, J. B. & Nathan, P. W. (1967). On the site of action of diazepam in spasticity in man. *J Neurol Sci*, **5**: 33–7.

Corbett, M., Frankel, H. L. & Michaelis, L. (1972). A double-blind cross-over trial of valium in the treatment of spasticity. *Paraplegia*, **10**: 19–22.

Costa, E. & Guidotti, A. (1979). Molecular mechanisms in the receptor action of the benzodiazepines. *Ann Rev Pharm Toxicol*, **19**: 531–45.

Coward, D. M. (1994). Tizanidine: neuropharmacology and mechanism of action. *Neurology*, **44** (Suppl. 9): S6–S11.

Curtis, D. R., Leah, J. D. & Peet, M. J. (1983). Spinal interneurone depression by DS103–282. *Br J Pharmacol*, **79**: 9–11.

Curtis, D. R., Gynther, B. D., Lacey & Beattie, D. T. (1997). Baclofen: reduction of presynaptic calcium influx in the cat spical cord in vivo. *Exp Brain Res*, **113**: 520–33.

Dall, J. T., Harmon, R. I. & Quinn, C. M. (1996). Use of clonidine for the treatment of spasticity arising from various forms of brain injury: a case series. *Brain Injury*, **10**: 453–8.

Das, T. K. & Park, D. M. (1989). Botulinum toxin in the treatment of spasticity. *Br J Pharmacol*, **87**: 1044–9.

Davidoff, R. A. (1985). Antispasticity drugs: mechanisms of action. *Ann Neurol*, **17**: 107–16.

Davies, J. (1982). Selective depression of synaptic transmission of spinal neurones in the cat by a new centrally acting muscle relaxant, 5-chloro-4-(2-imidazolin-2-yl-amino)-2,1,3-benzothiodazole (DS103–282). *Br J Pharmacol*, **76**: 473–81.

Davies, J., Johnston, S. E. & Lovering, R. (1983). Inhibition by DS 103–282 of D-(3H) aspartate release from spinal cord slices. *Br J Pharmacol*, **78**: 2P.

De Graaf, E. M., Oosterveld, M., Tjabbes, T. et al. (1996). A case of tizanidine-induced hepatic injury. *J Hepatol*, **25**: 772–3.

Delwaide, P. J. & Pennisi, G. (1994). Tizanidine and electrophysiologic analysis of spinal control mechanisms in humans with spasticity. *Neurology*, **44** (Suppl 9): S21–S28.

Demeurisse, G., Demol, O. & Robaye, E. (1980). Motor evaluation in vascular hemiplegia. *Eur Neurol*, **19**: 382–9.

Dicpinigaitis, P. V., Nierman, D. M. & Miller, A. (1993). Baclofen-induced bronchoconstriction. *Ann Pharmacother*, **27**: 883–4.

Donovan, W. H., Carter, R. E., Rossi, C. D. & Wilkerson, M. A. (1988). Clonidine effect on spasticity: a clinical trial. *Arch Phys Med Rehabil*, **69**: 193–4.

Duncan, G. W., Shahani, B. T. & Young, R. R. (1976). An evaluation of baclofen treatment for certain symptoms in patients with spinal cord lesions: a double blind cross over study. *Neurology*, **26**: 441–6.

Dunn, M. & Davis, R. (1974). Perceived effects of marijuana on spinal cord injured males. *Paraplegia*, 1974; **12**: 175.

Ellis, K. O. & Carpenter, J. F. (1974). Mechanisms of control of skeletal muscle contraction by dantrolene sodium. *Arch Phys Med Rehabil*, **55**: 362–9.

Engle, H. A. (1966). The effect of diazepam (Valium) in children with cerebral palsy: a double-blind study. *Dev Med Child Neurol*, **8**: 661–7.

Eyssette, M., Rohmer, F., Serratrice, G. et al. (1988). Multi-centre, double-blind trial of a novel antispastic agent, tizanidine, in spasticity associated with multiple sclerosis. *Curr Med Res Opin*, **10**: 699–708.

Faigle, J. W. & Keberle, H. (1972). The metabolism and pharmokinetics of Lioresal. Spasticity: A topical survey. In *An International Symposium, Vienna 1971*, ed. W. Birkmayer, pp. 94–100. Vienna: Huber.

Feldman, R. G., Kelly-Hayes, M., Conomy, J. P. & Foley, J. M. (1978). Baclofen for spasticity in multiple sclerosis: a double-blind crossover and three-year study. *Neurology*, **28**: 1094–8.

Foote, S. L., Bloom, F. E. & Aston-Jones, G. (1983). Nucleus locus coeruleus: new evidence of anatomical and physiological specificity. *Physiol Rev*, **63**: 844–914.

From, A. & Heltberg, A. (1975). A double blind trial with baclofen (Lioresal) and diazepam in spasticity due to multiple sclerosis. *Acta Neurol Scand*, **51**: 158–66.

Fromm, G. H. & Terrence, C. F. (1987). Comparison of L-baclofen and racemic baclofen in trigeminal neuralgia. *Neurology*, **37**: 1725–8.

Gelenberg, A. J. & Poskanzer, D. C. (1973). The effect of dantrolene sodium on spasticity in multiple sclerosis. *Neurology*, **23**: 1313–15.

Glass, A. & Hannah, A. (1974). A comparison of dantrolene sodium and diazepam in the treatment of spasticity. *Paraplegia*, **12**: 170–4.

Greenberg, H. S., Werness, A. S., Pugh, J. E. et al. (1994). Short-term effects of smoking marijuana on balance in patients with multiple sclerosis and normal volunteers. *Clin Pharmacol Ther*, **55**: 324–8.

Guidotti, A., Toffano, G. & Costa, E. (1978). An endogenous protein modulates the affinity of GABA and benzodiazepine receptors in rat brain. *Nature*, **257**: 553–5.

Hainaut, K. & Desmedt, J. E. (1975). Effect of dantrolene sodium on calcium movements in single muscle fibres. *Nature*, **252**: 728–9.

Haslam, R. H. A., Walcher, J. R., Lietman, P. S. et al. (1974). Dantrolene sodium in children with spasticity. *Arch Phys Med Rehabil*, **55**: 384–8.

Hassan, N. & McLellan, D. L. (1980). Double-blind comparison of single doses of DS103–282, baclofen, and placebo for suppression of spasticity. *J Neurol Neurosurg Psych*, **43**: 1132–6.

Hattab, J. R. (1980). Review of European clinical trials with baclofen. In *Spasticity: Disordered Motor Control*, ed. R. G. Feldman, R. R. Young & W. P. Koella pp. 71–86. Chicago: Year Book Medical Publishers.

Henry, J. L. (1980). Pharmacological studies on baclofen in the spinal cord of the cat. In *Spasticity: Disordered Motor Control*, ed. Feldman, R. G., Yong, R. R. & Koella, W. P., pp. 437–52. Chicago: Year Book Medical Publishers.

Herman, R., Mayer, N. & Mecomber, S. A. (1972). Clinical pharmaco-physiology of dantrolene sodium. *Am J Phys Med*, **51**: 296–311.

Hill, D. R. & Bowery, N. G. (1981). 3H-baclofen and 3H-GABA bind to bicuculline insensitive GABA-B sites in rat brain. *Nature*, **290**: 149–52.

Hoogstraten, M. C., Van der Ploeg, R. J. O., Van der Burg, W. et al. (1988). Tizanidine versus baclofen in the treatment of spasticity in multiple sclerosis patients. *Acta Neurol Scand*, **77**: 224–30.

Hudgson, P. & Weightman, D. (1971). Baclofen in the treatment of spasticity. *BMJ*, **4**: 15–17.

Hunt, S. M., McKenna, S. P. & McEwan, J. (1980). A quantitative approach to perceived health status: a validation study. *J Epidemiol Community Health*, **34**: 281–6.

Hwang, A. S. & Wilcox, G. L. (1989). Baclofen, gamma-aminobutyric acid B receptors and substance P in the mouse spinal cord. *J Pharmacol Exp Ther*, **248**: 1026–33.

Jami, L., Murthy, K. S. K., Petite, J. E. et al. (1983). Action of dantrolene sodium on single motor units of cat muscle in vivo. *Brain Res*, **261**: 285–94.

Johnston, G. A. R., Hailstone, M. H. & Freeman, C. G. (1980). Baclofen: stereoselective inhibition of excitant amino acid release. *J Pharm Pharmacol*, **32**: 230–1.

Katrak, P. H., Cole, A. M. D., Poulos, C. J. & McCauley, J. C. K. (1992). Objective assessment of spasticity, strength, and function with early exhibition of dantrolene sodium after cerebrovascular accident: a randomized double-blind controlled study. *Arch Phys Med Rehabil*, **73**: 4–9.

Katz, R. T. (1988). Management of spasticity. *Am J Phys Med & Rehabil*, **67**: 108–16.

Katz, R. T. & Rymer, W. Z. (1989). Spastic hypertonia: mechanisms and measurement. *Arch Phys Med Rehabil*, **70**: 144–55.

Kendall, H. P. (1964). The use of diazepam in hemiplegia. *Ann Phys Med*, **7**: 225–8.

Kennedy, P., Walker, L. & White, D. (1991). Evaluation of goal planning and advocacy in a rehabilitative environment for spinal cord injured people. Paraplegia. *Int J Spinal Cord*, **29**: 197–202.

Ketel, W. B. & Kolb, M. E. (1984). Long-term treatment with dantrolene sodium of stroke patients with spasticity limiting the return of function. *Curr Med Res Opin*, **9**: 161–9.

Ketelaer, C. J. & Ketelaer, P. (1972). The use of Lioresal in the treatment of muscular hypertonia due to multiple sclerosis. Spasticity: a topical survey. In *An International Symposium, Vienna 1971*, ed. W. Birkmayer, pp. 128–31. Vienna: Huber.

Khan, O. & Olek, M.J. (1995). Clonidine in the treatment of spasticity in patients with multiple sclerosis. *J Neurol*, **242**: 712–15.

Kiplinger, G. F., Manno, J. E., Rodda, B. E. & Forney, R. B. (1971). Dose-response analysis of the effects of tetrahydrocannabinol in man. *Clin Pharmacol Ther*, **12**: 650–7.

Knutsson, E., Lindblom, U. L. F., Martensson, A. (1974). Plasma and cerebrospinal fluid levels of baclofen (Lioresal) at optimal therapeutic responses in spastic paresis. *J Neurol Sci*, **23**: 473–84.

Ko Ko, C. & Ward, A. B. (1997). Management of spasticity. *Br J Hosp Med*, **58**: 401–5.

Lapierre, Y., Bouchard, S., Tansey, C. et al. (1987). Treatment of spasticity with tizanidine in multiple sclerosis. *Can J Neurol Sci*, **14**: (3 Suppl.): 513–17.

Leslie, G. C. & Part, N. J. (1981a). The effect of dantrolene sodium on intrafusal muscle fibres in the rat soleus muscle. *J Physiol (Lond)*, **318**: 73–83.

Leslie, G. C. & Part, N. J. (1981b). The action of dantrolene sodium on rat fast and slow muscle in vivo. *Br J Pharmacol*, **72**: 665–72.

Liversedge, L. A. (1960). Use of phenol in the relief of spasticity. *BMJ*, **242**: 31–3.

Lossius, R., Dietrichson, P. & Lunde, P. K. M. (1985). Effect of clorazepate in spasticity and rigidity: a quantitative study of reflexes and plasma concentrations. *Acta Neurol Scand*, **71**: 190–4.

Malec, J., Harvey, R. F. & Cayner, J. J. (1982). Cannabis effect on spasticity in spinal cord injury. *Arch Phys Med Rehabil*, **63**: 116–18.

Manyard, F. M. (1986). Early clinical experience with clonidine in spinal spasticity. *Paraplegia*, **24**: 175–82.

March, H. O. (1965). Diazepam in incapacitated cerebral palsied children. *JAMA*, **191**: 797–800.

Mathiowetz, V., Weber, K., Kashman, N. & Weber, K. (1985). Adult norms for the nine-hole peg test of finger dexterity. *Occup Ther J Res*, **5**: 24–37.

Medici, M., Pebet, M. & Ciblis, D. (1989). A double-blind, long-term study of tizanidine (Sirdalud) in spasticity due to cerebrovascular lesions. *Curr Med Res Opin*, **11**: 398–407.

Meinck, H. M., Schonle, P. W. & Conrad, B. (1989). Effect of cannabinoids on spasticity and ataxia in multiple sclerosis. *J Neurol*, **236**: 120–2.

Meyler, W. J., Bakker, H., Kok, J.J., Agoston, S. & Wesseling, H. (1981). The effect of dantrolene sodium in relation to blood levels in spastic patients after prolonged administration. *J Neurol Neurosurg Psych*, **44**: 334–9.

Milanov, I. (1992). Mechanisms of tetrazepam action on spasticity. *Acta Neurol Belg*, **92**: 5–15.

Miller, D. H. & Haas, L. F. (1984). Pneumonitis, pleural effusion and pericarditis following treatment with dantrolene. *J Neurol Neurosurg Psych*, **47**: 553–4.

Misgeld, U., Bijak, M. & Jarolimek, W. (1995). A physiological role for GABA B receptors and the effects of baclofen in the mammalian nervous system. Prog Neurol, **46**: 423–62.

Monster, A. W. (1974). Spasticity and the effect of dantrolene sodium. *Arch Phys Medi Rehabil*, **55**: 373–83.

Monster, A. W., Tamai, Y. & McHenry, J. (1974). Dantrolene sodium: its effects on extrafusal muscle fibres. *Arch Phys Med Rehabil*, **55**: 355–62.

Muramatsu, I. & Kigoshi, S. (1992). Tizanidine may discriminate between imidazoline-receptors and alpha-2–adrenoceptors. *Jpn J Pharmacol*, **59**: 457–9.

Naftchi, N. E. (1982). Functional restoration of the traumatically injured spinal cord in cats by clonidine. *Science*, **217**: 1042–4.

Nance, P. W. (1994). A comparison of clonidine, cyproheptadine and baclofen in spastic spinal cord injured patients. *J Am Para Soc*, **17**: 150–6.

Nance, P. W., Bugaresti, J., Shellengerger, K. et al. (1994). Efficacy and safety of tizanidine in the treatment of spasticity in patients with spinal cord injury. *Neurology*, **44** (Suppl. 9): S44–S52.

Nance, P. W., Shears, A. H. & Nance, D. M. (1985). Clonidine in spinal cord injury. *Can Med Assoc J*, **133**: 41–2.

Nance, P. W., Shears, A. H. & Nance, D. M. (1989). Reflex changes induced by clonidine in spinal cord injured patients. *Paraplegia*, **27**: 296–301.

Newman, P. M., Nogues, M., Newman, P. K. et al. (1982). Tizanidine in the treatment of spasticity. *Eur J Clin Pharmacol*, **23**: 31–5.

Nogen, A. G. (1976). Medical treatment for spasticity in children with cerebral palsy. *Child's Brain*, **2**: 304–8.

Noth, J. (1991). Trends in the pathophysiology and pharmacotherapy of spasticity. *J Neurol*, **238**: 131–9.

Olpe, H. R., Demieville, H., Baltzer, V., et al. (1978). The biological activity of D- & L-baclofen (Lioresal). *Eur J Pharmacol*, **52**: 133–6.

Olsen, R. W. (1987). GABA-benzodiazepine-barbiturate receptor interactions. *J Neurochem*, **37**: 1–13.

Pagano, M. A., Ferreiro, M. E. & Herskovits, E. (1988). Comparative study of tizanidine and baclofen in patients with chronic spasticity. *Rev Neurol Argent*, **14**: 268–76.

Palmeri, A. & Weisendanger, M. (1990). Concomitant depression of locus coerulus neurons and of flexor reflexes by an aplha-2–adrenergic agonist in rats: a possible mechanism for an alpha-2–mediated muscle relaxation. *Neuroscience*, **34**: 177–87.

Pedersen, E., Arlien-Soborg, P. & Mai, J. (1974). The mode of action of the GABA derivative of baclofen in human spasticity. *Acta Neurol Scand*, **50**: 665–80.

Penn, R. D., Savoy, S. M. & Corcos, D. (1984). Intrathecal baclofen alleviates spinal cord spasticity. *Lancet*, **1**: 1078.

Petite, J. E., Cameron, W. E. & Murthy, K. S. K. (1980). Effect of dantrolene sodium on the discharge of primary spindle afferents during fusimotor stimulation. *Soc Neurosci Abstr*, **6**: 218.

Petro, D. J. & Ellenberger, C. (1981). Treatment of human spasticity with delta-9-tetrahydrocannabinol. *J Clin Pharmacol*, **21**: 413S–416S.

Petusevsky, M. L., Faling, L. J., Rocklin, R. E. et al. (1979). Pleuropericardial reaction to treatment with dantrolene. *JAMA*, **242**: 2772–4.

Pinder, R. M., Brogden, R. N., Speight, T. M. & Avery, G. S. (1977). Dantrolene sodium: a review of its pharmacological properties and therapeutic efficacy in spasticity. *Drugs*, **13**: 3–23.

Pinto, O. D., Polikar, M. & Debono, G. (1972). Results of international clinical trials with Lioresal. *Postgrad Med J*, **48**: (Suppl 5): 18–23.

Polc, P., Mohler, H. & Haefely, W. (1974). Effect of diazepam on spinal cord activities: possible sites and mechanisms of action. *Naunyn-Schmiedeberg's Arch Pharmacol*, **284**: 319–37.

Price, G. W., Kelly, J. S., Bowery, N. G. (1987). The location of GABA-B receptor binding sites in mammalian spinal cord. *Synapse*, **1**: 530–8.

Price, G. W., Wilkin, G. P., Turnbull, M. J. & Bowery, N. G. (1984). Are baclofen-sensitive GABA-B receptors present on primary afferent terminals of the spinal cord? *Nature*, **307**: 71–3.

Putney, J. W. & Bianchi, C. P. (1974). Site of action of dantrolene in frog sartorius muscle. *J Pharmacol Exp Ther*, **189**: 202–12.

Rack, P. M. H. (1966). The behaviour of mammalian muscle during sinusoidal stretching. *J Physiol* (London). **183**: 1–17.

Rivas, D. A., Chancellor, M. B., Hill, K. & Freedman, M. K. (1993). Neurological manifestations of baclofen withdrawal. *J Urol*, **150**: 1903–5.

Ross, S. A. & Elsohly, M. A. (1995). Constituents of Cannabis sativa L.XXVIII. A review of the natural constituents: 1980–1994. *J Pharm Sci*, **4**: 1–10.

Roussan, M., Terrence, C. & Fromm, G. (1987). Baclofen versus diazepam for the treatment of spasticity and long-term follow-up of baclofen therapy. *Pharmatherapeutica*, **4**: 278–84.

Roy, C. W. & Wakefield, I. R. (1986). Baclofen pseudopsychosis: case report. *Paraplegia*, **24**: 318–21.

Rustemovic, N., Huic, M., Opacic, M. et al. (1994). Tizanidine-induced acute toxic hepatitis: case report. *Pharmaca*, **32**: 457–61.

Ryan, D. M. & Blumenthal, F. S. (1993). Baclofen-induced dyskinesia. *Arch Phys Med Rehabil*, 74: 766–7.

Sachais, B. A., Logue, J. N. & Carey, M. S. (1977). Baclofen, a new antispastic drug: a controlled, multicenter trial in patients with multiple sclerosis. *Arch Neurol*, 34: 422–8.

Sandford, P. R., Spengler, S. E. & Sawasky, K. B. (1988). Clonidine in the treatment of brainstem spasticity. *Am J Phys Med Rehabil*, 71: 301–3

Sawynok, J. & Dickson, C. (1985). D-baclofen is an antagonist at baclofen receptors mediating antinociception in the spinal cord. *Pharmacology*, 1985; 31: 248–59.

Sayers, A. C., Burki, H. R. & Eichenberger, E. (1980). The pharmacology of 5-chloro-4-(2-imidazolin-2-yl-amino)-2,1,3-benzothiadazole (DS 103–282), a novel myotonolytic agent. *Arzneimittel-Forsch*, 30: 793–803.

Schlosser, W. (1971). Action of diazepam on spinal cord. *Arch Int Pharmacodyn Ther*, 194: 93–102.

Schmidt, R. T., Lee, R. H. & Spehlman, R. (1976). Comparison of dantrolene sodium and diazepam in the treatment of spasticity. *J Neurol Neurosurg Psych*, 39: 350–6.

Schomburg, E. D. & Steffens, H. (1988). The effect of DOPA and clonidine on reflex pathways from group II afferents to alpha-motorneurons in the cat. *Exp Brain Res*, 71: 442–6.

Schwartz, M., Turski, L., Janiszewski, W. & Sontag, K. H. (1983). Is the muscle relaxant effect of diazepam in spastic mutant rats mediated through GABA-independent benzodiazepine receptors? *Neurosci Lett*, 36: 175–80.

Sierralta, F., Naquira, D., Pinardi, G. & Miranda, H. F. (1996). Alpha-adrenoceptor and opioid receptor modulation of clonidine-induced antinociception. *Br J Pharmacol*, 119: 551–4.

Skerritt, J. H. & Johnston, G. A. R. (1983). Enhancement of GABA binding by benzodiazepines and related anxiolytics. *Eur J Pharmacol*, 89: 193–8.

Skerritt, J. H., Willow, M. & Johnston, G. A. R. (1982). Diazepam enhancement of low affinity GABA binding to rat brain membranes. *Neurosci Lett*, 29: 63–6.

Smith, C. R., LaRocca, N. G., Giesser, B. S. & Scheinberg, L. C. (1991). High-dose oral baclofen: experience in patients with multiple sclerosis. *Neurology*, 41: 1829–31.

Smith, C., Birnbaum, G., Carter, J. L. et al. (1994). Tizanidine treatment of spasticity caused by multiple sclerosis: results of a double-blind, placebo-controlled trial. *Neurology*, 44: (Suppl. 9): S34–S43.

Smolenski, C, Muff, S. & Smolenski-Kautz, S. (1981). A double-blind comparative trial of a new muscle relaxant, tizanidine (DS103–282), and baclofen in the treatment of chronic spasticity in multiple sclerosis. *Curr Med Res Opin*, 7: 374–83.

Stein, R., Nordal, H. J., Oftedal, S. I. & Slettebo, M. (1987). The treatment of spasticity in multiple sclerosis: a double-blind clinical trial of a new anti-spasticity drug tizanidine compared with baclofen. *Acta Neurol Scand*, 75: 190–4.

Terrence, D. V. & Fromm, G. H. (1981). Complications of baclofen withdrawal. *Arch Neurol*, 38: 588–9.

Tolosa, E. S., Soll, R. W., Loewenson, J. W. (1975). Treatment of spasticity in multiple sclerosis with dantrolene. *JAMA*, 233: 1046.

Tremblay, L. E. & Bedard, P. J. (1986). Effect of clonidine on motor neuron excitability in spinalized rats. *Neuropharmacology*, 25: 41–6.

Ungerleider, J. T., Andyrsiak, T., Fairbanks, L. et al. (1987). Delta-9-THC in the treatment of spasticity associated with multiple sclerosis. *Adv Alcohol Subst Abuse*, 7: 39–50

United Kingdom Tizanidine Trial Group. (1994). A double-blind, placebo-controlled trial of tizanidine in the treatment of spasticity caused by multiple sclerosis. *Neurology*, 44: (Suppl. 9): S70–S78.

Unnerstall, J. R., Kopajtic, T. A. & Kuhar, M. J. (1984). Distribution of alpha-2 agonist binding sites in rat and human central nervous system: analysis of some functional, anatomic correlates of pharmacologic effects of clonidine and related adrenergic agents. *Brain Res*, 319: 69–101.

Utili, R., Boitnott, J. K. & Zimmerman, H. J. (1977). Dantrolene-associated hepatic injury: incidence and character. *Gastroenterology*, 72: 610–16.

Verrier, M., Ashby, P. & Macleod, S. (1977). Diazepam effect on reflex activity in patients with complete spinal lesions and in those with other causes of spasticity. *Arch Phys Med Rehabil*, 58: 148–53.

Wade, D. T. (1988). Neurological rehabilitation. *Int Dis Stud*, 9: 45–7.

Wagstaff, A. J. & Bryson, H. M. (1997). Tizanidine: a review of its pharmacology, clinical efficacy and tolerability in the management of spasticity associated with cerebral and spinal disorders. *Drugs*, 53: 435–52.

Wallace, J. D. (1994). Summary of combined clinical analysis of controlled clinical trial with tizanidine. *Neurology*, 44: (Suppl 9): S60–S69.

Wang, M. Y. & Dun, N. J. (1990). Phaclofen-insensitive presynaptic inhibitory action of +/− baclofen in neonatal rat motorneurons in vitro. *Br J Pharmcol*, 99: 413–21.

Ward, A., Chaffman, M. O. & Sorkin, E. M. (1986). Dantrolene: a review of its pharmacokinetic properties and therapeutic use in malignant hyperthermia, the neuroleptic malignant syndrome and an update of its use in muscle spasticity. *Drugs*, 32: 130–68.

Ward, A. B. (1999). The use of botulinum toxin type-A in spastic diplegia due to cerebral palsy. *Euro J Neurol*, 6 (Suppl. 4): S95–S98.

Ware, J. E. (1993). *SF-36 Heath Survey: Manual and Interpretation Guide*. Boston: The Health Institute, New England Medical Center.

Weingarden, S. I. & Belen, J. G. (1992). Clonidine transdermal system for treatment of spasticity in spinal cord injury. *Arch Phys Med Rehabil*, 73: 876–7.

Weiser, R., Terenty, T., Hudgson, P. et al. (1978). Dantrolene sodium in the treatment of spasticity in chronic spinal cord disease. *Practitioner*, 221: 123–7.

Whyte, J. & Robinson, K. M. (1990). Pharmacologic management. In *The Practical Management of Spasticity in Children and Adults*, ed. M. B. Glenn & J. Whyte, pp. 201–26. Philadelphia: Lea & Febiger.

Wilkinson, S. P., Portmann, B. & Williams, R. (1979). Hepatitis from dantrolene sodium. *Gut*, 20: 33–6.

Wilson, L. A. & McKechnie, A. A. (1966). Oral diazepam in the treatment of spasticity in paraplegia: a double-blind trial and subsequent impressions. *Scot Med J*, 11: 46–51.

Yablon, S. A. & Sipski, M. L. (1993). Effect of transdermal clonidine in spinal spasticity: a case series. *Am J Phys Med Rehabil*, 72: 154–7.

Young, R. R. & Delwaide, P. J. (1981). Spasticity. *N Engl J Med*, 304: 28–33, 96–9.

8

Chemical neurolysis in the management of spasticity

A. M. O. Bakheit

Introduction

In the mid-1950s destruction of peripheral nerves with chemical substances such as phenol and alcohol solutions (i.e. chemical neurolysis) was introduced as a novel method of treatment of severe pain associated with cancer (Maher, 1955; Brown, 1958). A few years later peripheral nerve blocks with local anaesthetics and neurolytic agents were found to be effective in the management of muscle spasticity and neurogenic bladder disorders, and more recently they have also been used to predict the outcome of certain surgical procedures such as selective dorsal rhizotomy.

An important therapeutic use of peripheral nerve and intrathecal blocks is in the treatment of severe or intractable pain – e.g. pain associated with cancer, trigeminal and post-herpetic neuralgia. Complete symptomatic relief is achieved in more than 70% of patients with chronic pain due to neurogenic causes or ischaemia (Hatangdi & Boas, 1975). Nerve blocks are also valuable in the management of bladder dysfunction due to spinal cord injury or disease. The selective chemical denervation of S3 sacral segment in patients with a hyperactive detrusor muscle increases bladder capacity and reduces the uninhibited contractions. Continence is usually achieved in these patients without sphincter disturbances or sexual dysfunction (Torrens, 1974; Rockswold & Bradley, 1977). Chemical neurolysis is also effective in the management of severe upper and lower limb muscle spasticity. In most patients it relieves the muscle spasticity without significantly affecting the voluntary muscle contraction (Brown, 1958; Khalili & Betts, 1967). This confers chemical neurolysis a major advantage over treatment with oral anti-spasticity drugs.

Chemical neurolysis can be achieved with peripheral nerve blocks, motor point (intramuscular) injections and the intrathecal administration of alcohol or phenol. These procedures are generally safe, effective and relatively easy to perform. They are preferred to oral anti-spasticity drugs which often cause systemic adverse effects and are non-selective in their action thus affecting both spastic and normal muscles. The latter adverse effect may lead to functional loss. In a study by Katrak et al. (1992) of patients recovering from stroke, dantrolene reduced muscle strength in the unaffected extremities without significantly reducing muscle tone or improving function in the spastic limbs. Another disadvantage of systemic anti-spasticity drugs is that their effectiveness diminishes with prolonged use. Tolerance to these drugs usually develops after a few weeks or months of treatment and progressive dosage increments are often required to maintain an optimal therapeutic response.

Chemical neurolysis is only one of many methods of treatment of muscle spasticity and the best clinical outcomes are achieved when it is utilized as part of an overall management strategy. Factors which precipitate or aggravate muscle spasticity such as urinary tract infections and faecal impaction should be identified and treated. Clinical experience also suggests that an intensive physiotherapy programme following the nerve blocks or motor point injections improves motor function. In some cases it is more useful to combine neurolysis with serial splinting of the spastic limb, the application of plaster casts or the use of an orthosis.

The effect of neurolytic agents is irreversible and their use should, therefore, only be considered when a clear treatment goal has been identified. There is a large variation in the way muscle spasticity affects patients depending on the site and chronicity of the upper motor neurone lesion, its underlying cause, the degree of neural recovery and the way the nervous system compensates for the functional loss. Frequently spasticity is functionally useful and an individualized approach to the management of this symptom is, therefore, essential.

Indications for treatment

Severe chronic muscle spasticity often causes constant gnawing pain. In addition, it is frequently associated with muscle spasms that occur spontaneously or when the patient attempts to move. In severe cases the spasms may even be precipitated by sudden noise. Spasms of the hip flexors, extensors or adductors may be accompanied by the involuntary bladder emptying and occasionally faecal incontinence. Other effects of severe muscle spasticity include impaired motor function and the development of deformities and contractures. Generally, treatment of spasticity is indicated to alleviate distressing symptoms such as pain or muscle spasms, to improve motor function, to facilitate activities of daily living – e.g. washing and dressing, urethral catheterization or perineal hygiene – or to prevent or reduce the complications which are often associated with muscle hypertonia such as contractures or difficulties in maintaining a comfortable position in bed or chair.

There is no research evidence at present to show which patients are most likely to benefit from nerve blocks and motor point injections. However, given the fact that the beneficial effect of these procedures usually lasts for several months and that good results cannot be relied upon after two or three injections (Bakheit et al., 1996a), it is likely that the technique is most helpful for those whose spasticity may be troublesome in the medium rather than the long term. This would include patients recovering from severe head injury or a recent relapse of multiple sclerosis in whom spasticity is so severe that splinting or the application of plaster casts is impracticable because of the risk of soft tissue damage. Another group of patients who are likely to benefit from chemical neurolysis are those in whom spasticity is preventing acquisition of motor skills, such as children with cerebral palsy establishing increased independence in walking. A third group is subjects who are likely to require future surgical treatment for the complications of spasticity such as the control of pain, the relief of muscle spasms or the surgical release of contractures but in whom there are clinical or technical advantages in delaying such surgery.

Indications for medial popliteal nerve blocks

Medial popliteal nerve blocks and motor point injections of the gastrosoleus muscles are indicated in cases of foot equinus resistant to serial casting or preventing the effective use of an ankle–foot orthosis and when sustained ankle clonus interferes with motor function or causes discomfort to the patient – e.g. when it prevents comfortable placement of the foot on the wheelchair footplate. They are also useful in the management of distal foot deformities in children with cerebral palsy. For example, by reducing the muscle imbalance in the lower limb a medial popliteal nerve block provides valuable information regarding the choice of the surgical procedure for the treatment of secondary foot deformities such as hallux valgus or metatarsal subluxations (Carpenter, 1983).

Indications for obturator nerve blocks

The main indications for obturator nerve blocks in ambulatory patients is 'scissoring gait'. In non-ambulatory patients this treatment may be considered when severe spasticity of the hip adductors interferes with urethral catheterization, washing and cleaning the perineal area and seating or positioning in bed. Occasionally, obturator nerve blocks are used to prevent the development of or to promote the healing of skin pressure sores on the medial aspect of the knees.

Obturator nerve blocks have also been used in the management of dislocation and subluxation of the hip joint. This complication occurs in 25% of patients with cerebral palsy and is often associated with severe pain. Treatment is usually effective in pain relief probably due to reduced stretching of the joint capsule and less friction of the femoral head against the periosteum of the acetabulum (Trainer et al., 1986).

Nerve blocks for upper limb muscle spasticity

In the upper limbs chemical neurolysis seldom improves motor function and is mainly indicated to facilitate activities of daily living. For example, the improved elbow extension following a successful musculo-cutaneous nerve block often makes dressing easier and in some cases also increases the patient's reach with the paretic hand. Reduction of spasticity of the finger flexors is sometimes necessary to facilitate hand hygiene and to prevent skin laceration in the palm of a claw hand. Percutaneous phenol nerve blocks are often successful in these cases but the procedure involves a higher risk than when it is used for lower limb spasticity. The median and ulnar nerves run in close proximity to the blood vessels of the upper limb and an attempt to infiltrate the nerves with the neurolytic agent may result in vascular damage. Furthermore, both nerves contain sensory fibres and the sensory loss following neurolysis may cause loss or deterioration of hand function and increase the risk of burns and injury. The use of botulinum toxin is probably more appropriate for management of upper limb spasticity.

The diagnostic use of nerve blocks

Diagnostic nerve blocks with local anaesthetics are sometimes necessary to assess the risk/benefit ratio of chemical neurolysis. Although the effect of local anaesthetics is not identical to that of phenol or alcohol, their use often yields clinically valuable information. Bupivacaine is best suited for this purpose as its effect lasts seven to eight hours when given in a dose of 1 mg/kg body weight (0.5% Marcain contains 5.28 mg/ml of bupivacaine HCl).

Diagnostic nerve blocks may be used to predict the effects of chemical neurolysis on motor function – e.g. when severe spasticity of the wrist and finger flexors is causing functional difficulties but the patient still has some voluntary muscle power in the affected hand. They may also be used to assess the effects of sensory loss on the patients' functional ability when injections of mixed sensory–motor nerves are being considered. Diagnostic nerve blocks have also been found valuable in predicting the functional outcome of surgical procedures for spasticity such as selective dorsal rhizotomy and in the management of foot dystonia (Bakheit et al., 1996b).

The pharmacological properties of neurolytic agents

Phenol (a benzene derivative of carbolic acid) and ethyl alcohol are the drugs most commonly used for peripheral nerve and intrathecal blocks. Other agents such as cresol and chlorocresol may also be used. Although these agents were initially thought to reduce muscle tone by the selective inhibition of gamma efferent pathways, their effect on muscle spasticity was subsequently shown to be due to their local anaesthetic and neurolytic properties. As with conventional local anaesthetics, nerve conduction is initially blocked in the small fibres within the nerve trunk

– i.e. sympathetic and sensory fibres – and then in the large motor axons. Braun et al. (1973) attributed this selective effect of dilute solutions of phenol or alcohol to the fact that fibres with a small diameter have more relative surface contact area for a given volume of nerve tissue than large alpha fibres. Typically, recovery of nerve conduction occurs in the reverse order.

Neurolytic agents also penetrate the nerve tissue and coagulate protein. The application of phenol and alcohol solutions causes nerve tissue destruction which is proportional to the concentration and volume of fluid injected. Interestingly, the myelin sheath is more susceptible than the axons to this neurolytic injury. The pathological changes resulting from chemical neurolysis occur in a predictable sequence. Histological changes consisting of a marked inflammatory reaction in the nerve tissue occur within hours of the application of the neurolytic agent (Nathan et al., 1965). These are followed in a few days by Wallerian degeneration that is maximal two weeks after the injection. In the event of severe damage the nerve fibres are often replaced by fibrous tissue. Finally, within a few weeks of the injection, evidence of partial nerve regeneration mainly by collateral sprouting is usually evident and by the fourteenth week regeneration is almost complete (Burkell & McPhee, 1970). The neurolytic effect is non-selective and involves both myelinated and non-myelinated nerve fibres. Very high concentrations of neurolytic agents, for example 15% phenol in saline or 10% phenol in iophendylate (Myodil), may also cause localized vasculitis, tissue infarction and arachnoiditis (Baxter & Schacherl, 1962).

Phenol is soluble in water, glycerine and other organic solvents. Aqueous phenol is suitable for peripheral nerve blocks and motor point injections whereas phenol in glycerine is preferred for intrathecal block. Phenol in glycerine has a higher specific gravity than cerebrospinal fluid (CSF). This allows the solution to be easily manipulated around the desired nerve roots by the appropriate careful positioning of the patient. Interestingly, chlorocresol in glycerine (1:50) is thought to be a better agent than phenol for the management of pain in cancer patients. It was claimed to provide a more reliable symptomatic relief presumably because it acts partly by diffusion and spreads to a greater length of the nerve root. Aqueous solutions of phenol have been shown to have a more potent neurolytic effect than phenol in glycerine.

Procedure

Nerve blocks

Chemical neurolysis is most frequently used for the medial popliteal, the obturator, the sciatic and the musculo-cutaneous nerve of the arm. Nerve blocks are usually carried out percutaneously as described below. However, occasionally 'open' blocks of the motor branches of mixed sensory–motor nerves are performed. Following the surgical exposure of the nerve, the motor division is identified with an electrical stimulator and 2–5 ml of the neurolytic agent are injected in a 2 cm segment of the nerve beneath the neural sheath. The most effective site of block depends on the course of the nerve in the limb and where it divides to innervate the muscles that are being considered for treatment.

An essential pre-requisite for the success of peripheral percutaneous nerve blocks is the accurate placement of the injection. This can be achieved easily with an electrical stimulator utilizing a teflon-coated needle electrode as a probe. Alternatively, a standard venflon connected to the cathode of the stimulator could be used. The electrode wire is wrapped around the needle shaft at the top and the plastic sheath is replaced to ensure that the needle is insulated except at the tip. Although some clinicians use anatomical landmarks as the guide for needle placement, this method is often inadequate and is associated with up to 40% treatment failure (Ferrer-Brechner & Brechner, 1976). Nerve blocks require full co-operation from the patient and the frequent discomfort that occurs afterwards means that children might require a light general anaesthetic.

Medial popliteal nerve block

The medial popliteal (tibial) nerve is a continuation of the sciatic nerve. It runs in the middle of the popliteal fossa where it gives off branches to the heads of the gastrocnemius from its proximal portion approximately 1 cm above the head of the fibula. Each of these divisions gives off three to five terminal branches in the proximal fifth of the muscle. The middle and distal branches enter deep into the muscle and supply the main muscle mass and the distal third, respectively. The branches to the soleus, popliteus and tibialis posterior muscles arise more distally. Further branches below the popliteal fossa innervate the flexor digitorum longus and flexor hallucis longus muscles. The terminal branches innervate the toe flexors and the small muscles of the foot.

The medial popliteal nerve may be blocked at the apex of the popliteal fossa or 2–3 cm lower, at the level of the popliteal crease (Figure 8.1). However, injection placement in the latter site is less effective than a more proximal block (Felsenthal, 1974). This is presumably because the nerve fibres are more dispersed distally. It is easier to do medial popliteal nerve blocks with the patient lying prone. Alternatively, the procedure could be performed with the patient lying on his/her side and the limb held in full extension by an assistant to prevent flexion withdrawal. The location of the medial popliteal nerve behind the knee can be easily identified at the level of the tibial epicondyles with an electrical stimulator, initially

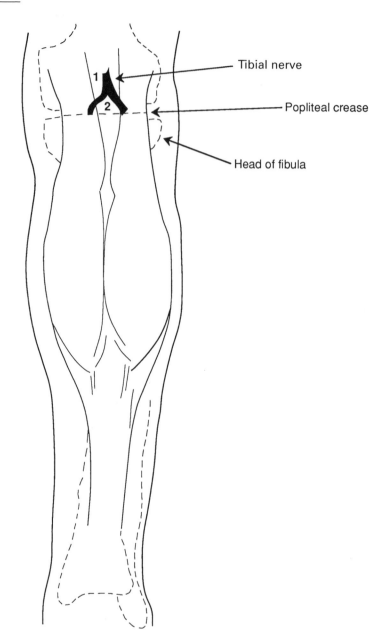

Fig. 8.1   Medial popliteal nerve block at the apex of the popliteal fossa (1) is more effective than a nerve block at the level of the popliteal crease (2).

using surface electrodes delivering 5–50 volt pulses of 0.1 msec duration. The skin
is then cleansed with iodine solution and infiltrated with 1% lignocaine. The needle
probe is then introduced and manoeuvred in the tissue using stimulus pulses of
decreasing strength until a contraction of the spastic muscles supplied by the nerve
is obtained in response to 0.5 mA electrical pulse with a stimulus duration of
0.05–0.1 msec. Between 3 and 5 ml of 4.5% phenol in water or 50% ethyl alcohol
is then injected over three to four minutes. Slowly the position of the needle tip is
readjusted in each plane to ensure that the twitch had been fully suppressed. If a
new site is found during this manoeuvre a further 1–2 ml of phenol should be
injected. Ankle clonus is immediately abolished or significantly attenuated with a
successful nerve block.

Obturator nerve blocks

The obturator nerve passes through the obturator foramen into the thigh in the
upper medial part of the femoral triangle. (The femoral triangle is formed by the
lateral border of the adductor longus, the sartorius muscle and the inguinal ligament.) The nerve emerges about 2 cm below the inguinal ligament and just lateral
to the origin of the tendon of the adductor longus muscle (Figure 8.2). It then
immediately divides into anterior (superficial) and posterior (deep) branches. It is
a predominantly motor nerve and supplies the hip adductors. It also gives off
branches to the hip and knee joints and a cutaneous branch to a restricted skin area
on the medial aspect of the middle of the thigh. In a third of subjects there is an
accessory obturator nerve which emerges from the pelvis above the superior pubic
ramus and joins the anterior branch of the main trunk approximately 4–5 cm
below the inguinal ligament.

Localization of the obturator nerve is made with the patient supine and both legs
slightly abducted. The tendon of the adductor longus muscle is usually easily palpable in patients with hip adductor spasticity. The femoral artery is approximately
2 cm lateral to the obturator nerve and femoral pulsation is another useful landmark. Stimulation of the nerve may initially be carried out using a surface probe
and then a needle electrode as described in the above section and is confirmed when
a significant contraction of the adductor muscles is seen. Following injection of the
anterior branch the needle is inserted 2 cm deeper and perpendicular to the coronal
plane to block the posterior branch. A total of 4–5 ml of phenol or alcohol equally
divided between the two sites is usually sufficient.

The obturator nerve can be blocked in the pelvis before it divides but this procedure is technically difficult in patients with spasticity of the hip flexors and/or
adductors. This difficulty arises because the needle has to pass through the obturator foramen into the pelvis in a direction parallel to the trunk.

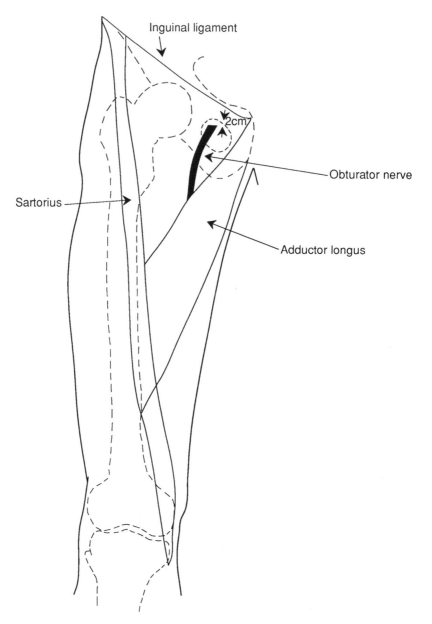

Fig. 8.2   A diagram showing the exit of the obturator nerve in the upper medial part of the femoral triangle, approximately 2 cm below the inguinal ligament.

Sciatic nerve block

The sciatic nerve exits the pelvis through the sciatic foramen and runs between the greater trochanter and the ischeal tuberosity. The nerve gives off branches to the hamstring muscles before it divides, usually at the level of mid-thigh, into the tibial (medial popliteal) and common peroneal nerves.

Sciatic nerve fibres to the hamstrings converge at the level of the gluteal fold (Felsenthal, 1974) and are easily localized with a nerve stimulator in the middle of a line joining the greater trochanter and the ischeal tuberosity. Sciatic nerve blocks are indicated for the relief of knee flexors spasticity.

Block of the musculo-cutaneous nerve of the arm

This nerve is a continuation of the lateral cord of the brachial plexus. It innervates the biceps brachii, brachialis and coraco-brachialis muscles and the skin of the lateral aspect of the forearm. With the patient supine and the upper limb abducted to 90° and externally rotated the nerve can be easily identified with an electrical nerve stimulator in the proximal third of the medial aspect of the arm. At this level the nerve runs in the groove formed by the biceps brachii and the short head of the brachialis muscles. Musculo-cutaneous nerve blocks may be used alone but a better response is usually obtained if it is combined with motor point injections of the brachioradialis muscle (Keenan et al., 1990).

Lumbar spinal nerve blocks

Multiple paravertebral lumbar spinal nerve blocks have been reported to reduce hip flexor spasticity for a period of 4–10 months in most cases (Meelhuysen et al., 1968). For an optimal therapeutic response the nerves of L2, L3 and L4 ipsilateral to the flexed hip need to be injected at a single treatment session.

The spinal nerves are blocked close to their point of exit from the vertebral foramina as follows. With the patients lying on their side and the spine flexed, the spinal nerve is localized in the appropriate intervertebral space 4 cm lateral to the midline. A useful surface landmark is the iliac crest which corresponds to L4–L5 vertebral interspace. The needle (which also acts as the stimulating electrode) is introduced perpendicular to the skin to a depth of 5 cm and then manipulated medially and inferiorly until responses from the iliacus and psoas muscles are observed. Good clinical results may be obtained by injecting as little as 0.2 ml of 5% aqueous phenol per each site.

Motor point injections

Clinical experience suggests that nerve blocks are more effective than motor point injections. The effect of motor point injections is usually incomplete and is of shorter duration in most cases. Nevertheless, because the technique of motor point injections is simple, inexpensive and does not require special equipment, this procedure still has a place in the management of muscle spasticity, especially when the appropriate equipment or expertise is not available or the financial cost of treatment is an important consideration.

The motor points of a muscle is the area of arborization of the motor nerve terminals and clustering of the motor end plates. These generally correspond to the sites used for placement of electrodes for conventional electromyography (EMG). Motor point blocks may be performed without EMG guidance using anatomical surface landmarks. A general rule of thumb is that the motor points of limb muscles lie in the muscle belly, half-way between the muscle origin and its point of insertion (Brash, 1955).

A modification of motor point injections known as the intramuscular alcohol (or phenol) wash is to infiltrate multiple sites in the muscle belly with the neurolytic agent which renders the accurate localization of the motor points unnecessary (Carpenter & Seitz, 1980). The beneficial effect of intramuscular alcohol wash is usually one to four weeks.

Motor point injections of the gastrosoleus muscles

Effective motor point blocks can be achieved by injecting the heads of the gastrocnemius just below the popliteal crease. An intramuscular alcohol or phenol wash of the gastrocnemius muscles is carried out as follows. The visible bulk of the calf muscle is divided into four equal parts and 2–4 ml of the neurolytic agent is infiltrated into the centre of each quadrant. The dose depends on the patient's age, muscle size and the desired effect on muscle tone. The soleus muscle is injected through the same points as those in the distal two quadrants of the gastrocnemius but the needle is passed deeper and directed medially towards the axis of the limb in order to penetrate the muscle bulk.

Motor point injections of the hip adductors

It is easier to identify each of the three hip adductor muscles with the patient supine and both legs slightly abducted. The adductor brevis runs diagonally from the inferior pubic ramus to the lesser trochanter of the femur below the adductor longus. All the motor points of this muscle are concentrated in the proximal and middle thirds (Brash, 1955).

In more than 80% of subjects the neurovascular hilum of the adductor longus is found in the proximal two-thirds of the muscle (Brash, 1955). This roughly corresponds to the motor points of the adductor brevis and in adults lies approximately 7–8 cm below the pubic tubercle (which can be located by palpating the tendon of the adductor longus). Infiltration of the motor points of both muscles can, therefore, be achieved through insertion of the needle at this point. After injecting

3–4 ml of the neurolytic agent into the muscle belly of the adductor longus, the needle should be advanced to a depth of 4–5 cm to reach the adductor brevis where a further 3–4 ml of the drug is released.

The adductor magnus receives nerve supply mostly from the deep division of the obturator nerve by a variable number of branches which enter the muscle in the proximal and middle thirds. This area lies halfway between the site of the muscle origin and its insertion – i.e. the pubic tubercle and the medial femoral epicondyle, respectively. This is the optimal site for the motor point injection. However, if the patient can tolerate a second injection the treatment effect is often enhanced by the additional infiltration of the proximal third of the muscle. The superficial placement of the injection may result in the denervation of the gracilis muscle (which, in addition to thigh adduction, rotates the tibia medially).

A more simple technique of intramuscular neurolysis of the hip adductors is to infiltrate each of the four quadrants of the muscle bulk in the upper third of the medial aspect of the thigh (Carpenter & Seitz, 1980). Up to 20 ml of alcohol may be required for a good response. However, this method is less likely to be as effective as the motor point injection of individual muscles.

Motor point blocks of the hip flexors

The main hip flexor is the psoas major muscle. Fibres of this muscle arise from T12 and L1–L5 vertebrae and converge as they descend into the pelvis. The muscle tendon passes beneath the inguinal ligament to its site of insertion on the lesser trochanter of the femur. Adjacent to the anterior surface of the psoas major lie the kidney, ureters, renal vessels, the common and external iliac artery and vein. Consequently infiltration of the psoas major with alcohol or phenol can result in damage to the aforementioned retroperitoneal structures. Furthermore, rectal, vesical and sexual dysfunction following this procedure may result from damage of sympathetic and parasympathetic nerve fibres. However, these risks are reduced if the procedure is carried out under ultrasound monitoring (Koyama et al., 1992). With the patient in the lateral position the inferior pole of the kidney and the psoas muscle are identified from the back with the ultrasound probe at the level of L1–L4. The thickness and width of the muscle are then determined. The block is made in the medial part of the muscle near the vertebral body avoiding the lumbar and femoral arteries.

The therapeutic effects of chemical neurolysis

A number of factors contribute to the motor functional disability associated with long-standing upper motor neurone lesions. Although muscle spasticity may interfere with motor function, abnormalities of the descending neural control, re-organization of reflex activity at the spinal segmental level and changes in the contractile and visco-elastic properties of muscle fibres are also important in the pathogenesis of the poor motor performance in these patients.

The clinical effect of nerve blocks with phenol or alcohol on spasticity is usually evident with the onset of denervation approximately two weeks after the injection. However, an immediate transient effect due to the anaesthetic properties of these agents may be observed. The patient develops hypotonia of the appropriate muscle group and reduced resistance to passive stretch. The corresponding deep tendon reflexes are diminished or abolished and impairment or loss of skin sensation occurs with neurolysis of mixed sensory–motor nerves. Painful dysaesthesiae may also develop. In most cases the voluntary muscle strength is not affected, presumably because of a compensatory increase in the recruitment of motor units (the force generated by a muscle partially depends on the number of motor units recruited). An immediate increase in motor function following nerve blocks has been reported in some patients with residual muscle strength and in a few cases active movements which were not present before the blocks were observed (Copp et al., 1970).

The optimal concentration and dosage of the neurolytic agents

Chemical neurolysis is most effective when spasticity is the main cause of the functional disability and the clinical effect of treatment depends on the concentration and the volume of the injected neurolytic agent. Functional gains are also more likely to occur in patients who had selective motor control – i.e. the ability to move part of the limb at will, before treatment (Braun et al., 1973). Spasticity may be functionally beneficial – e.g. when a primitive extensor pattern is utilized for ambulation. In these circumstances partial nerve blocks may be desirable and it is often necessary to 'titrate' the dose of the neurolytic agent in order not to abolish the useful effect of spasticity.

Various concentrations and dosage schedules of phenol have been used. Generally, the effect of phenol when used in concentrations less than 4.5% seems to be modest and short lived. This clinical observation is consistent with laboratory evidence. Even at 1% concentration phenol resulted in degeneration of nerve fibres in experimental animals but this neurolytic effect was considerably less than that of 5% and 7.5% phenol.

No prospective comparative studies of the effectiveness of the different concentrations of neurolytic agents have been carried out to date. In a retrospective study Bakheit et al. (1996a) have found that 4.5% aqueous phenol was more effective than the 3% solution for obturator and medial popliteal nerve blocks. Using a functional assessment scale based on predetermined treatment goals which have been identified for each patient, the results of 56 nerve blocks in 28 patients were evaluated over a follow-up period of up to 18 months. The treatment goals were achieved in 89% of those treated with 4.5% phenol compared to 18% of those who received the drug in the 3% concentration. The duration of effect was also shorter with 3% phenol.

Tardieu et al. (1968) attempted to establish the optimal concentration of ethyl alcohol for peripheral nerve blocks. They found that the stepwise increase in the concentration of alcohol up to 45% progressively increased the effectiveness of the injection of a given volume of fluid but that no additional benefit resulted from further increases in concentration. Generally the effect of 50% alcohol in peripheral nerve blocks is comparable to that of 4.5% phenol in water (Bakheit et al., 1996b).

In a study of 36 patients who received a total of 50 nerve blocks with 2–3 ml of 5% phenol, improvement in muscle tone by two or three grades on the Ashworth scale was achieved in just over half the patients at one month and this effect was still maintained at two months in only two-thirds of the respondents (Gunduz et al., 1992). By contrast, when an average of 3.2 ml of 6.7% phenol (range 1–6 ml) was given per medial popliteal nerve block, good results were obtained in all of the 92 nerve blocks performed and only 22 of them (37.2%) were repeated during a mean follow-up period of 16.8 months (Petrillo & Knoploch, 1988). In most patients the beneficial effects of treatment last three to four months and the effectiveness of the injection diminishes when the procedure is repeated more than two or three times (Bakheit et al., 1996a).

Complications

Chemical neurolysis is generally safe and effective when it is carried out by a physician experienced in the procedure. By far the commonest complication is treatment failure. This is usually due to poor localization of the nerve, inadequate dose or concentration of the neurolytic agent or the presence of heterotopic ossification of the muscle being treated.

Complications directly resulting from the injection technique such as soft tissue injury are rare. Occasionally, intramuscular haematomas due to vascular injury complicate motor point blocks. There is also a small risk of damage to blood vessels with the neurolytic agents. This has occasionally led to the development of ischaemic gangrene of the upper limb. Surgical exploration and the direct injection of phenol or alcohol into the motor branches of mixed peripheral nerves in the upper limbs has been suggested to safeguard against this complication. However, the use of botulinum toxin injections is a preferred alternative treatment in these circumstances. Infection at the site of the injection is very rare, probably because of the antiseptic properties of the neurolytic agents. Nerve blocks of mixed sensory–motor nerves often result in severe impairment of skin sensation and increase the risk of burns and injury. Some patients also develop painful dysaesthesiae which are often transient. Interestingly, phenol is less likely than alcohol to cause dysaesthesiae when used for neurolysis of mixed sensory–motor nerves. Occasionally, paroxysmal lancinating pain similar to that of trigeminal neuralgia develops in the area of the nerve block, but it usually resolves spontaneously in 7–10 days.

Lumbar paravertebral nerve blocks are generally safe. In one series of 12 patients who received a total of 31 treatments (Meelhuysen et al., 1968) the only complication reported was constipation and faecal impaction in one subject.

Following motor point blocks, pain at the injection site and a transient burning sensation may develop but these are usually uncommon and transient. However, in some cases they may last up to three months or more. Treatment with transcutaneous electrical stimulation and/or tricyclic antidepressants is usually effective but, in severe cases refractory to these measures a further nerve block or even neurectomy may be necessary (Braun et al., 1973). Some patients develop transient local hyperaemia and tenderness lasting one or two days. Contrary to common belief, local tissue necrosis with subsequent fibrous tissue formation does not seem to occur frequently. In a study by Carpenter & Seitz (1980) of patients treated with 50% alcohol in doses of 2–6 ml, no fibrosis was found on muscle biopsy four to six weeks after the motor point injections.

Intrathecal block

Adminstration of phenol or alcohol into the intrathecal space is generally reserved for severe cases of lower limb spasticity refractory to other methods of treatment. It is usually associated with serious morbidity and should be avoided in subjects with reasonable bladder and bowel control. It is contra-indicated in ambulatory patients and those with reasonable prognosis for functional recovery.

Procedure

Lumbar intrathecal block is best carried out with the patient in the lateral position on a tilt table and the roots to be treated lower most. It is sometimes necessary to carry out the procedure under radiographic control, as severe spasticity may be associated with spinal deformity and distortion of the surface anatomical landmarks which are commonly used to determine the site of the lumbar puncture. A lumbar puncture is performed in the usual way and once the CSF starts to flow the needle is pointed upwards at an angle of 45° with the horizontal. The neurolytic agent is then injected and the patient is immediately returned to the lateral position and rocked gently to allow the drug to run into the nerve root sleeve. It is advisable that a test injection with 0.5 ml of a local anaesthetic is given to ensure the correct placement of the needle in the subarachnoid space. The patient usually reports tingling or skin sensory loss in the distribution of the blocked nerve root within 40 seconds of a successful injection.

When alcohol is used, the foot of the bed should be raised 45 cm and remain elevated for 24 hours to prevent diffusion of alcohol rostrally into the spinal cord and brain stem (alcohol is lighter than CSF). Absolute alcohol is injected at a rate of 1 ml per minute until the limb is completely flaccid. The total effective dose is usually 7–12 ml. Sometimes 5–10% phenol in glycerine is used instead of alcohol, but alcohol is preferred as its effect is usually more permanent than phenol (Merritt, 1981). If phenol is used, the foot of the bed is lowered (the specific gravity of phenol in glycerine is 1.25 compared to 1.007 for CSF). Phenol is then manoeuvred around the desired nerve roots by the careful positioning of the patient and tilting of the table. A useful guide is the distribution of anaesthesia, reduction in muscle tone and loss of tendon reflexes. The patient's position must remain unchanged for at least an hour after the phenol injection.

Complications

Intrathecal block is usually painless because of the immediate anaesthetic effect of the neurolytic agents. Some patients experience headaches and vomiting but these symptoms are usually self-limiting and often resolve in a few hours. Either alcohol or phenol in glycerine may be used for intrathecal block.

Intrathecal block is often complicated by loss of bladder and bowel control and it is generally thought that this procedure should be considered only in patients with complete paraplegia and no prospects of functional recovery. The possibility of destruction of the nerve fibres to the bladder and rectal sphincters is particularly high with neurolysis of L5, S1–S3 roots which is necessary for the treatment of hamstring muscle spasticity. The risk is less when the hip flexors and adductors (L1–L4 roots) are treated.

The loss of muscle tone in the lower limbs, which occurs following intrathecal blocks predisposes to thrombosis of leg and pelvic veins and increases the risk of pulmonary embolism. However, neither the incidence of deep vein thrombosis, nor the frequency of pulmonary thrombo-embolism following intrathecal blocks is known.

Summary

- Chemical neurolysis is only one method of treatment of muscle spasticity and the best clinical outcomes are achieved when it is utilized as part of the overall management strategy.
- A clear functional goal must be identified before treatment is given.

- Treatment is generally indicated for the relief of the distressing symptoms associated with spasticity, to improve motor function or to facilitate activities of daily living.
- Accurate placement of the injection is essential for successful nerve blocks. The use of an electrical stimulator with a needle probe is advisable.
- The optimal concentration of aqueous phenol and ethyl alcohol for nerve blocks appears to be 4.5% and 50% respectively; 4–5 ml of the solution may be necessary for a successful nerve block. The duration of effect is usually three to four months and the beneficial effects of treatment often diminish when the procedure is repeated more than two or three times.
- Nerve blocks should be avoided in the upper limbs because of the associated loss of skin sensation and the risk of vascular damage. Botulinum toxin is a useful alternative for the treatment of upper limb spasticity.

REFERENCES

Bakheit, A. M. O., Badwan, D. A. H. & McLellan, D. L. (1996a). The effectiveness of chemical neurolysis in the treatment of lower limb muscle spasticity. *Clin Rehabil*, **10**: 40–3.

Bakheit, A. M. O., McLellan, D. L. & Burnett, M. E. (1996b). Symptomatic and functional improvement of foot dystonia with medial popliteal nerve block. *Clin Rehabil*, **10**: 347–349.

Baxter, D. W. & Schacherl, U. (1962). Experimental studies on the morphological changes produced by intrathecal phenol. *Can Med Assoc J*, **86**: 1200–6.

Brash, J. C. (1955). *Neurovascular Hila of Limb Muscles*. Edinburgh: E. & S. Livingstone.

Braun, R. M., Hoffer, M. M., Mooney, V., McKeever, J. & Roper, B. (1973). Phenol nerve block in the treatment of acquired spastic hemiplegia in the upper limbs. *J Bone Joint Surg*, **55A**: 580–5.

Brown, A. S. (1958). Treatment of intractable pain by subarachnoid injection of carbolic acid. *Lancet*, **2**: 975–8.

Burkell, W. E. & McPhee, M. (1970). Effect of phenol injection into peripheral nerve of rat: electron microscope studies. *Arch Phys Med Rehabil*, **51**: 391–7.

Carpenter, E. B. (1983). Role of nerve blocks in the foot and ankle in cerebral palsy: therapeutic and diagnostic. *Foot Ankle*, **4**: 164–6.

Carpenter, E. B. & Seitz, D. G. (1980). Intramuscular alcohol as an aid in management of spastic cerebral palsy. *Develop Med Child Neurol*, **22**: 497–501.

Copp, E. P., Harris, R. & Kennan, J. (1970). Peripheral nerve block and motor point block with phenol in the management of spasticity. *Proc R Soc Med*, **63**: 937–8.

Felsenthal, G. (1974). Nerve blocks in the lower extremities: anatomic considerations. *Arch Phys Med Rehabil*, **55**: 504–7.

Ferrer-Brechner, T. & Brechner, V. L. (1976). The accuracy of needle placement during diagnostic and therapeutic nerve blocks. In *Advances on Pain Research and Therapy*, ed. J. J. Bonica et al., pp. 679–83. New York: Raven Press.

Gunduz, S., Kalyon, T. A., Hursun, H., Mohur, H. & Bilgic, F. (1992). Peripheral nerve block with phenol to treat spasticity in spinal cord injured patients. *Paraplegia*, **30**: 808–11.

Hatangdi, V. S. & Boas, R. A. (1975). Management of intractable pain – the scope and role of nerve blocks: review of one year's experience. *New Zealand Med J*, **81**: 45–8.

Katrak, P. H., Cole, A. M. D., Poulos, C. J. & McCauley, J. C. K. (1992). Objective assessment of spasticity, strength, and function with early exhibition of the dantrolene sodium after cerebro-vascular accident: a randomised double-blind study. *Arch Phys Med Rehabil*, **73**: 4–9.

Keenan, M. A. E., Tomas, E. S., Stone, L. & Gersten, L. M. (1990). Percutaneous phenol block of the musculocutaneous nerve to control elbow flexor spasticity. *J Hand Surg*, **2**: 340–6.

Khalili, A. A. & Betts, H. B. (1967). Peripheral nerve block with phenol in the management of spasticity. *JAMA*, **200**: 1155–7.

Koyama, H., Murakami, K., Suzuki, T. & Suzuki, K. (1992). Phenol block for hip flexor muscle spasticity under ultrasonic monitoring. *Arch Phys Med Rehabil*, **73**: 1040–3.

Maher, R. M. (1955). Relief of pain in incurable cancer. *Lancet*, **1**: 18–20.

Meelhuysen, F. E., Halpern, D. & Quast, J. (1968). Treatment of flexor spasticity of hip by para-vertebral lumbar spinal nerve block. *Arch Phys Med Rehabil*, **49**: 36–41.

Meritt, J. (1981). Management of spasticity in spinal cord injury. *Mayo Clin Proc*, **56**: 614–22.

Nathan, P. W., Sears, T. A. & Smith, M. C. (1965). Effects of phenol solutions on the nerve roots of the cat: an electrophysiological and histological study. *J Neurol Sci*, **2**: 7–29.

Petrillo, C. R. & Knoploch, S. (1988). Phenol block of the tibial nerve. *Int Disability Studies*, **10**: 97–100.

Rockswold, G. L. & Bradley, W. E. (1977). The use of sacral nerve blocks in the evaluation and treatment of neurologic bladder disease. *J Urol*, **118**: 415–17.

Tardieu, G., Tardieu, C., Hariga, J. & Gagnard, L. (1968). Treatment of spasticity by injection of dilute alcohol at the motor point or by epidural route. *Develop Med Child Neurol*, **10**: 555–68.

Torrens, M. J. (1974). The effect of selective sacral nerve blocks on vesical and urethral function. *J Urol*, **112**: 204–5.

Trainer, N., Bowser, B. L. & Dahm, L. (1986). Obturator nerve block for painful hip in adult cerebral palsy. *Arch Phys Med Rehabil*, **67**: 829–30.

9

The use of botulinum toxin in spasticity

Elizabeth C. Davis and Michael P. Barnes

Introduction

Botulinum toxin (BTX) is the most potent neurotoxin known to humans and its clinical effects have been recognized since the end of the nineteenth century. The toxin is produced by the Gram negative anaerobic bacterium, *Clostridium botulinum* and ingestion of it can produce the rare and often fatal paralytic illness, botulism. The paralytic effect of the toxin is due to blockade of neuromuscular transmission (Burgen et al., 1949). Injection of BTX into a muscle causes irreversible chemodenervation and local paralysis. It was this discovery which led to the development of the toxin as a therapeutic tool. It is now used clinically for a wide range of conditions (Jankovic, 1994).

There has been a burgeoning of interest in the medical use of BTX, particularly since its efficacy and safety have now been demonstrated. Its use in the management of spasticity is one of its more recent applications and this chapter reviews its mode of action and current therapeutic use in spasticity.

Clinical pharmacology

There are seven immunologically distinct serotypes of botulinum toxin (labelled A–G); the only type in routine clinical use is BTX type A (BTXA). This chapter focuses on the use of BTXA. However, investigations into the clinical use of type B (Tsui et al., 1995; Lew et al., 1997), type C (Eleopra et al., 1997) and type F (Ludlow et al., 1992; Greene & Fahn, 1993; Houser et al., 1998) are currently taking place. Type B botulinum toxin should soon have a European license and be available for clinical use.

Botulinum toxin acts selectively on peripheral cholinergic nerve endings to inhibit the release of acetylcholine. It also inhibits transmitter release from pre- and post ganglionic nerve endings of the autonomic system but it does not affect the synthesis or storage of acetylcholine. Following the binding, internalization and activation of the toxin in the presynaptic nerve terminals of the neuromuscular junction, there is chemical denervation. This process is temporary because the muscle is progressively reinnervated by nerve sproutings.

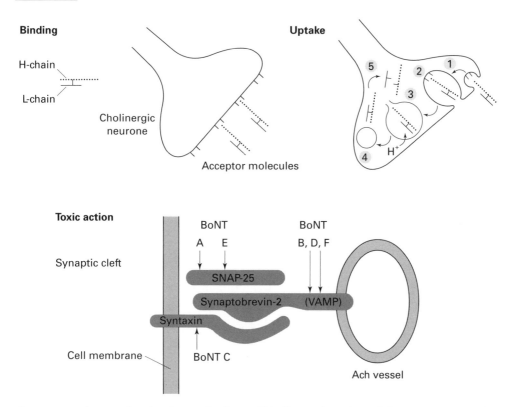

Binding

H-chain

L-chain

Cholinergic
neurone

Acceptor molecules

Uptake

Toxic action

BoNT
A E

BoNT
B, D, F

Synaptic cleft

SNAP-25

Synaptobrevin-2   (VAMP)

Syntaxin

Cell membrane

BoNT C

Ach vessel

Fig. 9.1   Diagram showing the mechanisms of binding and uptake and the toxic actions of the botulinum neurotoxins within the cholinergic nerve terminal. (Redrawn from *Handbook of Botulinum Treatment*, ed. P. Moore, p. 21. Oxford: Blackwell, 1995.)

The toxin is synthesized as a single polypeptide chain (molecular weight 150 kD). These molecules are relatively inactive until their structure is modified by cleavage into a light (50 kD) and a heavy (100 kD) chain which are linked by a disulphide bond.

Selective, high affinity binding of BTXA occurs at the presynaptic neurone of the neuromuscular junction. It is the C terminal of the heavy chain that determines cholinergic specificity and is responsible for this binding. After internalization, the disulphide bond is cleaved and the N terminal of the heavy chain promotes penetration and translocation of the light chain across the endosomal membrane into the cytosol. Here it interacts with, and cleaves the fusion protein SNAP 25 (synaptosomal associated protein) and inhibits the calcium mediated release of acetylcholine from the presynaptic nerve terminal, thereby weakening the muscle (Blasi et al., 1993). Chemical denervation is induced in both the alpha motor innervated extrafusal fibres and the gamma motor innervated intrafusal muscle fibre endings (Rosales et al., 1996). See Figure 9.1. Botulinum toxin types B and F act similarly, but cleave the fusion protein VAMP (vesicular associated membrane protein) and type C acts by cleaving syntaxin. This process is reversed within two to four months as a result of nerve sprouting and muscle reinnervation.

It is believed that the clinical effects of the toxin are due to the peripheral effects described above, however, retrograde axonal transport and intraspinal transfer of botulinum toxin have been shown in a mammalian model (Wiegand et al., 1976). This explanation is used with regard to the effects of the toxin that occur distant to the site of the injection.

There is a 24 to 72 hour delay between the administration of the toxin and the onset of clinical effects. This delay may be due to the time required for the enzymatic disruption of the acetylcholine release process by the toxin. The duration of response to BTXA is from two to six months and it is dependent on the dosage used, the condition being treated and the size and activity of the muscle injected. Adverse effects are primarily due to excessive weakening of the muscles being treated although there are reports of self-limiting fatigue, nausea, headache and fever (Greene et al., 1990). Unfortunately, immunoresistance to BTXA can also develop. The frequency of BTXA antibodies reported to occur varies from 3–5% (Zuber et al., 1993; Greene et al., 1994) with one study reporting 57% (Siatkowski et al., 1993). However, the latter were not specifically blocking antibodies and therefore did not affect the clinical response. Differences in antibody detection may relate to the methods used for their detection and it has been suggested that the only reliable method of detecting circulating neutralizing antibodies is by the mouse bioassay (Hatheway & Dang, 1994). It is not yet known in detail whether patients who develop secondary non-responsiveness to type A due to antibody formation will respond clinically to the other BTX types. However, there is now good evidence that type B toxin does have a positive effect in type A resistant people (Brin et al., 1999).

BTXA is commercially purified for clinical use and marketed as Dysport® (Ipsen) and Botox® (Allergan). A vial of Dysport® contains 500 units (1 unit = 0.025 ng) and a vial of Botox® contains 100 units (1 unit = 0.4 ng). However, there are significant differences between the observed potencies of these two distinct products in the clinical situation and suggestions of an equivalency ratio of Dysport®/Botox® ranging from 3:1 to 4:1 at standard vial dilutions have been made (Brin & Blitzer, 1993; Sampaio et al., 1997b; Odergren et al., 1998).

Botulinum toxin as a therapy for spasticity

BTXA was first used therapeutically for strabismus (Scott, 1979). It is now considered the treatment of choice in a variety of focal dystonias including blepharospasm (Jankovic & Schwartz, 1993), oromandibular dystonia (Brin et al., 1994), adductor spasmodic dysphonia (Truong et al., 1991; Whurr et al., 1993), cervical dystonia (Dauer et al., 1998), task specific dystonias (Tsui et al., 1993) and hemifacial spasm

(Jitpimolmard et al., 1998). In the last few years it has increasingly been recognized as an effective and useful tool for the treatment of spasticity.

Assessment

Prior to using botulinum toxin as a treatment for spasticity, it is important that there has been a full clinical assessment. This is necessary to ensure that any deformity which is present, can be reduced to some extent by slow passive extension. This is because the toxin is not able to free a joint that is fixed or stiff, nor in the main, is it believed that the toxin is able to lengthen muscles that are already shortened. It would therefore be an inappropriate use of resources to use BTXA in such cases. In some centres a physiotherapist and a medical doctor work together to carry out this assessment. The Spasticity Study Group have produced an algorithm for the use of botulinum toxin in adult onset spasticity (Brin & The Spasticity Group, 1997). This is a useful tool for any clinician intending to initiate the use of botulinum toxin as a therapy in the management of spasticity. It is also worthwhile establishing the objectives of treatment prior to its implementation. Examples of treatment goals include: the reduction of spasm frequency; the reduction of pain; to increase range of movement; to improve hygiene; to aid fitting of orthoses; to improve function; to delay or avoid surgery; to improve cosmesis; and to ease the burden on carers. Many of the studies discussed here do use some of these indices as outcome measures.

The injection technique

For the treatment of spasticity, botulinum toxin has to be injected into the involved muscles. The technique for injection is relatively simple – the toxin is diluted in normal saline and is then injected intramuscularly into the affected area.

The optimal site for injection into large muscles is unclear (Borodic et al., 1992). Using electromyography (EMG) as a guide in the identification and injection of the motor points of the muscle does not seem to convey any clinical advantage. One explanation is that the motor points, identified in this way, may be remote from the neuromuscular junction and the site of action of the botulinum toxin.

For this reason, although EMG is used for research purposes and in many of the studies cited in this chapter, it is not generally recommended in the clinical setting. In particular, it is not required if the muscles are easily identifiable and palpable.

Once injected, the toxin diffuses along the muscle planes. This process is dose dependent when the volume injected is fixed (Borodic et al., 1994). By giving the same dose in a larger volume, the spread of the toxin may be increased, despite a reduction in the concentration gradient. Practically, it appears that the effects of the toxin are more sensitive to the dose, rather than to the concentration of the toxin.

It has been suggested that multiple, small injections may be more effective than single injections (Park, 1995). Park also comments that if the muscle fibres are allayed in parallel, injections across the belly of the muscle may be most effective; in contrast injections along the length of the muscle may be more appropriate if the fibres are arranged longitudinally. However, there is no unequivocal evidence for these statements and further work in this area needs to be undertaken.

Botulinum toxin can be injected into a variety of muscle groups depending upon the clinical problem. For example, in the treatment of wrist and finger spasticity, the forearm flexor compartment is injected, in elbow flexion problems the biceps brachii and/or brachioradialis is injected. Other sites commonly injected include: the medial and lateral hamstrings for knee flexion difficulties; the gastrocnemii and posterior tibialis for spastic foot drop with inversion and plantarflexion of the foot; the hip adductors; and more recently the psoas group in hip flexion problems.

The dosage used varies considerably, depending upon the bulk of the muscle and the number of muscles to be injected. An average dose for unilateral injection of the leg adductors is 400–600 units of Dysport® (100–150 units Botox®). Some studies have also demonstrated that the effectiveness of doses varies considerably among patients (Pullman et al., 1996). The studies, which are discussed in this chapter, do use varying sites and dosage regimes and at present it is apparent that there is no universally accepted procedure for botulinum toxin injections in spasticity.

Clinical trials

The assessment of the efficacy and tolerability of BTXA in the treatment of spasticity is troublesome as other symptoms such as pain also influence outcome. The initial reports in the literature were difficult to compare as they included individuals with spasticity from varying aetiologies, with a variety of affected muscle groups and utilized a range of rating scales. Later studies, however, focus on more specific problems using homogeneous populations.

General use

Initial investigations into the use of BTXA in spasticity reported both subjective and objective improvements (Das & Park, 1989a,b). Six patients with severe stroke-related upper limb spasticity were injected into the biceps and forearm flexors using EMG guidance. The duration of effect in these cases was 16 weeks, the injections were well tolerated and there were no significant side-effects. The value of the toxin in reducing spasticity and helping to improve function was therefore recognized.

Several open-labelled studies went on to support these findings and to advocate the use of BTXA for the reduction of spasticity (Dengler et al., 1992; Memin et al., 1992; Hesse et al., 1992; Konstanzer et al., 1993; Dunne et al., 1995; Bhakta et al., 1996; Pullman et al., 1996; Sampaio et al., 1997a). Some of these use a heterogeneous population of cases including stroke, traumatic brain injury, MS (multiple sclerosis) and other causes of spasticity, and both upper and lower limbs were injected. Using such mixed samples makes it difficult to compare studies. Notwithstanding these difficulties, the use of the toxin in the management of spasticity is now well recognized (Hesse & Mauritz, 1997). Some of these series report benefits, in terms of spasticity, in all cases (Memin et al., 1992), while others describe improvements in terms of pain and hygiene (Konstanzer et al., 1993) and document no adverse effects. Others have used mixed populations while focusing on definite problems such as spastic foot drop (Dengler et al., 1992). Here, EMG guidance aided injection into the calf muscles and intensive physiotherapy was also utilized. Most cases showed improvement in some aspect of their problem but a side-effect of excessive muscle weakness was documented. However, the use of two treatment modalities in this study could arguably make interpretation of the results more difficult. Dunne looked at 40 patients with mixed diagnoses, and EMG guidance was employed for injections into both upper and lower limbs (Dunne et al., 1995). The results indicated that 85% of subjects derived worthwhile benefit in terms of posture and range of motion, pain reduction and increased function. The onset of action was four days with a peak effect at three weeks and an average duration of five months. The adverse effects included pain at the injection site, symptomatic weakness (one case) and local infection (one case). A placebo controlled cross-over study using BTXA (Grazko et al., 1995) in 12 patients demonstrated a significant reduction in tone, increase in function and ease of nursing care in eight of the cases. Five also benefited from alleviation of spasm. However, the sample was again mixed, with only three out of the 12 cases having spasticity secondary to stroke, and injections were given into both upper and lower limbs. The average duration of effect was two to four months and there were no reported side-effects.

Other reports lend support to the use of BTXA for obtaining functional improvements. In a retrospective analysis of 39 cases of spasticity secondary to a variety of pathologies, improvements in spasticity, range of motion, brace to tolerance, pain relief and subjective functional improvement were described (Pierson et al., 1996). In another series, BTXA improved the motor functional disability which is often associated with severe localized muscle spasticity (Watanabe et al., 1998). This mixed population included both adults and children.

Thus, in spasticity secondary to a number of aetiologies, BTXA appeared safe and effective in reducing spasticity and increasing function when injected into both upper and lower limbs. Further studies focused on spasticity secondary to specific causes, injecting specific muscle groups in order to provide more precise data.

Stroke

Open-label studies have investigated the use of BTXA in people with stroke-related upper limb spasticity and all support its use and provide evidence of its effectiveness in reducing muscle tone (Hesse et al., 1992; Bhakta et al., 1996; Sampaio et al., 1997a). The evidence regarding functional gains remains variable; one difficulty lies with the measurement of function.

Hesse found the use of higher dosages (1600 units of Dysport®) injected into a greater number of sites, using EMG guidance, to be most effective in reducing spasticity as rated on the Ashworth scale. If the spasticity was reduced, ease of personal care was reported to increase, although changes on the rating scales (Rivermead and Barthel) were not achieved.

Bhakta et al. (1996) and Sampio et al. (1997a) also studied the functional implications of using the toxin in spasticity secondary to stroke. Bhakta suggests that BTXA is safe and effective at reducing both disability and spasticity in those with severe upper limb spasticity. In this study, 17 patients with a non-functioning arm were assessed at baseline and two weeks after treatment; they were followed up until a loss of initial functional benefit was reported. Treatment consisted of a single course of injections into four upper limb muscle groups (biceps, and the hand and finger flexors) using one of the two preparations of BTXA. Outcome was assessed using the modified Ashworth scale, goniometer measurements and a rating scale based on a patient defined goals assessment. Significant improvements were obtained with regard to spasticity and range of movement, and overall 14 out of the 17 patients reported some functional benefit. The benefits were noted within two weeks and lasted from 1 to 11 months.

In contrast, Sampio confirmed improvements in spasticity but not in functional outcome. Nineteen patients were assessed at baseline, one week, and one, two and three months after treatment. EMG guidance was used in some cases and the hand and finger flexors were injected. A number of outcome tools were utilized including the Ashworth scale, passive joint mobility, spasm frequency, pain severity, Frenchay arm test and degree of satisfaction with functional outcome. The latter was only used on the final assessment. The results showed a significant improvement in spasticity, joint mobility and arm function. Disappointingly, two-thirds of this population rated their functional improvement as none or mild. Spasms and pain were not a significant problem in this group. The authors explain the discrepancy between the reduction in spasticity and lack of functional improvement as being related to the fact that only hand and finger flexors were injected, those with associated elbow flexion were therefore not completely treated and this would obviously affect their function.

A multicentre randomized, double-blind placebo controlled trial studied the use of the toxin in post-stroke severe upper extremity spasticity (Simpson et al., 1996). All 39 individuals, who were at least nine months post stroke, were randomized to receive either placebo or one of three different doses of the Botox® (75, 150, 300 units). EMG guidance was used for injecting into the elbow and wrist flexors. Only treatment with the highest dose resulted in a statistically significant mean decrease in muscle tone at two, four and six weeks after injection. These clinical and statistically significant improvements were derived from the Ashworth and global rating scales. There were no significant differences between placebo and treatment for motor functions, pain, caregiver dependency and competence in daily activities. The improvements peaked at two and lasted for six weeks with a return to baseline at 10 weeks. The highest dosing regime was found to be most effective and no serious adverse effects were documented. With regard to functional changes, the results of this study are not in accord with the results obtained in other series (Bhakta et al., 1996; Pierson et al., 1996) which do demonstrate an increased range of motion, facilitation of hand hygiene and improved motor function in stroke patients with a residual motor function.

The lack of demonstrable functional benefit was explained by the fact that most of the cases had a high function at baseline, with little scope for improvement and the global functional measures used may not have been sufficiently sensitive. It was thought that the standardized injection criteria meant that other involved muscles could not be treated thus limiting the functional gains. The authors comment that in an extension open label follow-up phase where additional affected muscles were injected, considerable functional gains were reported.

Many of the studies described above discuss the treatment of upper limb spasticity; however, lower limb problems have also been addressed. Following two open studies (Dengler et al., 1992; Hesse et al., 1994), a double-blind placebo controlled trial was conducted (Burbaud et al., 1996). Hesse specifically addressed lower limb extensor spasticity in 12 chronic hemiparetic patients. A statistically significant improvement on gait analysis parameters and a reduction in plantar flexion spasticity occurred when the calf muscles were injected under EMG guidance. The duration of effect was eight weeks. In the double-blind placebo controlled trial, 23 patients with spastic foot drop were injected into the calf muscles (soleus, gastrocnemius, tibialis posterior and flexor digitorum longus) under EMG guidance. A dose of 1000 units of Dysport® was used and a significant, clear subjective improvement in foot spasticity was reported after its administration. Significant changes on the Ashworth scale were also noted for ankle extensors, inverters and active ankle dorsiflexion. Gait velocity was slightly improved and the effects lasted for three months.

Recently studies have evaluated the efficacy of BTXA in combination with other treatment modalities (Reiter et al., 1998; Hesse et al., 1998). Reiter's group compared the effects of a combination of selective, lower dose (100 units of Botox®) BTXA injections into the tibialis posterior and ankle taping, with the currently used dose of toxin (190–320 units) into a number of calf muscles. Both groups showed a reduction in spasticity, as measured by the Ashworth scale. Although the duration of effect was less in the combination group, they both demonstrated increased gait velocity and step length and a change in the position of the foot, at rest and during passive movement. The only difference between the groups was less gain in passive dorsiflexion in the combination group. They concluded that both regimes were as effective in reducing foot inversion with a positive effect on the parameters of gait. This study supports previous suggestions that higher dosages of BTXA are more effective at correcting foot position and increasing the passive range of movements (Hesse et al., 1994; Dengler et al., 1992; Dunne et al., 1995; Burbaud et al., 1996). However, the specific problem of inversion can be satisfactorily controlled using the combination treatment. This may represent a more cost-effective approach to treating focal spasticity as suggested by Pierson et al. (1996). The use of smaller doses may also prevent the development of antibodies (Jankovic & Schwartz, 1995).

A randomized placebo controlled study assessed combination treatment with short-term electrical stimulation (Hesse et al., 1998). Four treatment groups were used in 24 stroke patients. Injections of either placebo or toxin (1000 units of Dysport®) into six upper limb flexor muscles was combined with additional electrical stimulation in two of the groups. The stimulation was given three times for half an hour for three days. Assessments of tone, limb position and difficulties with three upper limb motor tasks were carried out before, 2, 6, and 12 weeks after injection. Most improvements were seen in the combination group. Statistically significant improvement in palm cleaning occurred; differences in tone and placing the arm through a sleeve were noted. It was concluded that short-term electrical stimulation enhances the effectiveness of BTXA in the treatment of chronic upper limb flexor spasticity after stroke.

Overall, the evidence supports the use of BTXA in the treatment of post stroke spasticity. More work is needed to provide evidence on the efficacy with regard to functional gains. The optimal timing of the treatment, its dosage, the value of using combination approaches and the use of EMG remains to be clarified. Many of the reports highlight the need for detailed clinical evaluation and individualized treatment for achieving maximum benefits.

Multiple sclerosis

The beneficial effects of BTXA on focal spastic muscle contractions was demon-strated in a double-blind cross-over trial involving nine patients with chronic MS (Snow et al., 1990). Injections into the adductor muscle group resulted in a statis-tically significant reduction in spasticity (as measured by a spasm frequency score) and a statistically significant improvement in ease of nursing care (as measured by the hygiene score). Reports of decreased pain were also documented. There were no adverse effects with the standard dosage of 400 units of Botox®. Other uncon-trolled reports support these findings (Benecke, 1994). Here EMG-guided injec-tions into the adductor group resulted in decreased pain; benefits with regard to cleaning and catheterizing the patients were also noted. Again, the quantification of such benefits was noted to be problematical. The studies that use mixed cases often include spasticity secondary to MS (Konstanzer et al., 1993; Dunne et al., 1995; Grazko et al., 1995) and these lend further support regarding the effectiveness of botulinum toxin in decreasing lower limb spasticity in patients with MS.

Traumatic brain injury

There are few reports specifically addressing spasticity secondary to traumatic brain injury. In one open labelled study, 21 patients with severe spasticity in the wrist and finger flexors were injected using EMG guidance (Yablon et al., 1996). After the injections, passive range of movement exercises and casting were used as clinically indicated. Statistically significant improvements in the range of move-ment and spasticity (as measured by the modified Ashworth scale) were docu-mented in both the acutely (up to 12 months) and chronically (more than 12 months) injured. Although the use of BTXA was recommended the results of this study are confounded by the use of multiple forms of treatment.

The effect of the toxin on tone in the early stages of rehabilitation has also been evaluated (Pavesi et al., 1998). EMG guidance was used to inject into the upper limb muscles found to be contributing to the spasticity on clinical examination in six cases. Statistically significant improvements on the Ashworth scale and range of movements were found, and improvements in activities of daily living were also described. However, casting was also used and this may have confounded the result. A single subject kinesiological case study has demonstrated the efficacy of the toxin showing improvements in parameters on gait analysis (Wilson et al., 1997). Another case study (Palmer et al., 1998) also showed a significant reduction in tone and clonus with the use of toxin in lumbrical spasticity.

Together with the results from studies using heterogeneous samples including TBI (Dengler et al., 1992; Pierson et al., 1996; Watanabe et al., 1998), the use of BTXA in this condition is advocated. Although Pavesi et al. (1998) do recommend the earlier use of BTXA for optimal management, there is a need for more evidence in this area.

Spinal cord injury

A number of the earlier studies on spasticity management included cases of spinal cord injury (SCI) in the populations assessed. Although the numbers of such cases were small, there were no reported differences in their results compared with the other causes of spasticity (Dunne et al., 1995; Pierson et al., 1996; Watanbe et al., 1998).

A single case report describes functional gains when EMG-guided selective injection of BTXA was used in the hand muscles of a C5/6 incomplete spinal cord injury (Richardson et al., 1997). Certain functions were difficult to perform as a consequence of muscle imbalance. It was postulated that the use of BTXA in the agonists might allow improvements to occur in the antagonists. Functional goals were identified, and following treatment, gains were made in these areas; there was also a reduction in spasticity. Some resultant weakness did occur causing some functional losses but gains were made in the tasks originally identified. The improvements were sustained for 12 weeks.

This report suggests that the selective use of the toxin not only reduces spasticity but can help improve certain functions. The need for a multidisciplinary assessment and a clear definition of functional goals was emphasized.

Detrusor–sphincter–dyssynergia (DSD)

The involuntary contraction of the external urethral sphincter during the detrusor contraction is a particular problem in the high spinal cord injured patient and in other neurological conditions such as MS and will be included here as a form of spasticity. It results in voiding dysfunction and can lead to urological complications. Several treatments, including surgery are used and the use of BTXA has been evaluated. Some groups (Dykstra & Sidi, 1990; Schurch et al., 1996) showed that the toxin does relax the external urethral sphincter and reduce DSD in around 80% of cases. These studies used iterative injections (1–5 in one week/one month intervals) most of which were given cystoscopically. Others (Petit et al., 1998) showed a single cystoscopical injection of a lower dose of the toxin (150 units of Dysport®) to be effective. It significantly decreased the post voiding residual volume, the bladder pressure on voiding and the urethral pressure. This enabled an improvement in the modality of voiding. The effects lasted from two to three months and was well tolerated.

More recently, the use of a transperineal injection in five tetraplegic patients was shown to be effective in improving bladder function and reducing residual volumes (Gallien et al., 1998). Autonomic dysreflexia also decreased in intensity. The results

for this less invasive technique, using 100 units of Botox® also support consideration of the toxin as treatment for DSD. A controlled double-blind study is required
to substantiate these results.

Conclusions

The usefulness of BTXA in the management of spasticity secondary to a variety of
clinical conditions is increasing. Its use for the treatment of a number of movement
disorders is now well accepted (Jankovic & Brin, 1991) and it is licensed for the
treatment of blepharospasm, hemifacial spasm and cervical dystonia. It has
recently been licensed for use in equinus foot spasticity in cerebral palsy. Other
applications continue to be explored and it is likely that its use will increase.

It is increasingly being used for the management of focal spasticity, secondary to
a number of aetiologies, in the adult and in childhood cerebral palsy. It has been
suggested that functional benefits may be enhanced with careful patient selection
and individualized treatment. Although currently only licensed for use for spasticity secondary to cerebral palsy, it is increasingly being used clinically for the other
causes of spasticity. However, the indication for use in these categories remains
unlicensed.

The advantages of treatment with botulinum toxin over other forms of local
treatment can be listed as follows:
- Simplicity of injection technique.
- Lack of requirement for precise localization of motor end points.
- Absence of a sensory disturbance.
- Ease of dose adjustment according to previous response.
- Reversibility of overall effect after two to three months of treatment.
- Paucity of systemic side effects.

Its reversible yet long lasting action, ease of administration, favourable safety
and adverse effect profile are factors that contribute to its usefulness. Its safety
and efficacy are well established (National Institutes of Health Consensus
Development Conference, 1991) but the optimal time to initiate treatment, the
optimal dosage and the potential for combination treatment approaches need more
research. The average duration of effect is three months.

There are however a number of disadvantages including the cost, the need for
repeat injections and the potential for the development of antibodies. The cost of the
toxin is significant and is therefore a major limitation to the use of botulinum toxin.
With more widespread usage and increasing indications for use, it will begin to have
a more significant impact upon purchasers of health services. This is a problem now
in some parts of the UK and abroad and is likely to be more of a problem in the
future. The need for repeat injections at approximately three-monthly intervals will

mean that botulinum clinics will slowly but steadily increase with regard to the numbers of attendees. The botulinum clinic in Newcastle upon Tyne, UK, for example, started in 1992 as a monthly clinic run by one consultant in Rehabilitation Medicine/Neurology, but has grown to a clinic three times a week each run with the involvement of three doctors. One solution is the development of an outreach nurse practitioner who can be trained to inject either in an outpatient department or at the patient's home. A study in Newcastle upon Tyne has shown a nurse practitioner to be as efficacious and safe as the medical practitioners and able to provide a service that is much more appreciated by the patients given the increased time for consultation and increased flexibility of a home visiting system (Whitaker et al., 2000). This was, however, for the treatment of dystonia.

Another disadvantage is the possibility of the development of antibodies. Although so far there has been no evidence of a diminishing response to the effect of botulinum toxin with years of treatment (Jankovic & Schwartz, 1993), the problem of immunoresistance may increase with the more widespread use of BTXA. However, treatment with other immunologically distinct serotypes may overcome this (Greene & Fahn, 1993). It is therefore important that research into the development of other serotypes continues such that effective relief from clinically treatable conditions can be maintained in the future.

Clinicians should be aware of its mode of action, the local anatomy of the area to be injected, the potential side effects that are usually related to local weakness, and the potential contra-indications to treatment. The latter include myasthenia gravis, Lambert Eaton Syndrome, pregnancy and the use of aminoglycoside antibiotics.

The use of botulinum toxin for spasticity caused by a variety of neurological disorders is continuing to be investigated. In the future, clearly defined treatment goals should be outlined, and regular assessments, using reliable and valid measures should be made in an effort to improve clinical outcome. Botulinum toxin has been shown to be safe and efficacious for a wide range of spasticity related problems and it is becoming an increasingly important tool for the clinician involved in the management of this disabling condition.

REFERENCES

Benecke, R. (1994). Botulinum toxin for spasms and spasticity in the lower extremities. In *Therapy with Botulinum Toxin*, ed. J. Jankovic & M. Hallett, pp. 557–65. New York: Marcel Dekker.

Bhakta, B. B., Cozens, J. A., Bamford, J. M. & Chamberlain, M. A. (1996). Use of botulinum toxin in stroke patients with severe upper limb spasticity. *J Neurol Neurosurg Psychiatry*, **61**: 30–5.

Blasi, J., Chapman, E., Link, E. et al. (1993). Botulinum neurotoxin A selectively cleaves the synapse protein SNAP-25. *Nature*, **265**: 160–3.

Borodic, G. E., Ferrante, R., Pearce, B. L. & Smith, K. (1994). Histologic assessment of dose-related diffusion and muscle fiber response after therapeutic botulinum-A toxin injections. *Mov Disord*, **9**: 31–9.

Borodic, G. E., Ferrante, R., Wiegner, A. W. & Young, R. R. (1992). Treatment of spasticity with botulinum toxin. *Ann Neurol*, **31**: 113.

Brin, M. F. & Blitzer, A. (1993). Botulinum toxin: dangerous errors (letter). *J R Soc Med*, **86**: 493–4.

Brin, M. F., Blitzer, A., Herman, S. & Stewart, C. (1994). Oromandibular dystonia: treatment of 96 patients with Botulinum Toxin Type A. In *Therapy with Botulinum Toxin*, ed. J. Jankovic & M. Hallet, pp. 429–35. New York: Marcel Dekker.

Brin, M. F., Lew, M. F., Adler, C. H. et al. (1999). Safety and efficacy of Neurobloc (botulinum toxin type B) in type A resistant cervical dystonia. *Neurology*, **53**: 1431–8.

Brin, M. F. and the Spasticity Study Group (1997). Dosing, administration, and a treatment algorithm for use of botulinum toxin A for adult-onset spasticity. *Muscle Nerve*, **20** (Suppl. 6): S208–S220.

Burbaud, P., Wiart, L., Dubos, J. L. et al. (1996). A randomized, double blind, placebo controlled trial of botulinum toxin in the treatment of spastic foot in hemiparetic patients. *J Neurol Neurosurg Psychiatry*, **61**: 265–9.

Burgen, A. S. V., Dickens, F. & Zatman, L. J. (1949). The action of botulinum toxin on the neuromuscular junction. *J Physiol*, **109**: 10–24.

Das, T. K. & Park, D. M. (1989a). Botulinum toxin in treating spasticity. *Br J Clin Pract*, **43**: 401–2.

Das, T. K. & Park, D. M. (1989b). Effect of treatment with botulinum toxin on spasticity. *Postgrad Med J*, **65**: 208–10.

Dauer, W. T., Burke, R. E., Greene, P. & Fahn, S. (1998). Current concepts on the clinical features, aetiology and management of idiopathic cervical dystonia. *Brain*, **121**: 547–60.

Dengler, R., Neyer, U., Wohlfarth, K., Bettig, U. & Janzik, H. H. (1992). Local botulinum toxin in the treatment of spastic foot drop. *J Neurol*, **239**: 375–8.

Dunne, J. W., Heye, N. & Dunne, S. L. (1995). Treatment of chronic limb spasticity with botulinum toxin A. *J Neurol Neurosurg Psychiatry*, **58**: 232–5.

Dykstra, D. D. & Sidi, A. A. (1990). Treatment of detrusor–sphincter–dyssynergia with botulinum A toxin: a double blind study. *Arch Phys Med Rehab*, **71**: 24–6.

Eleopra, R., Tugnoli, V., Rossetto, O., Montecuccu, C. & De Grandis, D. (1997). Botulinum neurotoxin serotype C: a novel effective botulinum toxin therapy in human. *Neurosci Lett*, **224**: 91–4.

Gallien, P., Robineau, S., Verin, M., Le Bot M. P., Nicholas, B. & Brissot, R. (1998). Treatment of detrusor–sphincter–dyssynergia by transperineal injection of botulinum toxin. *Arch Phys Med Rehab*, **79**: 715–17.

Grazko, M. A., Polo, K. B. & Bhaman, J. (1995). Botulinum toxin for spasticity, muscle spasms, and rigidity. *Neurology*, **45**: 712–17.

Greene, P. E. & Fahn, S. (1993). Use of Botulinum toxin type F injections to treat Torticollis in patients with immunity to botulinum toxin type A. *Mov Disord*, **8**: 479–83.

Greene, P., Fahn, S. & Diamond, B. (1994). Development of resistance to Botulinum toxin type A in patients with Torticollis. *Mov Disord*, **9**: 213–17.

Greene, P., Kang, U., Fahn, S., Brin, M., Moskowitz, C. & Flaster E. (1990). Double blind placebo controlled trial of botulinum toxin injections for the treatment of spasmodic torticollis. *Neurology*, **40**: 1213–18.

Hatheway, C. L. & Dang, C. (1994). Immunogenicity of the neurotoxins of *Clostridium botulinum*. In *Therapy with Botulinum Toxin*, ed. J. Jankovic & M. Hallet, pp. 93–108. New York: Marcel Dekker.

Hesse, S., Friedrich, H., Domasch, C. & Mauritz, K. H. (1992). Botulinum toxin therapy for upper limb spasticity: preliminary results. *J Rehab Sci*, **5**: 98–101.

Hesse, S., Lucke, D., Malezic, M., Bertelt, C., Friedrich, H., Gregoric, M. & Mauritz, K. H. (1994). Botulinum toxin treatment for lower limb extensor spasticity in chronic hemiparetic patients. *J Neurol Neurosurg Psychiatry*, **57**: 1321–4.

Hesse, S. & Mauritz, K. H. (1997). Management of spasticity. *Curr Opin Neurol*, **10**: 498–501.

Hesse, S., Reiter, F., Konrad, M. & Jahnke, M. T. (1998). Botulinum toxin type A and short term electrical stimulation in the treatment of upper limb flexor spasticity after stroke: a randomized, double blind, placebo controlled trial. *Clin Rehab*, **12**: 381–8.

Houser, M. K., Sheean, G. L. & Lees, A. J. (1998). Further studies using higher doses of botulinum toxin type F for torticollis resistant to botulinum toxin type A. *J Neurol Neurosurg Psychiatry*, **64**: 577–580.

Jankovic, J. (1994). Botulinum toxin in movement disorders. *Curr Opin Neurol*, **7**: 358–66.

Jankovic, J. & Brin, M. F. (1991). Therapeutic uses of botulinum toxin. *N Engl J Med*, **3224**: 1186–94.

Jankovic, J. & Schwartz, K. (1993). Longitudinal experience with botulinum toxin injections for treatment of blepharospasm and cervical dystonia. *Neurology*, **43**: 834–6.

Jankovic, J. & Schwartz, K. (1995). Response and immunoresistance to botulinum toxin injections. *Neurology*, **45**: 1743–6.

Jitpimolmard, S., Tiamkao, S. & Laopaiboon, M. (1998). Long-term results of botulinum toxin type A (Dysport) in the treatment of hemifacial spasm: a report of 175 cases. *J Neurol Neurosurg Psychiatry*, **64**: 751–7.

Konstanzer, A., Ceballos-Baumann, A. O., Dressnandt & Conrad, B. (1993). Botulinum toxin A treatment in spasticity of arm and leg. *Nervenarzt*, **64**: 517–52.

Lew, M. F., Adornato, B. T., Duane, D. D. et al. (1997). Botulinum toxin type B (BotB): a double blind, placebo controlled, safety and efficacy study in cervical dystonia. *Neurology*, **49**: 701–7.

Ludlow, C. L., Hallett, M., Rhew, K. et al. (1992). Therapeutic uses of Type F botulinum toxin (letter). *N Engl J Med*, **326**: 349–50.

Memin, B., Pollak, P., Hommel, M. & Perret, J. (1992). Treatment of spasticity with botulinum toxin. *Rev Neurol (Paris)*, **148**: 212–14.

National Institutes of Health Consensus Development Conference. Clinical Use of Botulinum toxin. *Arch Neurol*, **48**: 1294–8.

Odergren, T., Hjaltson, H., Kaakkola, S. et al. (1998). A double blind, randomised, parallel group study to investigate the dose equivalence of Dysport® and Botox® in the treatment of cervical dystonia. *J Neurol Neurosurg Psychiatry*, **64**: 6–12.

Palmer, D. T., Horn, L. J. & Harmon, R. L. (1998). Botulinum toxin treatment of lumbrical spasticity: a brief report. *Am J Phys Med Rehabil*, **77**: 348–50.

Park, D. M. (1995). Spasticity in adults. In *Handbook of Botulinum Toxin Treatment*, ed. P. Moore, pp. 209–21. Oxford: Blackwell Science.

Pavesi, G., Brianti, R., Medici, D., Mammi, P., Mazzucchi, A. & Mancia, D. (1998). Botulinum toxin type A in the treatment of upper limb spasticity among patients with traumatic brain injury (letter). *J Neurol Neurosurg Psychiatry*, **64**: 419–20.

Petit, H., Wiart, L., Gaujard, E. et al. (1998). Botulinum A toxin treatment for detrusor–sphincter–dyssynergia in spinal cord disease. *Spinal Cord*, **36**: 91–4.

Pierson, S. H., Katz, D. I. & Tarsy, D. (1996). Botulinum A toxin in the treatment of spasticity: functional implications and patient selection. *Arch Phys Med Rehab*, **77**: 717–21.

Pullman, S. L., Greene, P., Fahn, S. & Pederson, S. F. (1996). Approach to the treatment of limb disorders with Botulinum toxin A. Experience with 187 patients. *Arch Neurol*, **53**: 617–24.

Reiter, F., Lagalla, G., Ceravolo, G. & Provinciali, L. (1998). Low dose botulinum toxin with taping for the treatment of spastic equinovarus foot after stroke. *Arch Phys Med Rehab*, **79**: 532–5.

Richardson, D., Edwards, S., Sheean, G. L., Greenwood, R. J. & Thompson, A. J. (1997). The effect of botulinum toxin on hand function after incomplete spinal cord injury at the level of C5/6: a case report. *Clin Rehab*, **11**: 288–92.

Rosales, R., Arimura, K., Takenaga, S. & Osame, M. (1996). Extrafusal and intrafusal muscle effects in experimental botulinum toxin A injection. *Muscle Nerve*, **19**: 488–96.

Sampaio, C., Ferreira, J. J., Pinto, A. A., Crespo, M., Ferro, J. M. & Castro-Caldas, A. (1997a). Botulinum toxin type A for the treatment of arm and hand spasticity in stroke patients. *Clin Rehab*, **11**: 3–7.

Sampaio, C., Ferreira, J. J., Simoes, F. et al. (1997b) A. DYSBOT: a single blind, randomized parallel study to determine whether any differences can be detected in the efficacy and tolerability of the formulations of botulinum toxin type A-Dysport and Botox assuming a ratio of 4:1. *Mov Disord*, **12**: 1013–18.

Schurch, B., Hauri, D., Rodic, B., Curt, A., Meyer, E. & Rossier, A. B. (1996). Botulinum A toxin as a treatment of detrusor–sphincter–dyssynergia: a prospective study in 24 spinal cord injury patients. *J Urol*, **155**: 1023–9.

Scott, A. B. (1979). Botulinum toxin injection into extraocular muscles as an alternative to strabismus surgery. *Ophthalmology*, **87**: 1044–9.

Siatkowski, R. M., Tyotyunikow, A. & Biglan, A. W. (1993). Serum antibody production to Botulinum A toxin. *Ophthalmology*, **100**: 1861–6.

Simpson, D. M., Alexander, D. N., O'Brien, C. F. et al. (1996). Botulinum toxin type A in the treatment of upper extremity spasticity: a randomized, double blind, placebo controlled trial. *Neurology*, **46**: 1306–1310.

Snow, B. J., Tsui, J. K. C., Bhatt, M. H., Varelas, M., Hashimoto, S. A. & Calne, D. B. (1990). Treatment of spasticity with botulinum toxin: a double blind study. *Ann Neurol*, **28**: 512–15.

Truong, D. D., Rontal, M., Rolnick, M., Aronson, A. E. & Mistura, K. (1991). Double-blind controlled study of botulinum toxin in adductor spasmodic dysphonia. *Laryngoscope*, **101**: 630–4.

Tsui, J. K. C., Bhatt, M., Calne, S. & Calne, D. B. (1993). Botulinum toxin in the treatment of writer's cramp: a double-blind study. *Neurology*, **43**: 183–5.

Tsui, J. K. C., Hayward, M., Mak, E. K. M. & Schulzer, M. (1995). Botulinum Toxin type B in the treatment of cervical dystonia: a pilot study. *Neurology*, **45**: 2109–10.

Watanabe, Y., Bakheit, A. M. O. & McLellan, D. L. (1998). A study of the effectiveness of botulinum toxin type A (Dysport) in the management of muscle spasticity. *Disabil Rehabil*, **20**: 62–5.

Whitaker, J., Butler, A., Semylen, J. & Barnes, M. P. (2000). Botulinum toxin for people with dystonia treated by an outreach nurse practitioner. *Arch Phys Med Rehabil*. (In press.)

Whurr, R., Lorch, M., Fontana, H., Brookes, G., Lees, A. & Marsden, C. D. (1993). The use of botulinum toxin in the treatment of adductor spasmodic dysphonia. *J Neurol Neurosurg Psychiatry*, **56**: 526–30.

Wiegand, H., Erdmann, G. & Wellhoner, H. H. (1976). [125] I-Labelled botulinum A neurotoxin: pharmacokinetics in cats after intramuscular injection. *Arch Pharmacol*, **292**: 161–5.

Wilson, D. J., Childers, M. K., Cooke, D. L. & Smith, B. K. (1997). Kinematic changes following botulinum toxin injection after traumatic brain injury. *Brain Inj*, **11**: 157–67.

Yablon, S. A., Agana, B. T., Ivanhoe, C. B. & Boake, C. (1996). Botulinum toxin in severe upper extremity spasticity among patients with traumatic brain injury: an open labeled trial. *Neurology*, **47**: 939–44.

Zuber, M., Sebald, M., Bathien, N., De Recondo, J. & Rondot, P. (1993). Botulinum antibodies in dystonic patients treated with type A botulinum toxin: frequency and significance. *Neurology*, **43**: 1715–18.

10

Intrathecal baclofen for control of spinal and supraspinal spasticity

David N. Rushton

Introduction

Intrathecal baclofen (ITB)

Penn and Kroin in 1985 first described the benefits to be obtained from long-term infusion of baclofen into the spinal subarachnoid space, with their report of the treatment of six patients with severe continuing spasticity and spasms resulting from spinal injury or demyelinating diseases. They found a dramatic dose-related benefit which was highly valued by patients, who reported functional improvements in their activities of daily living and reduced discomfort, as well as improvement in sleep patterns, continence and nocturia. Voluntary power did not improve, but one patient in the initial series was enabled to walk, provided the dose was carefully titrated so that her spasticity and spasms were controlled, while some lower limb rigidity remained. The authors found that the optimum dose varied widely, and that the effects were strongly dose-related. There was evidence of some drug tolerance; during the first few months the average daily dose rose from 100–150 µg to something less than 500 µg. Because they were so much improved, patients were unwilling to take part in controlled trials involving placebo infusions. All of the significant findings put forward in this initial report have been amply confirmed during the following years, in subsequent larger and longer trials undertaken by the same authors and in many other centres. Although the initial and many subsequent trials were open, double-blind randomized placebo-controlled trials of intrathecal baclofen (ITB) have more recently been conducted in spinal spasticity, finding the same magnitude of benefit (Ordia et al., 1996).

Pharmacology of baclofen

Baclofen and gamma-aminobutyric acid (GABA)

Baclofen is an agonist to the bicuculline-insensitive variety of GABA receptor, known as $GABA_B$. There is a high density of $GABA_B$ receptors in the dorsal horn, particularly in lamina II (substantia gelatinosa) and III. Unlike the $GABA_A$ receptor, $GABA_B$ is not a complete ionic channel, but is coupled indirectly to calcium (Ca^{2+}) channels. Activation of presynaptic $GABA_B$ receptors therefore causes an inhibition of calcium-mediated inward current, so inhibiting the release of excitatory neurotransmitters such as aspartate and glutamate in the polysynaptic pathways of the dorsal horn. This alters and reduces the excitability of monosynaptic and polysynaptic reflexes. Baclofen is thought also to exert a postsynaptic action which also acts to reduce reflex excitability (Azouvy et al., 1993). This may be the basis of its reduction of H-reflex amplitude in patients with spinal lesions.

Baclofen and pain

Perhaps not surprisingly given its site of action, there is also pharmacological evidence that baclofen exerts anti-nociceptive effects. These are not mediated by opiate receptors and are not antagonized by naloxone. There is evidence of a carbamazepine-like suppression of excitatory neurotransmission in the cat trigeminal nucleus, and baclofen has been used successfully in the clinical treatment of trigeminal neuralgia (Fromm et al., 1992).

Pharmacokinetics of intrathecal baclofen

Baclofen in cerebrospinal fluid (CSF)

Baclofen is hydrophilic and crosses the blood–brain barrier poorly so that spinal intrathecal administration, which bypasses the blood–brain barrier, allows effective treatment of spasticity with a dose range that is 100–1000 times smaller than that required for oral treatment. It also allows a higher baclofen concentration to be achieved in the spinal cord than in the brain, because of the characteristics of the circulation of the CSF from the ventricles to the spinal subarachnoid space. The effective distribution volume of intrathecally-administered baclofen approximates to the volume of spinal CSF (about 75 ml), rather than total CSF volume. This explains why more effective treatment of spasticity of limbs and trunk is possible, without side-effects resulting from central actions of baclofen on the brain.

Localization of ITB

When the catheter is placed at lumbar level, the concentration of baclofen in the lumbar CSF is several times higher than at cervical level (Kroin & Penn, 1992), so it is possible preferentially to address spasticity in the lower limbs. Nevertheless, spinal CSF mixes quite quickly, while baclofen being hydrophilic penetrates the spinal cord tissue slowly, so that the response is always more widespread than the location of the catheter tip. The clinical response to a bolus infusion or injection of baclofen into the spinal theca suggests that the drug takes about one hour to diffuse to the relevant locations in the substantia gelatinosa of the cord.

Excretion of ITB

The plasma levels of baclofen in patients undergoing intrathecal infusion have been found to be vanishingly low (Muller et al., 1988). This is simply because the quantity is so small; intrathecal baclofen, like orally administered baclofen, is not metabolized, but is mainly excreted unchanged in the urine.

Neurophysiological effects of ITB

Spasticity

Spasticity has been defined (Lance, 1980) neurophysiologically as a

'motor disorder characterised by a velocity-dependent increase in tonic stretch reflexes (muscle tone) with exaggerated tendon jerks, resulting from hyperexcitability of the stretch reflex, as one component of the upper motor neurone syndrome.'

Unfortunately, the changes classified clinically as spasticity also often include components which when examined electromyographically are found not to be stretch-reliant, and which often accompany stretch-sensitive responses.

Spasticity score

ITB reduces spasticity as clinically assessed using the Ashworth scale, which in its modified form and in defined circumstances is a reliable six-point scale of spastic increase in tone (Bohannon & Smith, 1987). It should not be used in the presence of dystonia, rigidity or extrapyramidal disorders, and it cannot be used to assess hypotonia. ITB has been found to result in a diminution of two points or more in Ashworth scores, in spasticity of both spinal and supraspinal origin (discussed below).

Spasm score

Flexion or extension spasms, more common in the lower limbs, may occur spontaneously or in response to cutaneous stimuli in spasticity. The clinical spasm frequency score is a five-point scale of self-reported spasm frequency; it has been found to respond in a dose-related and predictable way to ITB (Penn et al., 1989).

Flexion reflex excitability

The threshold of the electrically-induced flexion reflex in the lower limb (stimulate sural nerve, record biceps femoris using electromyography) has been found to be reduced in spinal spasticity, and the response amplitude to be increased. The response is normalized in some cases with ITB, a change which did not necessarily correlate with changes in Ashworth or spasm frequency scores (Parise et al., 1997).

Anterior horn cell excitability

The effect of ITB on the anterior horn cell in spasticity has been assessed using F-wave amplitude as an index. The F-wave is usually of low threshold, increased amplitude and increased duration in spasticity. Latency is not significantly abnormal. The abnormal F-wave amplitude and duration was found to be reduced by 40–80% following ITB, either as a bolus or a continued infusion (Dressandt et al., 1995).

Effects of ITB on function and quality of life

Functional Independence Measure (FIM)

In one study series (Albright et al., 1995), average FIM scores rose during the post-implantation follow-up period by 18 points; in those with good upper limb function the rise was larger (25 points) and covered most of the items apart from eating and stairs; in those with poor upper limb function the rise was less (4.8), and mainly focused on eating and wheelchair function. However, comfort was improved, nursing easier and care burden reduced.

Quality of life

Patients who previously had been institutionalized on account of spasticity are often enabled to return to live in the community following the start of ITB. In one study (Becker et al., 1995), a group of nine patients who had between them spent 755 days in acute care hospitals during the year before implantation, spent only 259 days in hospital during the year after surgery. A larger randomized placebo-controlled multicentre trial of 22 patients (Middel et al., 1997) examined the response on the sickness impact profile (SIP) and the Hopkins symptom checklist (HCSL). After three months of randomized placebo-controlled study, all patients were switched to ITB. After one year there were moderate but significant benefits of ITB on some dimensions of the SIP ('mobility'; 'body care and movement'), and of health behaviour ('sleep and rest'; 'recreation and pastimes'), but not in psychosocial behaviour, in comparison with the pre-operative condition.

Cost-benefit analysis

There have been few studies of the cost-benefit impact of ITB. A comparison of ITB and selective functional posterior rhizotomy over one year in 19 children with cerebral palsy showed that the cost of ITB was nearly four times higher (Albright et al., 1995). No attempt was made to compare the efficacy of the two treatment methods.

Indications and patient screening for ITB

General considerations

ITB may affect function, care or comfort; it may help more than one of these, and occasionally it may benefit all three. However, it is an elaborate, invasive and expensive form of treatment. It calls for regular follow-up for pump refills, which have to be done several times a year. The pump itself, if it is battery powered and not rechargeable, has to be replaced every five to six years. It is therefore fortunate that only a minority of patients with spasticity require ITB. Which ones are they?

Indications for ITB

ITB is used in patients with widespread spasticity, in whom alternative methods of management of their spasticity are ineffective or inadequate, or cause unacceptable side-effects. In all patients with spasticity, remediable aggravating factors such as urinary retention or infection, skin infection or pressure sores, uncomfortable seating and poor posture will have been addressed in their own right. Passive muscle stretching, active physiotherapy, hydrotherapy and active exercise all are important aids to controlling and minimizing spasticity, particularly during the stage when spasticity is developing. Oral anti-spastic agents such as baclofen, dantrolene, diazepam or tizanidine will have been introduced and titrated to find the optimum drug combination and dose range. This leads to a protocol whereby ITB is considered only in those patients in whom severe spasticity has developed in spite of preventive measures, and who cannot be adequately controlled in any less invasive way.

Alternatives to ITB in widespread spasticity

In many centres dealing with patients with severe spasticity, the use of unselective dorsal rhizotomy and intrathecal phenol as treatments for spasticity have been largely supplanted by ITB. Unselective rhizotomy often results in significant loss of sensory function, and non-reflex spasticity and spasms may recur. The effects of intrathecal phenol are found to be unpredictable in all but the most experienced hands, and it can be used only in patients who have already lost bladder and bowel control. Selective posterior rhizotomy has been used extensively at some centres for the treatment of spasticity, particularly in cerebral palsy. It has been compared with ITB in one centre, and found to be about equally effective; relative indications for one or the other form of treatment have been described (Albright et al., 1995). Epidural spinal stimulator implants are used, often in patients who have pain as well as spasticity, although the efficacy has not been compared with ITB (Barolat et al., 1995). Cerebellar stimulation is used for control of spasticity, and found to be effective particularly in cerebral palsy, but again no comparison with ITB for efficacy has been made (Sutcliffe, 1997).

Indications for botulinum toxin

Patients whose spasticity is focal and involves accessible muscles will have been offered local treatments such as intramuscular botulinum toxin, and are usually better managed in that way. Some patients with focal spasticity are managed with nerve blocks, but neuro-destructive injections are much less used now that botulinum toxin is available.

Implantation techniques and precautions

Trial dose

A trial dose of ITB is done for two reasons. Firstly, it is necessary to demonstrate that ITB will make a significant impact on the level of spasticity and spasms. Secondly, it is necessary to demonstrate that it will as a result significantly benefit function, comfort or hygiene. In order to achieve these demonstrations, the patient must be taken through a functional assessment as well as bedside tests of tone and spasms. The patient must therefore be mobilized, into walking or wheelchair as appropriate, during the action of the single intrathecal dose, which typically lasts for several hours. The period of bedrest following the lumbar puncture must therefore be not more than an hour or so. It is therefore considered to be advantageous to use as fine a needle as possible, preferably of the non-cutting fibre-splitting type, so as to minimize the risk of low-pressure headache.

An initial intrathecal trial dose of 25 or 50 μg of baclofen is used. The smaller initial trial dose should be used if the patient is not on oral baclofen, in case of sensitivity. If the response to the initial trial is inadequate, a second trial dose of 75 μg can be given the next day. The maximum single bolus trial dose recommended is 100 μg. Opinions vary as to whether oral baclofen should be continued unchanged through the trial. It is probably better to do so, on the grounds that to alter it would complicate the assessment; the bolus dose response is in any case a poor guide to the likely daily infusion rate which will subsequently be needed. ITB infusion is often found to improve bladder and sphincter function, and has been found to improve urodynamic parameters such as bladder capacity, reflex detrusor contractions, bladder compliance and detrusor-sphincter dyssynergia (Bushman et al.,

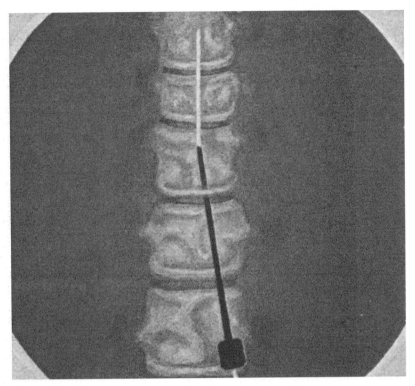

Fig. 10.1   Advancing the spinal catheter under fluoroscopic control. (Reprinted with permission of Medtronic Inc.)

1993). However, any bladder effects are often difficult to evaluate during the time available in the pre-implantation trials.

Implant surgery

After exposing the laminae, the subarachnoid space is accessed at L2/3 or L3/4 level using a Tuohy needle. Paramedian location of the needle helps avoid catheter kinking later, as the spine moves. The catheter is passed up to about T10. It is screened to ensure that it is not kinked in location (Figure 10.1). It is tunnelled through paraspinal muscle, which is sutured around it to help avoid CSF leakage past the catheter. The catheter is anchored to prevent slippage, and it is tunnelled through to the selected pump-pocket location, usually in the right iliac fossa deep to the external oblique muscle. The guide-wire is removed, and CSF should ooze from the catheter. The catheter is then trimmed to length (with sufficient surplus to ensure that it will never be stretched), and it is joined to the pump according to the manufacturer's instructions using the correct connector and strain-relief fairing. Programmable powered pumps are filled and started before implantation.

Postoperative procedure

The patient is managed in the recumbent position for the first 7–10 postoperative days. This is in order to discourage the development of a CSF leakage alongside the catheter. Subsequently, the dosage rate is adjusted according to response, to achieve the desired degree of spasticity reduction. The rate will need further adjustments as the patient mobilizes. The oral baclofen treatment, if given, will be tailed off as part of the same process; it should not be stopped precipitately.

Follow-up organization and procedures

The follow-up of patients with implanted pumps should preferably be managed at centres where a clinic can be set up for the purpose. This enables continuity of care, appointments for pump refills can be planned efficiently, and medical and patient time is not wasted waiting in the ward or theatre.

Dosage adjustments

For the manual pumps (Cordis 'Secor' or Pudenz-Schulte systems), patients decide for themselves when to pump, although a daily routine is preferred. After the pump is activated, it cannot be activated again until after a delay. This is to prevent accidental or deliberate overdosage. For the constant-infusion pumps (Therex 3000 or Infusaid 400), the dosage rate can be adjusted only by emptying the pump and refilling it with a different concentration of drug. For the programmable pumps such as the Medtronic Synchro Med range (Figure 10.2), the rate can be adjusted using the external programmer, which interrogates and reprogrammes the chip in the pump (Figure 10.3). The pump can be set to deliver different dosage rates by day and by night; currently, up to six different dosing rates can be set up for the 24 hours.

Pump refills

The programmable pumps emit a low-reservoir alarm sound when a preset level (usually 2 ml of their 18 ml capacity) remains. When telemetered after filling, they give the date on which their alarm will sound, and this facilitates setting the next appointment.

Results in clinical practice

Multiple sclerosis (MS)

In most series (Penn, 1992; Pattersen et al., 1994), MS patients have been implanted for the relief of severe lower limb spasticity and flexor spasms. The goals then are improved comfort and wheelchair posture, improved transfers and ease of personal hygiene. Most patients reported have been wheelchair-bound by the time they were

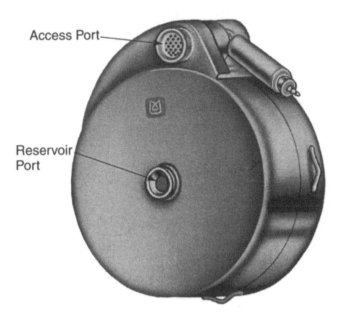

Access Port

Reservoir
Port

Fig. 10.2   Programmable pump implant (Medtronic SynchroMed). (Reprinted with permission of Medtronic Inc.)

implanted, and restoration of gait was not an issue. There are few reports of implantation in patients who are ambulant or near-ambulant with earlier disease; this may be because of a reluctance to perform elective implantation surgery in this group. However, there is a report that following five years of ITB in a group of 27 MS patients, treatment could be stopped in seven and greatly reduced in a further 10, without recurrence of spasticity. It is suggested that there may therefore be preventive value in earlier treatment of MS patients with ITB.

Spinal cord injury (SCI)

ITB is widely considered to be the treatment of choice for SCI patients who suffer from widespread spasticity that is inadequately controlled using conventional antispastic medication. This may represent about 5% of the SCI population (Soni, 1997). Conventional spasticity management will be fully employed during their primary spinal rehabilitation, including passive stretching, active physiotherapy, control of nociceptive stimuli, effective bladder and bowel management, and oral antispastic drug treatment. The majority are successfully managed in these ways. Not surprisingly, the longest follow-ups of ITB treatment have been achieved in this stable, often youthful, group. Besides abolishing spasticity, ITB has been found to alleviate pain of musculoskeletal origin in SCI (i.e. pain resulting from spasticity), though not neurogenic pain (Loubser & Akmann, 1996). For SCI patients, as for

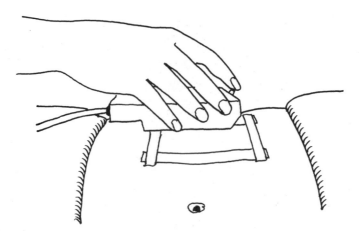

Fig. 10.3   Reprogramming the pump using the external radiofrequency controller. (Reprinted with permission of Medtronic Inc.)

MS patients, FIM score is found to improve more in paraplegia than in tetraplegia (Azouvi et al., 1996), but scores relating to the quality of life are improved in both groups (Albright et al., 1995; Middel et al., 1997).

Traumatic brain injury (TBI)

The effect of ITB on spasticity and spasm scores in patients with TBI has been found to be marked (Meythaler et al., 1996). Function was gained with long-term infusion (Meythaler et al., 1997), and there were no untoward side-effects. Early consideration for implantation has been recommended for TBI patients with severe spasticity (Becker et al., 1997). However, the dosage required for the treatment of supraspinal spasticity seems to be about twice that required for spinal spasticity (Saltuari et al., 1992), and there have been occasional reports of seizures apparently precipitated by ITB in this group (Rifici et al, 1994).

Cerebral palsy (CP)

ITB is effective against spasticity in this group, but it does not significantly influence athetosis or dystonia (Muller, 1992). It should be considered as an alternative to tenotomy, muscle lengthening or posterior rhizotomy where appropriate. In those who are able to walk, the main goal is to improve gait quality. Some residual extensor spasticity may need to be retained, if there is significant lower limb weakness. In those who are wheelchair-bound, the main goals are to improve wheelchair posture and comfort, without compromising trunk stability or head control. A small minority may achieve a functional gait with the assistance of ITB. Upper limb function and speech may be significantly improved in both walking and non-walking groups (Albright et al., 1993; Middel et al., 1997). The average ITB dose rate required is lower for the walking group than for the non-walking group. As for other patient groups, the dose rate often needs to be increased during the first year or two; it tends to remain unchanged thereafter.

ITB and the rehabilitation programme

Physical and occupational therapists need to be aware of the role and limitations of ITB treatment. Often, therapists will be the first to become aware of functional limitations attributable to spasticity, and may need to initiate the process of consideration for ITB. Patients may hear about ITB, and discuss the question with their therapist rather than their doctor. Charting of range and function before and after a trial dose is usually done by the therapist. The charts concerned are not standardized; they often focus more on impairment-based variables such as passive range of motion, and less on functional variables. There are reasons for this – the functional variables are more individual and more subjective. However, there is a need for a manageable, broadly-based assessment protocol (Campbell et al., 1995). After implantation, there may be complex functional changes requiring expert therapy advice. For example, if orthoses are discarded as a result of ITB, then gait and movement re-education may be needed. An increased level of physical functional independence may call for additional aids or instruction, in order to take safe advantage of the gain.

Complications of ITB

Catheter failure

Spinal catheters can become blocked, kinked, leaky, disconnected, dislodged or their outlet encased in secondary dura. The likelihood of catheter failure is minimized by care in checking the course and location of the catheter at the time of operation. It should be arranged so that it will not be pinched or kinked by the full range of lumbar motion. The catheter should be firmly fixed to paraspinal muscles using the fixing anchor devices provided, to prevent it from being dislodged. If symptom control is lost and catheter failure is suspected, then the problem should be investigated, rather than dealing with it by turning up the pump rate. An increased pump rate followed by spontaneous unkinking of a kinked catheter may result in a drug overdosage. Catheter faults are particularly likely to occur in children (Albright, 1996; Armstrong et al., 1997), probably because they are more active than adults, and have less paraspinal muscle bulk.

Baclofen overdosage

Minor degrees of ongoing overdosage are dealt with by adjusting the dose rate. Major bolus overdosage is usually caused by operator error, usually either inadvertently programming a bolus, or attempting to fill the reservoir through the flushing port, or wrong calculation of a bridging bolus. The patient may become weak, apnoeic or unconscious. The development of such symptoms requires immediate transfer to an intensive therapy unit so that ventilatory support can be given if required. The pump should be stopped until the patient recovers. Supportive therapy is usually adequate; there are no specific antagonists to baclofen which are clinically available, though mild respiratory depression may be reversed with physostigmine 1–2 mg iv (Muller-Schwefe & Penn, 1989; Saltuari et al., 1990). Both baclofen bolus dosage (Kofler et al., 1994) and sudden baclofen withdrawal (Rivas et al., 1993) have occasionally been associated with seizures. There has been a case report of hyperthermia, rhabdomyolysis and disseminated intravascular coagulation associated with sudden withdrawal of ITB due to catheter disconnection. The clinical condition improved only when the catheter was reconnected. A causative relation was presumed (Reeves et al., 1998).

CSF leakage

The pressure of the lumbar CSF rises to 20–30 mm Hg in the upright position, and is further raised on coughing or straining. In these circumstances CSF may find a way along the outside of the catheter, and accumulate in the potential space around the pump, forming a palpable or visible fluid swelling. Rapid escape of CSF from the theca in this way can lead to low-pressure headache which is therefore usually postural. If such a CSF leak occurs in the early postoperative period, it may often be cured by a period of recumbent nursing. If it persists, the fistula will have to be repaired. If a leak begins late, it is unlikely to resolve spontaneously. A CSF leak to the exterior (for example through the stitches closing the pump pocket) is dangerous and must be repaired immediately. It would be preferable for future designs of intrathecal catheter to incorporate a sealing system to prevent CSF from flowing along their outer surface. This precaution has been incorporated with success in other lumbar intrathecal implant devices (Brindley et al., 1986).

Implant infection

In skilled hands, and where correct procedures are followed, implant infection is rare. When it occurs, the whole implant should be removed. Perioperative infection may not become evident for weeks or months, particularly if a low-grade skin commensal is involved. The risk of perioperative infection of neurological implants may be reduced by preoperative antibiotic coating of the implant (Rushton et al., 1989). Haematogenous infection of an implant is excessively rare, but is a theoretical risk for example in association with bacterial endocarditis. Strict precautions have to be taken against introducing infection when the implant is refilled. Infection could be introduced either from the drug solution or atmospheric air, causing infection within the pump reservoir; or else from the needle, causing infection in the potential space around the pump. Both of these spaces are immunologically privileged, and infection in them is therefore to be rigorously avoided. Implantable pumps do incorporate bacterial filters so that any infection within their reservoir cannot be spread via the pump and catheter to the subarachnoid space. Refill systems also incorporate a bacterial filter as an added precaution.

Implant limitations and failures

Different types of pump have different limitations, failure rates and failure modes (Gardner et al., 1995; Teddy, 1997). The Medtronic range of programmable pumps, while expensive, has been found to be highly reliable within its lifetime; but its internal non-rechargeable battery fails predictably in three to five years, so that the pump then has to be replaced. The manually operated Cordis Secor is cheap, but has been associated with a higher complication rate. Also, if implanted too deep it is difficult to operate; if too shallow it tends to erode through the skin. The fixed-rate gas–liquid powered pumps (Therex, Infusaid) are simple and reliable, but offer no scope for adjusting the drug dosage rate other than by varying the concentration of the drug solution with which they are filled. Also, the flow rate varies with body temperature and atmospheric pressure.

REFERENCES

Albright, A. L. (1996). Baclofen in the treatment of cerebral palsy. *J Child Neurol*, **11**: 77–83.

Albright, A. L., Barron, W. B., Fasick, M. P., Polinko, P. & Janosky, J. (1993). Continuous intrathecal baclofen infusion for spasticity of cerebral origin. *JAMA*, **270**: 2475–7.

Albright, A. L., Barry, M. J., Fasick, M. P. & Janosky, J. (1995). Effects of continuous intrathecal baclofen infusion and selective posterior rhizotomy on upper extremity spasticity. *Pediatr Neurosurg*, **23**: 82–5.

Armstrong, R. W., Steinbok, P., Cochrane, D. D., Kube, S. D., Fife, S. E. & Farrell, K. (1997). Intrathecally administered baclofen for treatment of children with spasticity of cerebral origin. *J Neurosurg*, **87**: 409–14.

Azouvy, P., Mane, M., Thiebaut, J. B., Deny, P., Remy-Neris, O. & Bussel, B. (1996). Intrathecal baclofen administration for control of severe spinal spasticity: functional improvement and long-term follow-up. *Arch Phys Med Rehabil*, **77**: 35–9.

Azouvy, P., Roby Brami, A., Biraben, A., Thiebaut, J. B., Thurel, C. & Bussel, B. (1993). Effect of intrathecal baclofen on the monosynaptic reflex in humans: evidence for a postsynaptic action. *J Neurol Neurosurg Psychiatry*, **56**: 515–19.

Barolat, G., Singh-Sahni, K., Staas, W. E. Jr, Shatin, D., Ketcik, B. & Allen, K. (1995). Epidural spinal cord stimulation in the management of spasms in spinal cord injury: a prospective study. *Stereotact Funct Neurosurg*, **64**: 153–64.

Becker, R., Alberti, O. & Bauer, B. L. (1997). Continuous intrathecal baclofen infusion in severe spasticity after traumatic or hypoxic brain injury. *J Neurol*, **244**: 160–6.

Becker, W. J., Harris, C. J., Long, M. L., Ablett, D. P., Klein, G. M. & DeForge, D. A. (1995). Long term intrathecal baclofen therapy in patients with intractable spasticity. *Can J Neurol Sci*, **22**: 208–17.

Bohannon, R. W. & Smith, M. B. (1987). Interrater reliability of a modified Ashworth scale of muscle spasticity. *Phys Ther*, **67**: 206–7.

Brindley, G. S., Polkey, C. E., Rushton, D. N. & Cardozo, L. (1986). Sacral anterior root stimulators for bladder control in paraplegia: the first 50 cases. *J Neurol Neurosurg Psychiatry*, **49**: 1104–14.

Bushman, W., Steers, W. D. & Meythaler, J. M. (1993). Voiding dysfunction in patients with spastic paraplegia: urodynamic evaluation and response to continuous intrathecal baclofen. *Neurourol Urodyn*, **12**: 163–70.

Campbell, S. K., Almeida, G. L., Penn, R. D. & Corcos, D. M. (1995). The effects of intrathecally administered baclofen on function in patients with spasticity. *Phys Ther*, **75**: 352–62.

Dressandt, J., Auer, C. & Conrad, B. (1995). Influence of baclofen upon the alpha-motoneuron in spasticity by means of F-wave analysis. *Muscle Nerve*, **18**: 103–7.

Fromm, G. H., Terrence, C. F. & Chatta, A. S. (1992). Baclofen in the treatment of trigeminal neuralgia: double blind study and long-term follow-up. *Ann Neurol*, **15**: 240–4.

Gardner, B., Jamous, A., Teddy, P., Bergstrom, E., Wang, D., Ravichandran, G., Sutton, R. & Urquart, S. (1995). Intrathecal baclofen – a multicentre clinical comparison of the Medtronics Programmable, Cordis Secor and Constant Infusion Infusaid drug delivery systems. *Paraplegia*, **33**: 551–4.

Kroin, J. S. & Penn, R. D. (1992). Cerebrospinal fluid pharmacokinetics of lumbar intrathecal baclofen. In *Parenteral Drug Therapy in Spasticity and Parkinson's Disease*, ed. J. P. W. F. Lakke, E. M. Delhaas, A. W. F. Rutgers, pp. 67–77. New York: Parthenon.

Kofler, M., Kronenberg, M. F., Rifici, C., Saltuari, L. & Bauer, G. (1994). Epileptic seizures associated with intrathecal baclofen application. *Neurology*, **44**: 25–7.

Lance, J. W. (1980). Symposium synopsis. In *Spasticity: Disordered Motor Control*, ed. R. G. Feldman, R. R. Young & W. P. Koella, pp. 485–94. Chicago: Year Book Medical Publishers.

Loubser, P. G. & Akmann, N. M. (1996). Effects of intrathecal baclofen on chronic spinal cord injury pain. *J Pain Symptom Manage*, **12**: 241–7.

Meythaler, J. M., DeVivo, M. J. & Hadley, M. (1996). Prospective study on the use of bolus intrathecal baclofen for spastic hypertonia due to acquired brain injury. *Arch Phys Med Rehabil*, **77**: 461–6.

Meythaler, J. M., McCary, A. & Hadley, M. N. (1997). Prospective assessment of continuous intrathecal infusion of baclofen for spasticity caused by acquired brain injury: a preliminary report. *J Neurosurg*, **87**: 415–19.

Middel, B., Kuipers-Upmeijer, H., Bouma, L., Staal, M., Oenema, D., Postma, T., Terpstra, S. &

Stewart, R. (1997). Effect of intrathecal baclofen delivered by an implanted programmable pump on health related quality of life in patients with severe spasticity. *J Neurol Neurosurg Psychiatry*, **63**: 204–9.

Muller, H. (1992). Treatment of severe spasticity: results of a multicentre trial conducted in Germany involving the intrathecal infusion of baclofen by an implantable drug delivery system. *Dev Med Child Neurol*, **34**: 739–45.

Muller, H., Zierski, J., Dralle, D., Krauss, D. & Mutschler, E. (1988). Pharmacokinetics of intrathecal baclofen. In *Local Spinal Therapy of Spasticity*, ed. H. Muller, J. Zierski & R. D. Penn, pp. 223–6. Berlin: Springer Verlag.

Muller-Schwefe, G. & Penn, R. D. (1989). Physostigmine in the treatment of intrathecal baclofen overdose: report of three cases. *J Neurosurg*, **71**: 273–5.

Ordia, J. I., Fischer, E., Adamski, E. & Spatz, E. L. (1996). Chronic intrathecal delivery of baclofen by a programmable pump for the treatment of severe spasticity. *J Neurosurg*, **85**: 452–7.

Parise, M., Garcia-Larrea, L., Mertens, P., Sindou, M. & Mauguiere, F. (1997). Clinical use of polysynaptic flexion reflexes in the management of spasticity with intrathecal baclofen. *Electroencephalogr Clin Neurophysiol*, **105**: 141–8.

Patterson, V., Watt, M., Byrnes, D., Crowe, E. & Lee, A. (1994). Management of severe spasticity with intrathecal baclofen delivered by a manually operated pump. *J Neurol Neurosurg Psychiatry*, **57**: 582–5.

Penn, R. D. (1992). Intrathecal baclofen for spasticity of spinal origin: seven years of experience. *J Neurosurg*, **77**: 236–40.

Penn, R. D. & Kroin, J. S. (1985). Continuous intrathecal baclofen for severe spasticity. *Lancet*, **2**: 125–7.

Penn, R. D., Savoy, S. M., Corcos, D. C. et al. (1989). Intrathecal baclofen for severe spinal spasticity. *N Engl J Med*, **320**: 1517–18.

Reeves, R. K., Stolp-Smith, K. A. & Christopherson, M. W. (1998). Hyperthermia, rhabdomyolysis and disseminated intravascular coagulation associated with baclofen pump catheter failure. *Arch Phys Med Rehabil*, **201**: 353–6.

Rifici, C., Kofler, M., Kronenberg, M., Kofler, A., Bramanti, P. & Saltuari, L. (1994). Intrathecal baclofen application in patients with supraspinal spasticity secondary to severe traumatic brain injury. *Funct Neurol*, **9**: 29–34.

Rivas, D. A., Chancellor, M. B., Hill, K. et al. (1993). Neurological manifestations of baclofen withdrawal. *J Urol*, **150**: 1903–5.

Rushton, D. N., Brindley, G. S., Polkey, C. E. & Browning, G. V. (1989). Implant infections and antibiotic-impregnated silicone rubber coating. *J Neurol Neurosurg Psychiatry*, **52**: 223–9.

Saltuari, L., Baumgartner, H., Kefler, M. et al. (1990). Failure of physostigmine in treatment of acute severe intrathecal baclofen intoxication. *N Engl J Med*, **322**: 1535.

Saltuari, L., Kronenberg, M., Marosi, M. J., Kofler, M., Russegger, L., Rifici, C., Bramanti, P & Gerstenbrand, F. (1992). Long-term intrathecal baclofen treatment in supraspinal spasticity. *Acta Neurol Napoli*, **14**: 195–207.

Soni, B. M. (1997). Management of spasticity using intrathecal baclofen therapy. In *Proceedings, European Spasticity Management Meeting, Rome, December 1997*. (Unpublished.)

Sutcliffe, J. (1997). Cerebellar stimulation for spasticity. In *Neuroprostheses, Neuromodulators and Rehabilitation. A Report of the British Society of Rehabilitation Medicine*, ed. A. Ward, D. Rushton, J. Graham & N. Donaldson, pp. 27–8. London: British Society of Rehabilitation Medicine.

Teddy, P. (1997). Intrathecal Drug Delivery Systems. In *Neuroprostheses, Neuromodulators and Rehabilitation. A Report of the British Society of Rehabilitation Medicine*, ed. A. Ward, D. Rushton, J. Graham & N. Donaldson, pp. 47–9. London: British Society of Rehabilitation Medicine.

11

Surgical management of spasticity

Patrick Mertens and Marc Sindou

Introduction

Spasticity is one of the commonest sequelae of neurological diseases. In most patients spasticity is useful in compensating for lost motor strength. Nevertheless, in a significant number of patients it may become excessive and harmful leading to further functional losses. When not controllable by physical therapy, medications and/or botulinum toxin injections, spasticity can benefit from neurostimulation, intrathecal pharmacotherapy or selective ablative procedures.

Neurostimulation procedures

Stimulation of the spinal cord was developed in the 1970s on the basis of the 'gate control theory' of Melzach & Wall (1974) for the treatment of neurogenic pain. This method has been found to be partially effective in the treatment of spastic syndromes, such as those encountered in multiple sclerosis (Cook & Weinstein, 1973; Gybels & Van Roost, 1987) or spinal cord degenerative diseases, such as Strumpell–Lorrain syndrome. However, this method is generally most effective when spasticity is mild and when the dorsal column has sufficient functional fibres, as assessed by somatosensory evoked potentials. Stimulation electrodes are implanted, either percutaneously through a Tuohy needle under X-ray fluoroscopy or surgically via an open interlaminar approach, in the extradural space posteriorly to the dorsal column, at the level of the thoraco-lumbar spinal cord for spasticity in the lower limbs of paraparetic patients, or at the level of the cervical spinal cord for spasticity in the upper and/or lower limbs of quadriparetic patients. The electrodes are connected by means of flexible electrical wires to a generator inserted in the subcutaneous tissue and located under the abdominal skin for electrostimulation of the thoraco-lumbar spinal cord, or under the skin of the subclavicular region for cervical stimulation.

Cerebellar stimulation has been extensively and seriously tried for spasticity from cerebral palsy (Davis et al., 1982). For most of the studies, cerebellar stimulation did not prove to be sufficiently effective for it to be widely adopted (Seigfried & Lazorthes, 1985).

Deep brain stimulation, which yields positive results in patients with tremor, dystonia, akinesia, dyskinesia and/or non-spastic hypertonia (i.e. rigidity) especially in patients with Parkinson's disease, is not effective for the treatment of spasticity.

We have recently found *precentral cortical stimulation*, which was indicated for post-stroke pain in hemiplegic patients, to have some effect on spasticity in some patients (unpublished data).

Neuro-ablative procedures

When spasticity cannot be controlled by conservative methods or by botulinum toxin injections, ablative procedures must be considered. The surgery should be performed so that excessive hypertonia is reduced without suppression of useful muscular tone or impairment of the residual motor and sensory functions. Therefore, neuro-ablative techniques must be as selective as possible. Such selective lesions can be performed at the level of peripheral nerves, spinal roots, spinal cord or the dorsal root entry zone.

Peripheral neurotomies (PN)

Selective PN were introduced first for the treatment of spastic deformities of the foot by Stoffel (1913). Later, Gros et al. (1977) and Sindou & Mertens (1988) advocated making neurotomies more selective by using microsurgical techniques and intra-operative electrical stimulation for better identification of the function of the fascicles constituting the nerve. Selectivity is required to suppress the excess of spasticity without producing excessive weakening of motor strength and severe amyotrophy. To achieve this goal, preserving at least one-fourth of the motor fibres is necessary.

Neurotomies are *indicated when spasticity is localized* to muscles or muscular groups supplied by a single or a few peripheral nerves that are easily accessible. To help the surgeon decide if neurotomy is appropriate, temporary local anaesthetic block of the nerve (with xylocaine or with long-lasting bupivacaine) can be useful. Such a test can determine if articular limitations result from spasticity or musculo-tendinous contractures and/or articular ankyloses (only spasticity is decreased by the test). In addition, these tests give the patient an idea of what to expect from the operation. Botulinic toxin injections may also act as a 'prolonged' test for several weeks or months.

Lower limbs

For spasticity in the lower limbs (Mertens & Sindou, 1991), neurotomies of the tibial nerve at the popliteal region (Figure 11.1) and of the obturator nerve just

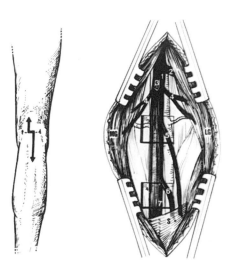 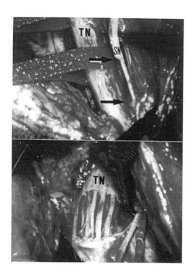

Fig. 11.1   Selective tibial neurotomy. *Left:* Skin incision in the right popliteal fossa. *Centre:* Dorsal
view showing tibial (1), and peroneal (2) nerves, Sural (sensory) nerve (3), medial
gastrocnemius and lateral gastrocnemius branches (4), soleus nerve (5), posterior tibialis
nerve (6). The distal trunk of the tibial nerve, just above the soleus arch (S), contains
fifteen to eighteen fascicles averaging 1 mm in diameter each – two-thirds are sensory.
Equinus and ankle clonus require section of the soleus nerve (5) and, if necessary, of the
medial and lateral gastrocnemius nerve (4). Varus necessitates interruption of the
posterior tibialis nerve (6). Tonic flexion of the toes requires section of the flexor fascicles
situated inside the distal trunk of the tibial nerve (7); their precise identification apart
from the sensory fascicles by electrical stimulation is of paramount importance to avoid
hypoaesthetic and dysaesthetic disturbances, as well as trophic lesions of the plantar skin.
Upper right: Operative view of the resection, over 7 mm in length (between the two
arrows), of two-thirds of the soleus nerve (SN). *Lower right:* Operative view of five
dissected fascicles inside the distal part of the tibial nerve (TN) at the level of the soleus
arch, after the epineural envelope has been opened.

below the subpubic canal (Figure 11.2) are the most common for the so-called
spastic foot and for spastic flexion-adduction deformity of the hip, respectively.

Tibial neurotomy is performed as follows. After exposure of the tibial nerve from
the popliteal region down to the soleus muscular arcade under general anaesthesia
not using curare, all the branches are individualized and identified one by one,
using the operating microscope and bipolar stimulation. Each branch (or fascicle)
considered as supporting harmful spasticity on the basis of stimulation is then partially resected over a 5 mm length to prevent regeneration. Conservation of one-
third to one-fifth of the fibres of each branch is sufficient to avoid loss of motor
function and amyotrophy. Comparing the results of stimulation of the distal and
proximal parts of the resected fibres, proved useful in controlling the effects of the
operation on muscular contraction. The particular branches of the nerve to be

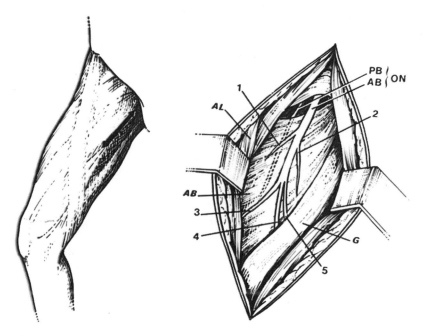

Fig. 11.2   Obturator neurotomy. Skin incision on the relief of the adductor longus muscle. Dissection of the anterior branch (AB) of right obturator nerve (ON). The adductor longus muscle (AL) is retracted laterally and the gracilis muscle (G) medially. The nerve is anterior to the adductor brevis muscle (AB). The adductor brevis nerve (1 and 2), adductor longus nerve (3), and the gracilis nerve (4 and 5) are shown. The posterior branch (PB) of the obturator nerve lies under the adductor brevis muscle (AB).

operated on are determined preoperatively by analysing all the components of the spastic disorder, according to the following schedule: (1) equinus and/or ankle clonus requires sectioning of the soleus nerve(s) and, if necessary, the two gastroc-nemius branches; (2) varus necessitates interruption of the posterior tibial nerve; and (3) tonic flexion of the toes requires sectioning of the flexor fascicles situated inside the distal trunk of the tibial nerve. Their precise identification, avoiding sensory fascicles, is of paramount importance in avoiding hypoaesthesia and dysaesthetic disturbances as well as trophic lesions of the plantar skin.

In 180 patients, 82% of tibial PN resulted in suppression of the disabling spasticity with improvement of the residual voluntary movements (P. Mertens & M. Sindou, unpublished data).

In contrast to the adult, in the spastic hemiplegic child the effects of tibial PN may be only transient. In our series of 13 paediatric cases, 8 cases had a recurrence (Berard et al., 1998).

Selective neurotomy of the branches to the knee flexors (hamstrings) can also be performed at the level of the sciatic trunk through a short skin incision in the

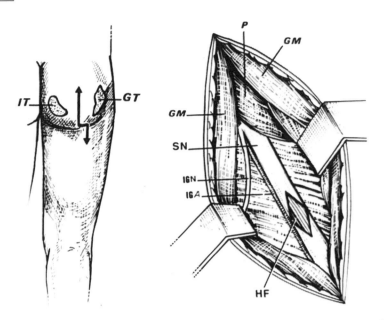

Fig. 11.3   Hamstring neurotomy. Skin incision between the ischial tuberosity (IT) and the greater trochanter (GT). Dissection of the right sciatic nerve (SN), under the piriformis muscle (P), after passing through the fibres of the gluteus maximus muscle (GM). The epineurium of the nerve is opened and fascicles for hamstring muscles (HF) are located in the medial part of the nerve. IGN: inferior gluteal nerve; IGA: inferior gluteal nerve artery.

buttock (Figure 11.3). For spastic hyperextension of the first toe (so-called permanent Babinski sign), a selective neurotomy of the branch(es) of the deep fibular nerve to the hallux extensor can be useful.

Upper limbs

Neurotomies are also indicated for spasticity in the upper limbs (Mertens & Sindou, 1991). Selective fascicular neurotomies can be performed in the musculocutaneous nerve for spastic elbow flexion (Figure 11.4), and in the median (and ulnar) nerve for spastic hyperflexion of the wrist and fingers (Figure 11.5).

The last procedure, which consists of sectioning the branches to the forearm pronators, wrist flexors and extrinsic finger flexors, is indicated for spasticity in the wrist and the hand – the aim being to open the hand and improve prehension. As the fascicular organization of the median and ulnar nerves does not allow for differentiation of motor from sensory fascicles at the level of their trunks, it is necessary to dissect the motor branches after they have left the nerve trunk in the forearm. Special care must be taken with the sensory fascicles to avoid painful manifestations.

Neurotomies of brachial plexus branches have now been developed for treating

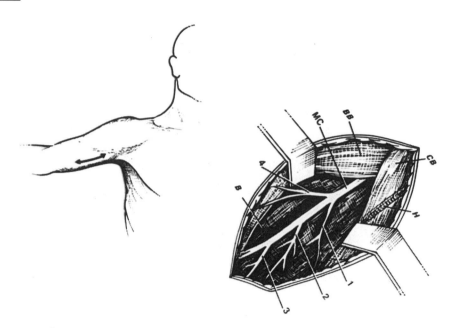

Fig. 11.4   Musculocutaneous neurotomy brachialis. Skin incision along the medial aspect of the biceps brachii. Dissection of the right musculocutaneous nerve (MC) in the space between the biceps brachii (BB) laterally, the coracobrachialis (CB) medially, and the brachialis (B) posteriorly. Branches to brachialis (1 and 2) and to biceps brachii (3 and 4). The humeral artery (H) and the median nerve are situated medially (they are not dissected).

the spastic shoulder (Decq et al., 1997). The pectoralis major muscle and teres major muscle are the main muscles implicated in this condition. This excess of spasticity restrains the active (and passive) abduction and external rotation of the shoulder. The pectoralis major nerve can be easily reached via an anterior approach of the shoulder. With the patient supine and the upper limb lying alongside the body, an incision is made at the innermost part of the delto-pectoral sulcus and curves along the clavicular axis. The teres major nerve can be approached posteriorly to the shoulder. With the patient in procubitus position and the upper limb lying alongside the body, a vertical incision is made along the inner border of the teres major. Decq et al. (1997) found a significant increase in amplitude and speed in the active mobilization of the spastic shoulder, leading to better functional use in five patients after surgery.

Improvement of motor function

Basically, selective neurotomies are able not only to reduce excess of spasticity and deformity, but also to improve motor function by reequilibrating the tonic balance

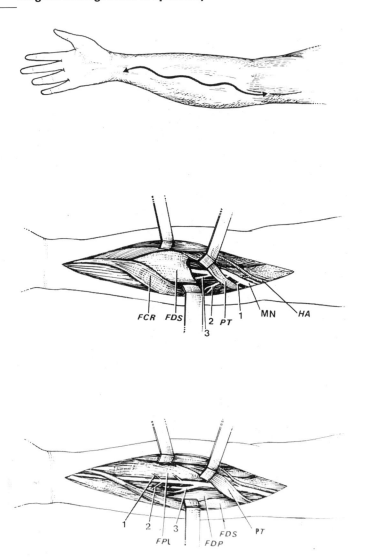

Fig. 11.5   Median neurotomy. Median neurotomy (slightly modified from Brunelli's technique). *Top:*
Skin incision on the right forearm from the medial aspect of the biceps brachii at the level
of the elbow to the midline above the wrist. *Centre:* First stage of the dissection; the
pronator teres (PT) is retracted upward and laterally, and the flexor carpi radialis (FCR) is
retracted medially. Branches from the median nerve (MN), before it passes under the
fibrous arch of the flexor digitorum superficialis (FDS), are dissected. These branches are
(1) to the pronotor teres and (2,3) two nerve trunks to the flexor carpi radialis, palmaris
longus and flexor digitorum superficialis. *Bottom:* Second stage of the dissection; the
fibrous arch of the FDS is sectioned to allow more distal dissection of the median nerve.
The FDS is retracted medially, and branches from the median nerve are identified to the
(1) flexor pollicis longus (FPL); (2) flexor digitorum profundus (FDP); and (3) the
interosseous nerve and its proper branches to these muscles.

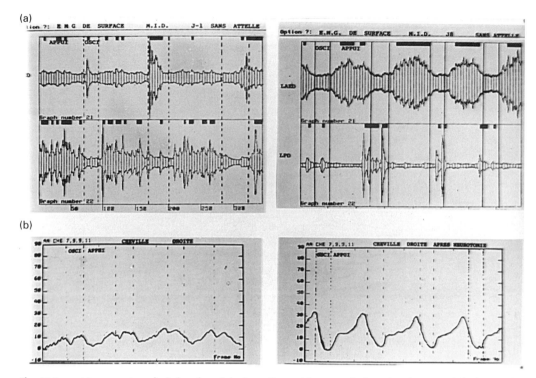

Fig. 11.6   Movement analysis in a hemiplegic patient with a spastic foot (equino-varus) before and
after selective tibial neurotomy. (a): Surface polyelectromyography of the tibialis anterior
(LAED) and the triceps surae (LPD) muscles on the spastic leg during walking. *Left:*
preoperative recordings showing desynchronized activities of the triceps surae, with
abnormal co-contractions of antagonist muscles – triceps surae and tibialis anterior. *Right:*
after selective tibial neurotomy there is a reappearance of muscular activities in the tibialis
anterior muscle, a clear decrease in triceps surae activities, and normal alternance of
contractions of these muscles (i.e. triceps surae at the end of the stance phase and tibialis
anterior during the swing phase). (b): Tridimensional movement analysis of the ankle
flexion-extension amplitude during the gait with VICON system. *Left:* preoperatively, the
amplitude of the spastic ankle is limited to 18 degrees of dorsal flexion. *Right:* after
selective tibial neurotomy, the dorsal flexion increased to 32°. Thus the tonic balance of
the ankle has been re-equilibrated by the selective tibial neurotomy; consequently, motor
function and gait have been improved.

between agonist and antagonist muscles (Figure 11.6). This was certainly true for
82% of 180 adult patients operated on for spastic foot using tibial PN. In our experience – since 1980 and more than 300 operations – tibial neurotomy has been the
most frequently used PN (Mertens & Sindou, unpublished data).

With regard to the spastic hand which is a very difficult problem to deal with, a
functional benefit in prehension can only be achieved if patients retain a residual

motor function in the extensor and supinator muscles, together with a sufficient residual sensory function. If these conditions are not present, only better comfort and better cosmetic aspect can be achieved.

We recently performed twenty-five median (and ulnar) neurotomies combined with tenotomies (predominantly of the epicondyle muscles) in the forearm (namely a Page–Scaglietti operation) (Brunelli & Brunelli, 1983) to treat spastic flexion of the wrist and fingers, with tendinous contractures. All patients in this special group – who did not have any voluntary effective motor function pre-operatively – had a better comfort and good cosmetic effect, but without any significant functional benefit.

Posterior rhizotomies

Posterior rhizotomy was performed by Foerster for the first time in 1908 to modify spasticity (Foerster, 1913), after Sherrington had demonstrated in 1898 using an animal model that decerebrate rigidity could be abolished by sectioning the dorsal roots, that is, by interruption of the afferent input to the monosynaptic stretch and polysynaptic withdrawal reflexes. Its undesired effects on sensory and sphincter functions limited its application in the past. To diminish these disadvantages, several surgeons in the 1960s and 1970s attempted to develop more selective operations, especially for the treatment of children with cerebral palsy.

Posterior selective rhizotomy

To reduce the sensory side-effects of the original Foerster method, Gros et al. (1967) introduced a technical modification that consisted of sparing one rootlet in five of each root, from L1 to S1. Using similar principles, Ouaknine (1980), a pupil of Gros, developed a microsurgical technique that consisted of resectioning one-third to two-thirds of each group of rootlets of all the posterior roots from L1 to S1.

Sectorial posterior rhizotomy

In an attempt to reduce the side-effects of rhizotomy on postural tone in ambulatory patients, Gros (1979) and his pupils Privat et al. (1976) and Frerebeau (1991) proposed a topographic selection of the rootlets to be sectioned. Firstly, a pre-operative assessment is done to differentiate the 'useful spasticity' (i.e. the one sustaining postural tone – abdominal muscles, quadriceps, gluteus medius) from the 'harmful spasticity' (i.e. the one responsible for vicious posture – hip flexors, adductors, hamstrings, triceps surae). This is followed by mapping the evoked motor activity of the exposed rootlets, from L1 to S2, by direct electrostimulation of each posterior group of rootlets. Finally, the rootlets to be sectioned are determined according to this pre-operative programme.

Partial posterior rhizotomy

Fraioli & Guidetti (1977) reported on a procedure for dividing the dorsal half of each rootlet of the selected posterior roots a few millimetres before its entrance into the posterolateral sulcus. Good results were obtained, without significant sensory deficit. This can be explained by the fact that partial sectioning leaves intact a large number of fibres of all types.

Functional posterior rhizotomy

The neurological search for specially organized circuits responsible for spasticity led Fasano et al. (1976) to propose the so-called functional posterior rhizotomy. This method is based on bipolar intra-operative stimulation of the posterior rootlets and analysis of the types of muscle responses by electromyography (EMG). Responses characterized by a permanent tonic contraction, an after-discharge pattern or a large spatial diffusion to distant muscle groups, were considered to belong to disinhibited spinal circuits responsible for spasticity. This procedure, which was especially conceived for use with children with cerebral palsy, has been also used by other outstanding surgical teams, each one having brought its own technical modifications to the method (Peacock & Arens, 1982; Cahan et al., 1987; Storrs, 1987; Abbott et al., 1989).

Personal technique

Our personal adaptations of these methods are summarized below. Selection of candidates for surgery was done in a multidisciplinary way, with the rehabilitation team, the physiotherapist, the orthopaedic surgeon and the neurosurgeon being present, as well as of course the patient's family. Candidates were retained only if spasticity was responsible for a halt in motor skill acquisitions and/or evolutive orthopaedic deformities in spite of intensive physiotherapy. The main goals of the surgery were clearly defined for every patient: improvement in comfort; decrease in orthopaedic risks; improvement for sitting, standing and/or walking; and improvement in urinary function. The muscles in which there was a harmful excess of tone and their – anatomically – corresponding lumbo-sacral roots (i.e. those to be resected, as well as the degree of their resectioning according to amount of spasticity to be reduced) were determined by the multidisciplinary team. The surgical procedure used is detailed in Figure 11.7. Until recently, we have only operated on very severely affected children – quadriplegic not able to locomote by their own. The results are reported in Hodgkinson et al. (1996) and summarized in Table 11.1. Since 1995 we have extended the indications to diplegic children able to walk; the effects are good but follow-up in this group is not yet sufficient to report on the results in detail.

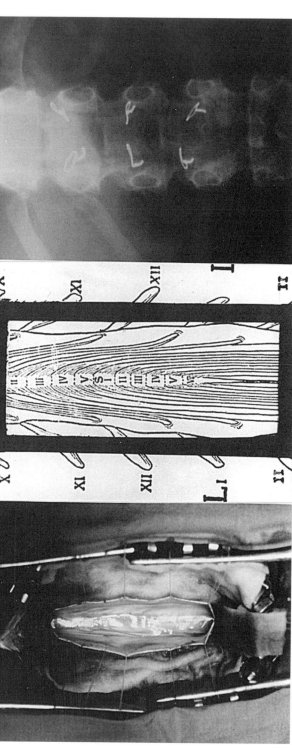

Fig. 11.7　Lumbo-sacral posterior rhizotomy for cerebral palsy children. Our personal technique consists of performing a limited osteoplastic laminotomy using a power saw, in one single piece, from T11 to L1 (left). The laminae will be replaced at the end of the procedure and fixed with wires (right). The dorsal (and ventral) L1, L2 and L3 roots are identified by electrical stimulation performed intradurally just before entry into their dural sheaths. The dorsal sacral rootlets can be seen at the entrance into the dorso-lateral sulcus of the conus medullaris. The landmark between S1 and S2 medullary segments is located 30 mm approximately from the exit of the tiny coccygeal root from the conus. The dorsal rootlets of S1, L5 and L4 are identified by their evoked motor responses. The sensory roots for bladder (S2–S3) can be identified by monitoring vesical pressure, and those for the anal sphincter (S3–S4) can be identified by rectomanometry (or simply using a finger introduced into the patient's rectum) or electromyography recordings. Surface spinal cord SEP recordings from tibial nerve (L5–S1) and pudendal nerve (S1–S3) stimulation may also be helpful.

For the surgery to be effective a total amount of 60% of dorsal rootlets must be cut, of course with a different quantity cut according to the level and function of the roots involved. Also, of course, the correspondence of the roots with the muscles having harmful spasticity or useful postural tone must be considered in determining the amount of rootlets to be cut; in most cases L4 (which predominantly gives innervation to the quadriceps femoris) has to be preserved.

Table 11.1. Results according to whether or not principal goal is reached

Principal goal	Number of cases	Goal reached	Goal not reached
Improvement in comfort	2	1	1
Orthopaedic risks	6	2	4
Improvement of sitting position	1	1	–
Improvement of standing and walking	8	6	2
Improvement of vesical function	1	0	1
Total	18	10	8

The results of posterior rhizotomies

The results obtained in children with cerebral palsy, whatever the technical modality of surgery may be, have been extensively reported in the literature. See Hodgkinson et al., 1996 for a review of the literature. Briefly, these publications show that about 75% of the patients, at one year or more after surgery, had nearly normal muscle tone that no longer limited the residual voluntary movements of limbs. After a serious and persisting physical therapy and rehabilitation programme, most children demonstrated improved stability in sitting and/or increased efficiency in walking. In most cases with installed contractures, deformities were not retrocessive, so that complementary orthopaedic surgery was justified.

Percutaneous thermorhizotomies and intrathecal chemical rhizotomies

Percutaneous radiofrequency rhizotomy, initially performed for the treatment of pain (Uematsu et al., 1974), was later applied to the treatment of neurogenic detrusor hyperreflexia (Young & Mulcachy, 1980) and of spasticity in the limbs (Herz et al., 1983; Kenmore, 1983; Kasdon & Lathi, 1984). The procedure in the lumbar spine is generally performed in the lateral recumbent position, the affected side uppermost, because the prone position would be very uncomfortable due to fixed tendons and joint resulting in abnormal postures. The entry point is about 7 cm from the midline just below the level of the intervertebral space. The needle is pushed obliquely upwards to the corresponding foramen under fluoroscopy so as to reach the target root tangentially. The radiofrequency (RF) probe is placed through the stylet and a stimulation current is applied with an increasing voltage until a motor response is obtained in the appropriate muscular group. The probe must be readjusted if a good motor response is not obtained with a threshold of less than 0.5 volts. The RF lesion is made at 90°C for two minutes. A stimulation test is then applied; an increase in threshold of at least 0.2 volts is desired to be certain of a significant relief of spasticity. Otherwise the procedure must be repeated. For the placement of the electrode at S1, the needle is inserted in the midline between the spinous processes of L5 and S1 and pushed laterally towards the elbow of the S1 nerve root (without penetration of the dura). RF–sacral rhizotomies can be performed at the foramen of S1 to S4 with cystometric monitoring for neurogenic bladder with detrusor hyperactivity. RF–thermorhizotomy can be also performed in the cervical spine. The patient is in the supine position. The tip of the needle is placed in the posterior compartment of the vertebral foramen to avoid damage to the vertebral artery. Percutaneous rhizotomies have the advantage of being less aggressive than the open procedures in very debilitated patients. The procedure seems more appropriate for spastic disturbances limited to a few muscular groups that correspond to a small number of spinal roots (as occurs in spastic hip, which can be treated by thermorhizotomy of L2–L3). The effects are most often temporary. In long-term follow-up, a high rate of recurrent spasticity is observed (five to nine months on average) but the preoperative level of spasticity is most often not totally reached and the procedure can be repeated.

Intrathecal injection of alcohol was first introduced for cancer pain (Dogliotti, 1931), and only later was it used for hypertonia in patients with severe spastic paraplegia (Guttman, 1953). Alcohol was then replaced by phenol (a hyperbaric solution), which is easier to control (Maher, 1955; Kelly & Gauthier-Smith, 1959; Nathan, 1959). The best candidates for phenol intrathecal injections are paraplegic patients suffering from severe spasms who do not have useful residual motor, sensory, or sphincter, function below the level of the lesion (see Chapters 8 and 10).

Longitudinal myelotomy

Longitudinal myelotomy was introduced by Bischof (1951) and was made more selective by Pourpre (1960) and later by Laitinen & Singounas (1971). The method consists of a frontal separation between the posterior and anterior horns of the lumbo-sacral enlargement from T11 to S2 performed from inside the spinal cord after a posterior commisural incision that reaches the ependymal canal. Laitinen & Singounas (1971) found that of 25 patients, 60% had complete relief of spasticity while 36% showed some residual spasticity in one or both legs. Within one year, some muscular tone returned in most patients, but it seldom produced troublesome spasticity. A harmful effect, however, on bladder function was present in 27% of the patients. Longitudinal myelotomy is indicated only for spastic paraplegias with flexion spasms, when the patient has no residual useful motor control and no bladder and sexual function.

Surgery in the dorsal root entry zone

Surgery in the dorsal root entry zone was introduced in 1972 (Sindou, 1972) to treat intractable pain. Because of its inhibitory effects on muscular tone, it has been applied to patients with focalized hyperspasticity (Sindou et al., 1974, 1982, 1985a,b). This method – named microDREZotomy (MDT) – attempts to selectively interrupt the small nociceptive and the large myotatic fibres (situated laterally and centrally, respectively), while sparing the large lemniscal fibres which are regrouped medially. It also enhances the inhibitory mechanisms of Lissauer's tract and dorsal horn (Eccles et al., 1961) (Figure 11.8).

MDT (Sindou et al., 1986, 1991a; Sindou & Jeanmonod, 1989) consists of microsurgical incisions that are 2–3 mm deep and at a 35° angle at the cervical level and at a 45°angle at the lumbo-sacral level followed by bipolar coagulations performed ventro-laterally at the entrance of the rootlets into the dorso-lateral sulcus, along all the cord segments selected for operation (Figure 11.8, right). For patients with paraplegia (Sindou & Jeanmonod, 1989), the L2–S5 segments are approached through a T11–L2 laminectomy (Figure 11.9), whereas for the hemiplegic upper limb (Sindou et al., 1986), a C4–C7 hemilaminectomy with conservation of the spinous processes is sufficient to reach the C5–T1 segments (Figure 11.8). Identification of the cord levels related to the undesirable spastic mechanisms is achieved by studying the muscle responses to bipolar electrical stimulation of the anterior and/or posterior roots. The motor threshold for stimulation of anterior roots is one-third that of the threshold for posterior roots. The lateral aspect of the DREZ is now exposed so that the microsurgical lesions can be performed, 2–3 mm in depth and at 35°–45° angles in the ventro-lateral aspect of the sulcus all along the selected segments of the spinal cord. Intra-operative neurophysiological monitoring may be of some help to identify cord levels, quantify the extent of MDT and avoid impairing long fibre tracts.

MDT is indicated in paraplegic patients, especially when they are bedridden as a result of disabling flexion spasms, and in hemiplegic patients with irreducible and/or painful hyperspasticity in the upper limb (Sindou et al., 1986, 1991a; Sindou & Jeanmonod, 1989; Beneton et al., 1991; Sindou, 1997). MDT also can be used to treat neurogenic bladder with uninhibited detrusor contractions resulting in voiding around a catheter (Beneton et al., 1991).

Our studies to date consist of 45 cases of unilateral cervical (C5–T1) MDT for harmful spasticity in the upper limb, 121 cases of bilateral lumbo-sacral MDT (L2 to S1 or S5) for disabling spasticity in the lower limbs and 12 cases of bilateral sacral S2–S3 (S4) MDT for hyperactive neurogenic bladder only. Effects on muscular tone can be judged only after a three-month follow-up. A 'useful' result on spasticity allowing withdrawal of antispasmodic medications, was obtained in 78% of

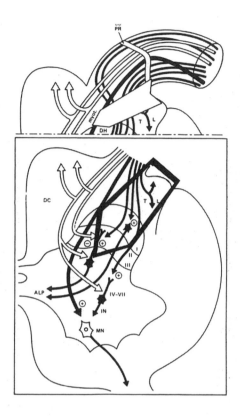
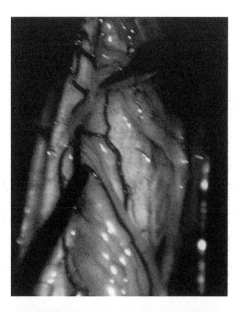
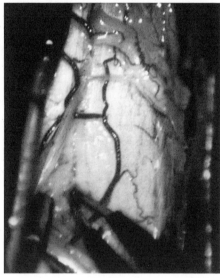

Fig. 11.8   Micro-drezotomy (MDT). *Left:* Organization of fibres at the dorsal root entry zone (DREZ) in humans. The large arrow shows the proposed extent of the MDT, that is, the lateral and central bundles formed by the nociceptive and myotatic fibres, as well as the excitatory medial part or the TL and the upper layers of the dorsal horn. *Right:* Principles of the technique of the MDT. Example at the cervical level through a right cervical hemilaminectomy (the procedure for the lumbo-sacral roots is the same). The right C6 posterior root has been retracted toward the inside to make the ventrolateral region of the DREZ accessible. The incision is performed into the dorsolateral sulcus using a small piece of razor blade (upper photograph). The incision is 2–3 mm deep and is made at 35° angle (at 45° angle for the lumbo-sacral level). Then microcoagulations are created with a very sharp and graduated bipolar microforceps down to the apex of the dorsal horn (lower photograph).

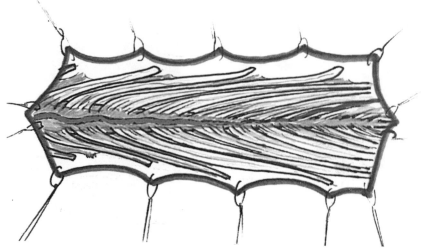

(a)   (b)

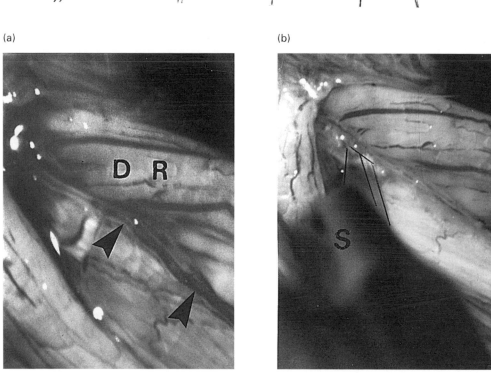

Fig. 11.9   MDT technique at the lumbo-sacral level. *Top:* For paraplegia, the conus medullaris is
approached through a (T10) T11–L2 laminectomy. Exposure of the left dorsolateral aspect
of the conus medullaris on the left side. *Bottom:* Exposure of the left posterolateral aspect
of the conus medullaris. (a) The rootlets of the selected lumbo-sacral dorsal roots (D) are
displaced dorsally and medially to obtain proper access to the ventrolateral aspects of the
dorsal root entry zone in the posterolateral sulcus. Only the tiny pial vessels (arrows) will
be coagulated with a thin, pointed, graduated bipolar microforceps. (b) Microscalpel (S)

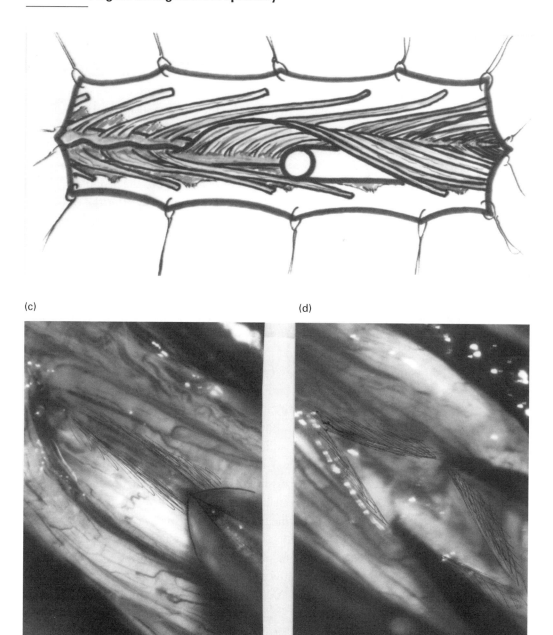

(c)   (d)

made from a small, elongated fragment of a razor blade mounted on a holder is ready to
start the incision, which will be at an angle of 45° ventromedially and 2–3 mm deep
(arrows, posterolateral sulcus). (c) Microcoagulations are performed inside the incision, 2
to 3 mm in depth, down the upper layers of the dorsal horn. (d) The line of incision is
opened (between the two tips of the bipolar forceps) and reveals its depth and the apex
of the dorsal horn.

patients with a spastic upper limb. A similarly useful effect was obtained in 75% of patients with spasticity in the lower limbs.

When spasms were present in paraplegic patients, they were suppressed or markedly decreased in 88% of cases. The results were better in spasticity (and spasms) caused by pure spinal cord lesions (in the order of 80% useful effects), followed by multiple sclerosis (75%). The least improvement was observed in patients with spasticity resulting from cerebral lesions (60%). Reduction in spasticity usually leads to a significant improvement of abnormal postures and articular limitations. This was achieved in about 90% of our patients. For the hemiplegic upper limb, the increase in articular amplitude was most remarkable for the elbow and shoulder (when not 'frozen') but was much more limited for the wrist and fingers, especially if there was retraction of the flexor muscles and no residual voluntary motor activity in the extensors. For the lower limb(s) with abnormal postures in flexion, the increase in articular amplitude was dependent on the degree of the preoperative retractions. When the post-MDT gains were deemed insufficient because of persistent joint limitations, complementary orthopaedic surgery was indicated. With regard to the five patients who had paraplegia with irreducible hyperextension, all were completely relieved.

In the patients with some voluntary movements hidden behind spasticity, reduction in the hypertonia results in an improvement in voluntary motor activity. Of the patients operated on for spasticity in the upper limb 50% had better motor activity of the shoulder and arm, but only half of those with some preoperative distal motor function obtained additional hand prehension. Only 10% of the patients with spasticity in the lower limb(s) had significant motor improvement after surgery, because most patients in this group had no functional preoperative motor function. In these very severely affected patients the main benefit was better comfort, less pain, ability to resume physical therapy and less dependence in their daily lives (Figure 11.10). See Sindou (1997) for pre- and postoperative assessment of patients (with details on the functional scores used). (Tables 11.2 and 11.3.)

Bladder capacity was significantly improved in 85% of the 38 patients who had hyperative neurogenic bladder with urine leakage around the catheter. These 32 improved patients were those in whom the detrusor was not irreversibly fibrotic. Pain when present was in general favourably influenced. MDT constantly produced a marked decrease in sensation.

Because most patients were in a precarious general and neurological state, death occurred in five (4%) patients, resulting from respiratory problems in four and bed sores in one. Two multiple sclerosis patients presented with an acute but transient increase in their pre-existing neurological symptoms during the postoperative period, whereas two others had a new postoperative clinical manifestation of the disease.

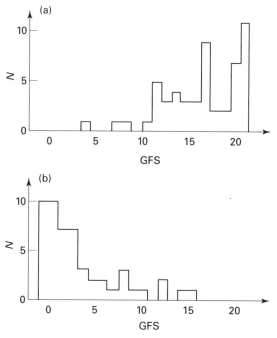

Fig. 11.10   Distribution of pre- (a) and postoperative (b) global functional scores (GFS) in patients with spasticity in the lower limbs. *N:* number of patients. (See Table 11.3 for explanation of the scoring system.)

Finally, mention should be made of one patient who had been operated on at the cervical level and who continued to have a persistent motor deficit in the ipsilateral leg after surgery.

With *rigorous selection* of patients, MDT can be very effective in relieving pain and suppressing excess spasticity. Good long-lasting relief of excess spasticity had been achieved in 80% of our patients. As a result, MDT, sometimes combined with complementary orthopaedic surgery, resulted in significant improvement in patient comfort and articular deformities and even enhancement of residual voluntary motility hidden preoperatively behind hypertonicity.

Orthopaedic surgery

Orthopaedic procedures can reduce spasticity by means of muscle relaxation that results from tendon lengthening and may help in restoring articular function when deformities have become irreducible. Current techniques for correcting excessive shortness of the muscle tendon assembly are muscular desinsertion, myotomy, tenotomy and lengthening-tenotomy. The lengthening operations most often used are: (1) the muscular desinsertion of the epicondylian muscles for flexed wrist and

Table 11.2. Functional score for hemiplegic patients with spasticity in the upper limb

Grade	Description
I	Absence of useful active mobility and uneasy and painful passive mobilization, making it difficult to dress and wash
II	Easy passive mobilization but without any useful voluntary movements
III	Slight but useful voluntary motor function
IV	Good active mobility with the possibility of prehension in the hand and fingers

fingers (Scaglietti's procedure); (2) the flexor digitorum lengthening for the hemiplegic hand; (3) the tendon lengthening of the heel cord for foot equinism; and (4) the hamstring-tendon lengthening associated with patellar-tendon shortening. Such techniques aim to obtain a more functional position for the limb or limbs involved. Excessive lengthening can lead to a decrease in muscular strength.

Tendon transfer has a different goal – to normalize articular orientation when it has been distorted by muscular imbalance. Transfer of spastic muscles must be avoided. If necessary, suppression of spasticity must be achieved by neurosurgical procedure before tendon transfer. A frequently indicated tendon transfer is the fixation of the distal tendon of the peroneus brevis onto the tibialis anterior for equino-varus foot (i.e. Bardot's procedure).

Osteotomies aim to correct bone deformity resulting from growth distorsion in a child (e.g. femoral derotation osteotomy to correct excessive anteversion in patients with cerebral palsy) or to treat stiffened joints (e.g. supracondylar femoral osteotomy for irreducible flexed knee). Articular surgery is indicated only when osteo-articular deformity cannot be corrected by osteotomy or tendon surgery alone. When a foot varus deformity is very severe and fixed, one can have recourse to a triple hind-foot arthrodesis – subtalar and midtarsal; with this technique the ankle remains free. Arthrodesis must not be performed in children until they have stopped growing.

Orthopaedic surgery can be undertaken to correct or even prevent irreducible deformities, to increase comfort in the more severely affected patients or to improve function in those who have recovered a sufficient level of voluntary motor function, but only after spasticity has been reduced.

Indications for surgery

In adults

Intrathecal baclofen (ITB) administration is indicated for para- or tetraplegic patients with severe and diffuse spasticity especially when from spinal origin.

Table 11.3. Global functional score for paraplegic patients with spasticity in the lower limb(s)

Pain
0   absent
1   rare and mild
2   frequent: minimal disability
3   marked and frequent: marked disability
4   permanent and severe

Spasms
0   absent
1   rare and mild spasms only during mobilizations: no disability
2   frequent, spontaneous but moderate spasms: moderate disability
3   frequent
4   almost constant and severe spasms: severe disability, major problems for sitting or lying

Sitting position
0   normal
1   mild difficulty
2   moderate to marked difficulty, causing reduction of sitting periods
3   severe difficulty: patient has to be tied down in position
4   impossible

Body transfers
0   normal
1   mild difficulty
2   moderate difficulty
3   marked difficulty, need for a person helping
4   severe difficulty, need for two persons helping

Washing and dressing
0   normal
1   mild difficulty
2   moderate difficulty
3   marked difficulty, need for a person helping
4   severe difficulty, need for two persons helping

Notes:

This score developed by Millet et al. (1981) cited in Sindou et al. (1991b) quantifies five components that are directly influenced by spasticity, abnormal postures and articular limitations and are parts of the patient's everyday life. The score goes from 0 to 4 for each component, with a total of 20/20 denoting a bedridden and totally dependent patient. A score of 10/20 was seen to correspond to the threshold between a decent condition and an unacceptable condition and thus as the lowest position at which to consider surgery.

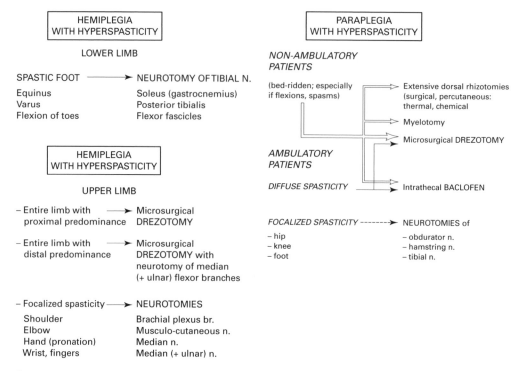

Fig. 11.11   A summary of the guidelines for surgical indications.

Because of its reversibility, this method has to be considered before considering an ablative procedure. However, the range is very narrow between excess of hypotonia with loss of strength and an insufficient effect. An intrathecal test through a temporary access port can be useful before indicating permanent implantation.

Neuro-ablative techniques are indicated for severe focalized spasticity in the limbs of paraplegic, tetraplegic or hemiplegic patients.

Neurotomies are preferred when spasticity is localized to muscle groups innervated by a small number of nerves, or a single, peripheral nerve. When spasticity affects an entire limb, MDT is preferred. Several types of neuro-ablative procedures can be combined in the treatment of one patient, when needed.

Whatever the situation and the aetiology may be, orthopaedic surgery must be considered only after spasticity has been reduced by physical and pharmacological treatments and, when necessary, by neurosurgical procedures.

Guidelines for surgical indications have been detailed elsewhere (Sindou & Mertens, 1991; Sindou et al., 1991b) and are summarized in Figure 11.11. The general rule is to *tailor individual treatments* as much as possible to the particular problems of the patient.

In children with cerebral palsy

In children, surgical indications depend on pre-operative abilities and disabilities and the eventual functional goals. As guidelines we have adopted the classification of six groups as defined by Abbott (1991).

(1)   In independent ambulatory patients, the goal is to improve efficiency and cosmesis in walking by eliminating as many abnormally responsive neural circuits as can be identified through functional posterior rhizotomy. Surgery is best performed as soon as possible after the child has demonstrated the ability to work with a therapist, usually between ages three and seven years, and frequently must be done in conjunction with operations on tendons because of concomitant shortened muscles.

(2)   For ambulatory patients dependent on assistance devices (i.e. canes, crutches, rollators, walkers), the goal is to lessen that dependence. A child with poor trunk control or lack of protective reaction but with good underlying strength in the antigravity muscles can safely undergo a functional posterior rhizotomy. In children dependent on hypertonicity in the quadriceps to bear weight, a limited sectorial rhizotomy is preferable. For children who are in the process of developing ambulatory skills and need an assistance device only temporarily, it is important to delay surgery until they have perfected these skills.

(3)   For quadriped crawlers (or bunny hoppers) the goal is to achieve assisted ambulation during mid-childhood to early adolescence. A functional posterior rhizotomy will decrease hypertonicity in the leg musculature and allow better limb alignment in the standing position for a child with adequate muscular strength. However, a child who exhibits quadriceps weakness can be considered for a sectorial posterior rhizotomy. Children in this group can present at a young age with progressive hip dislocation. The goal is to stop the progressive orthopaedic deformity by using obturator neurotomy with adductor tenotomies or functional posterior rhizotomy.

(4)   For commando (or belly) crawlers disabled by severe deficiencies in postural control, the goal of posterior rhizotomy is only to improve functioning in the sitting position by increasing stability.

(5)   In totally dependent children, with no locomotive abilities, the goals are simply to improve comfort and facilitate care. As with group 4, the preferred treatment is posterior rhizotomy, but there is also a need for exploring the efficacy of ITB.

(6)   For asymmetrical spasticity, selective peripheral neurotomies must be considered, especially obturator and tibial for the spastic hip and foot, respectively. For upper limb spasticity, the MDT procedure and/or selective neurotomies of the flexor muscles of wrist and fingers can be considered.

In summary, for children, the main goal is to stop and prevent progressive and irreversible orthopaedic deformities. Lumbo-sacral posterior rhizotomies can be indicated for reducing the excessive general level of spasticity in diplegic (and even quadriplegic, thanks to distant effects in upper limbs) patients. ITB is an alternative, but the range between an insufficient effect and an excessive effect responsible for a global decrease in tone impairing gait and reducing muscular strength, is often very narrow. In cases with localized hyperspasticity threatening a joint, peripheral neurotomy(ies) can be the solution, as for instance obturator neurotomy for hip spasticity. Frequently orthopaedic surgery can be usefully performed in conjunction with neurological surgery to lengthen tendons.

Conclusion

Spasticity is often a useful substitute for deficiency of motor strength, and therefore to that extent must be preserved. However, not infrequently, it may become harmful, leading to an aggravation of motor disability. When excessive spasticity is not sufficiently controlled by physical therapy and pharmacological means, patients can have recourse to surgery, especially neurosurgical procedures. By suppressing excessive spasticity, correcting abnormal postures and relieving the frequently associated pain, surgery for spasticity allows physiotherapy to be resumed and it sometimes results in the reappearance of, or improvement in, useful voluntary motility. When dealing with these patients, the surgeon must know the risks of the available treatments. To minimize those risks, the surgeon needs: a strong anatomic, physiological and chemical background; rigorous methods to assess and quantify the disorders; and the ability to work in a multidisciplinary team (Sindou et al., 1991b).

REFERENCES

Abbott, R. (1991). Indications for surgery to treat children with spasticity due to cerebral palsy. In *Neurosurgery for Spasticity: A Multidisciplinary Approach*, ed. M. Sindou, R. Abbott & Y. Keravel, pp. 215–17. New York: Springer Verlag.

Abbott, R., Forem, S. L. & Johann, M. (1989). Selective posterior rhizotomy for the treatment of spasticity. *Child's Nerv Syst*, **5**: 337–46.

Beneton, C., Mertens, P., Leriche, A. & Sindou, M. (1991). The spastic bladder and its treatment. In *Neurosurgery for Spasticity: A Multidisciplinary Approach*, ed. M. Sindou, R. Abbott & Y. Keravel, pp. 193–9. New York: Springer-Verlag.

Berard, C., Sindou, M., Berard, J. & Carrier, H. (1998). Selective neurotomy of the tibial nerve in the spastic hemiplegic child: an exploration of the recurrence. *J Pediatr Orthop*, **7**: 66–70.

Bischof, W. (1951). Die longitudinale Myelotomie. *Zentralbl Neurochir*, **2**: 79–88.

Brunelli, G. & Brunelli, F. (1983). Hyponeurotisation sélective microchirurgie dans les paralyses spastiques. *Ann Chir Main*, **2**: 277–80.

Cahan, L. D., Kundi, M. S., McPherson, D., Starr, A. & Peacock, W. J. (1987). Electrophysiologic studies in selective dorsal rhizotomy for spasticity in children with cerebral palsy. *Appl. Neurophysiol*, **50**: 459–682.

Cook, A. W. & Weinstein, S. P. (1973). Chronic dorsal column stimulation in multiple sclerosis. *NY J Med*, **73**: 2868–72.

Davis, R., Engle, H., Kudzma, J., Gray, E., Ryan, T. & Dusnak, A. (1982). Update of chronic cerebellar stimulation for spasticity and epilepsy. *Appl Neurophysiol*, **45**: 44–50.

Decq, P., Filipetti, P., Fevet, A., Djindjian, M., Saraoui, A. & Keravel, Y. (1997). Peripheral selective neurotomy of the brachial plexus collateral branches for the treatment of the spastic shoulder: anatomical study and clinical results on five patients. *J Neurosurg*, **86**: 648–53.

Dogliotti, A. (1931). Traitement des syndromes douloureux de la périphérie par l'alcoolisation sous-arachnoïdienne des racines postrieures à leur émergence de la moelle épinière. *Presse Médicale*, **39**: 1249–52.

Eccles, J., Eccles, R. & Magni, F. (1961). Central inhibitory action attributable to presynaptic depolarization produced by muscle afferent volleys. *J Physiol*, **159**: 147–66.

Fasano, V. A., Barolat-Romana, G., Ivaldi, A. & Sguazzi, A. (1976). La radicotomie postérieure fonctionnelle dans le traitement de la spasticité cérébrale. *Neurochirurgie*, **22**: 23–34.

Foerster, O. (1913). On the indications and results of the excision of posterior spinal nerve roots in men. *Surg Gynecol Obstet*, **16**: 463–74.

Fraioli, B. & Guidetti, B. (1977). Posterior partial rootlet section in the treatment of spasticity. *J. Neurosurg*, **46**: 618–26.

Frerebeau, P. (1991). Sectorial posterior rhizotomy for the treatment of spasticity in children with cerebral palsy. In *Neurosurgery for Spasticity: A Multidisciplinary Approach*, ed. M. Sindou, A. Abbott & Y. Keravel, pp. 145–7. New York: Springer-Verlag.

Gros, C. (1979). Spasticity: clinical classification and surgical treatment. In *Advances and Technical Standards in Neurosurgery*, ed. Krayenbühl, vol. 6, pp. 55–97. New York: Springer-Verlag.

Gros, C., Frerebeau, P., Benezech, J. & Privat, J. M. (1977). Neurotomie radiculaire selective. In *Actualités en Rééducation Fonctionnelle et Réadaptation*, ed. L. Simon, série 2, pp. 230–5. Paris: Masson.

Gros, C., Ouaknine, G., Vlahovitch, B. & Frerebeau, P. (1967). La radicotomie sélective postérieure dans le traitement neurochirurgical de l'hypertonie pyramidale. *Neurochirurgie*, **13**: 505–18.

Guttman, L. (1953). The treatment and rehabilitation of patients with injuries of the spinal cord. In Cope 2 (ed.): *History of the Second World War*, ed. Sir Zachary Cope, Surgery, pp. 422–516. London: HMSO.

Gybels, J. & Van Roost, D. (1987). Spinal cord stimulation for spasticity. In *Advances and Technical Standards in Neurosurgery*, ed. L. Symon, vol. 15, pp. 63–96. New York: Springer-Verlag.

Herz, D. A., Parsons, K. C. & Learl, L. (1983). Percutaneous radiofrequency foraminal rhizotomies. *Spine*, **8**: 729–32.

Hodgkinson, I., Berard, C., Jindrich, M. L., Sindou, M., Mertens, P. & Berard, J. (1996).

Radicotomie postérieure fonctionnelle chez l'enfant IMC. Résultats à un an post-opératoire sur 18 cas. *Ann Réadaptation Med Phys*, **39**: 103–11.

Kasdon, D. L. & Lathi, E. S. (1984). A prospective study of radiofrequency rhizotomy in the treatment of post-traumatic spasticity. *Neurosurgery*, **15**: 526–9.

Kelly, R. E. & Gauthier-Smith, P. C. (1959). Intrathecal phenol in the treatment of reflex spasms and spasticity. *Lancet*, **11**: 1102–5.

Kenmore, D. (1983). Radiofrequency neurotomy for peripheral pain and spasticity syndromes. *Contemp Neurosurg*, **5**: 1–6.

Laitinen, L. V. & Singounas, E. (1971). Longitudinal myelotomy in the treatment of spasticity of the legs. *J Neurosurg*, **35**: 536–40.

Maher, R. (1955). Relief of pain in incurable cancer. *Lancet*, **1**: 18–20.

Melzach & Wall, P. D. (1974). Presynaptic control of impulse at the first central synapse in the cutaneous pathway. *Prog Brain Res*, **12**: 92–118.

Mertens, P. & Sindou, M. (1991). Selective peripheral neurotomies for the treatment of spasticity. In *Neurosurgery for Spasticity: A Multidisciplinary Approach*, ed. M. Sindou, R. Abbott & Y. Keravel, pp. 119–32. New York: Springer-Verlag.

Nathan, P. W. (1959). Intrathecal phenol to relieve spasticity in paraplegia. *Lancet*, **11**: 1099–102.

Ouaknine, G. (1980). Le traitement chirurgical de la spasticité. *Union Med Can*, **109**: 1–11.

Peacock, W. J. & Arens, L. J. (1982). Selective posterior rhizotomy for the relief of spasticity in cerebral palsy. *S Afr Med J*, **62**: 119–24.

Pourpre, M. H. (1960). Traitement neurochirurgical des contractures chez les parapléques post-traumatiques. *Neurochirurgie*, **6**: 229–36.

Privat, J. M., Benezech, J., Frerebeau, P. & Gros, C. (1976). Sectorial posterior rhizotomy. A new technique of surgical treatment of spasticity. *Acta Neurochir*, **35**: 181–95.

Siegfried, J. & Lazorthes, Y. (1985). La neurochirurgie fonctionnelle de l'infirmité motrice d'origine cérébrale. *Neurochirurgie*, **31** (Suppl. 1): 1–118.

Sindou, M. (1972). *Etude de la Jonction Radiculo-Medullaire postérieure: La Radicellotomie Postérieure Sélective dans la Chirurgie de la Douleur.* Med. Thesis, Lyon.

Sindou, M. (1997). Spinal entry zone interruption for spasticity. In *Textbook of Stereotactic and Functional Neurosurgery*, ed. R. R. Tasker & P. Gildenberg, pp. 1257–66. New York: McGraw Hill.

Sindou, M., Abbott, R. & Keravel, Y. (Eds) (1991b). *Neurosurgery for Spasticity: A Multidisciplinary Approach.* New York: Springer-Verlag.

Sindou, M., Abdennebi, B. & Sharkey, P. (1985b). Microsurgical selective procedures in the peripheral nerves and the posterior root-spinal cord junction for spasticity. *Appl Neurophysiol*, **48**: 97–104.

Sindou, M., Fischer, G., Goutelle, A., Schott, B. & Mansuy, L. (1974). La radicellotomie postérieure sélective dans le traitement des spasticités. *Rev Neurol*, **130**: 201–15.

Sindou, M. & Jeanmonod, D. (1989). Microchirurgical-DREZ-otomy for the treatment of spasticity and pain in the lower limbs. *Neurosurgery*, **24**: 655–70.

Sindou, M., Jeanmonod, D. & Mertens, P. (1991a). Surgery in the dorsal root entry zone: microsurgical DREZ-tomy (MDT) for the treatment of spasticity. In *Neurosurgery for Spasticity: A Multidisciplinary Approach*, ed. M. Sindou, R. Abbott & Y. Keravel, pp. 165–82. New York: Springer-Verlag.

Sindou, M. & Mertens, P. (1988). Selective neurotomy of the tibial nerve for treatment of the spastic foot. *Neurosurgery*, **23**: 738–44.

Sindou, M. & Mertens, P. (1991). Indication for surgery to treat adults with harmful spasticity. In *Neurosurgery for Spasticity: A Multidisciplinary Approach*, ed. M. Sindou, R. Abbott & Y. Keravel, pp. 211–13. New York: Springer-Verlag.

Sindou, M., Mifsud, J. J., Boisson, D. & Goutelle, A. (1986). Selective posterior rhizotomy in the dorsal root entry zone for treatment of hyperspasticity and pain in the hemiplegic upper limb. *Neurosurgery*, **18**: 587–95.

Sindou, M., Millet, M. F., Mortamais, J. & Eyssette, M. (1982). Results of selective posterior rhizotomy in the treatment of painful and spastic paraplegia secondary to multiple sclerosis. *Appl Neurophysiol*, **45**: 335–40.

Sindou, M., Pregelj, R., Boisson, D., Eyssette, M. & Goutelle, A. (1985a). Surgical selective lesions of nerve fibers and myelotomies for the modification of muscle hypertonia. In *Recent Achievements in Restorative Neurology: Upper Motor Neuron Functions and Dysfunctions*, ed. Sir J. Eccles & M. R. Dimitrijevic, pp. 10–26. Basel: S. Karger.

Stoffel, A. (1913). The treatment of spastic contractures. *Am J Orthop Surg*, **10**: 611–19.

Storrs, B. (1987). Selective posterior rhizotomy for treatment of progressive spasticity in patients with myelomeningocele. *Pediatr Neurosci*, **13**: 135–7.

Uematsu, S., Udvarhelyi, G. B., Benson, D. W. & Siebens, A. A. (1974). Percutaneous radio-frequency rhizotomy. *Surg Neurol*, **2**: 319–25.

Young, B. & Mulcachy, J. J. (1980). Percutaneous sacral rhizotomy for neurogenic detrusor hyperreflexia. *J Neurosurg*, **53**: 85–7.

12

Management of spasticity in children

Marinis Pirpiris and H. Kerr Graham

Management of spasticity in children

Spasticity in children is a common and an important clinical problem. Despite this, clinicians have difficulty in agreeing with a definition of spasticity and there are no validated clinical measures that will quantify spasticity in children (Lance, 1980; see Chapter 2). The Ashworth scale (Ashworth, 1964), derived for adults and only validated in the upper limb, is of limited utility in quantifying spasticity in children (Bohannon & Smith, 1987; see Chapter 3).

Spasticity is only one feature of the upper motor neuron syndrome (UMN syndrome). Although clinicians tend to concentrate on the positive features of the UMN syndrome (spasticity, clonus, hyper reflexia) it is the negative features (weakness, loss of selective motor control, sensory impairment) that ultimately may limit function and determine prognosis (Gans & Glenn, 1982).

Spasticity can be defined as a velocity dependent resistance to passive movement of a joint and its associated musculature (Lance, 1980; Rymer & Powers, 1989; Massagli, 1991). However, patients do not complain about spasticity, they are more likely to be aware of stiffness, deformity and limitations in functional abilities. 'Stiffness' is a useful term because it is widely understood by both clinicians and by patients and it does not imply a specific causation (Boyd et al., 2000). It is also useful in terms of describing the limb pathology in children with spasticity. Although spasticity may be an early problem in the child with cerebral palsy, true muscle shortening or contracture also appears at an early stage and the majority of children will have a mixture of spasticity and contracture, the proportions varying with time. In any discussion of spasticity management in children, an agreed terminology is important in recognizing and describing two principal components of muscle stiffness:

- 'Dynamic' shortening or contracture, mainly caused by movement disorders such as spasticity (but not excluding mixed movement disorders). Typically 'dynamic' contracture is recognized in younger children with cerebral palsy or spasticity of recent onset. Such children are likely to exhibit hyperreflexia, clonus

Table 12.1. Aetiology of spasticity in 341 children (cerebral palsy, orthopaedic and spasticity clinics)

Aetiology of condition	Number of cases (%)
Cerebral palsy	79
Traumatic brain injury	6
Spina bifida	5
Spinal cord injury	2
Miscellaneous	8

and a velocity dependent resistance to passive joint motion. Children who exhibit 'dynamic' calf shortening may walk on their toes with an equinus gait but on the examination couch, the range of passive ankle dorsiflexion will be full or almost full.

- 'Fixed' shortening or 'myostatic' contracture describes the typical stiffness found in muscles of older children with cerebral palsy or spasticity of longer duration. The stiffness is much less velocity dependent, is still present during couch examination and, crucially, is present under anaesthesia.

The entire philosophical approach to management of spasticity and its sequelae in this chapter are predicated on this simple concept.

Causes of spasticity in children

With the eradication of poliomyelitis and the dramatic fall in the prevalence of spina bifida, the most common motor disorder in children in developed countries is cerebral palsy. The incidence of cerebral palsy in developed countries is static or even rising. The reductions in the prevalence of kernicterus due to neonatal jaundice has been overshadowed by improved survival of very low birth weight and premature infants, many of whom suffer from spastic diplegia and quadriplegia (Stanley & Alberman, 1984; Petterson et al., 1993a,b; Pellegrino & Dormans, 1998).

Other common causes of spasticity in children are traumatic brain injury and spinal cord injury. Table 12.1 shows the cause of spasticity in a consecutive sample of 341 children seen at some of the clinics at the Royal Children's Hospital in Melbourne, Australia, in 1998.

Spasticity in children will continue to be a common and challenging problem for the foreseeable future. Whilst reduction in the incidence of cerebral palsy would have the most impact in reducing the overall incidence of spasticity in children, prevention of traumatic brain injury and spinal cord injury is probably more realistic (Glasgow & Graham, 1997).

The pathology of spasticity

Given that the most common cause of spasticity in our clinics is cerebral palsy, subsequent discussion on pathology and management will focus mainly but not exclusively on spasticity in the context of juvenile cerebral palsy.

The pathology of spasticity cannot be separated from the pathology of the UMN syndrome. The child with diplegia who walks on his or her toes because of calf spasticity, may also be unable to voluntarily control the dorsiflexors of the ankle during gait. No matter how effective management of the calf spasticity is, gait may remain impaired because toe clearance cannot be achieved during the swing phase of gait (Perry, 1985, 1992). Indeed there is virtually always an effective solution to calf spasticity/stiffness/shortening but inability to control the ankle dorsiflexors during swing phase may mean lifelong dependence on an orthosis.

The limb pathology in cerebral palsy is acquired during childhood. Children with cerebral palsy do not have contractures, dislocated hips or scoliosis at birth. These common deformities are acquired during childhood. Muscle growth in children is a race between the pacemakers – i.e. the physes of the long bones, and the muscle-tendon units, in which the muscles are doomed to second place.

The prerequisite for normal muscle growth is frequent stretching of relaxed muscle. In children with cerebral palsy the muscles do not readily relax, because of spasticity and they are infrequently stretched because of reduced activity. Spasticity plus reduced activity leads to failure of longitudinal muscle growth, contractures and fixed deformities (Cosgrove & Graham, 1994; Ziv et al., 1984).

For convenience, the limb pathology can be considered in three stages (Figure 12.1):

- **Stage 1**: typically the younger child with cerebral palsy, the deformities are all dynamic or reversible. This is the phase when spasticity management, gait training and the use of orthoses may have a useful role.
- **Stage 2**: there are fixed contractures, which may require surgical lengthening of muscles or tendons.
- **Stage 3**: in addition to spasticity and contractures, there are changes in bones and joints, including torsion of the long bones and joint instability. The most common torsional problems are medial femoral torsion and lateral tibial torsion. Joint instability problems include hip subluxation and subtalar collapse in the hindfoot.

Despite the undoubted value of Mercer Rang's longitudinal view of limb pathology in the child with cerebral palsy (Rang, 1990), additional factors should be considered. Firstly, there is no smooth transition from stage 1 to stage 3. Spasticity, dynamic and fixed contractures coexist in varying proportions in most children. The transition from dynamic to fixed contracture occurs at different rates in different topographical types of cerebral palsy and at different rates in different

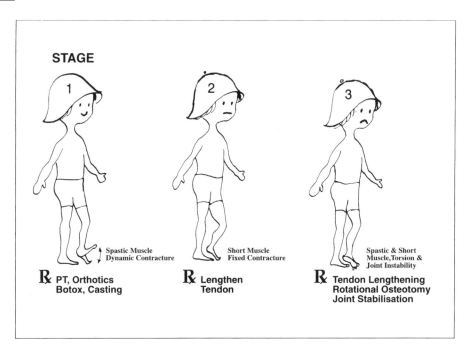

STAGE

1

2

3

Spastic Muscle
Dynamic Contracture

Short Muscle
Fixed Contracture

Spastic & Short
Muscle, Torsion &
Joint Instability

℞ PT, Orthotics
   Botox, Casting

℞ Lengthen
   Tendon

℞ Tendon Lengthening
   Rotational Osteotomy
   Joint Stabilisation

Fig. 12.1   The stages of lower limb pathology in the child with cerebral palsy (Modified after Rang.)

limb segments and even in different muscle groups in the same limb segment. There appears to be a 'biological clock' running at different speeds for different muscles in children with cerebral palsy, governing the timing of the transition from dynamic to fixed contracture (Boyd & Graham, 1997; Eames et al., 1999).

In hemiplegia, there is an earlier transition from dynamic to fixed contracture than in diplegia. The dynamic component to the contracture can be exploited by spasticity management (Eames et al., 1999). Also, in hemiplegia, fixed contracture develops in the lower limb earlier than in the upper limb. Spasticity management may be appropriate in the upper limb at an age when surgery is required for a fixed equinus deformity. In the hemiplegic upper limb, the first muscle to develop a fixed contracture is almost invariably the pronator teres (Boyd & Graham, 1997). This may result more from the absence of active supination than increased spasticity in the pronator teres. A useful strategy may be to combine a lengthening or re-routing of the pronator teres, with spasticity management of the wrist and finger flexors using botulinum toxin A (BTXA).

Recognition of these types of patterns may greatly improve the outcome of both spasticity and contracture management and lead to the development of creative strategies to deal with common clinical presentations (Boyd & Graham, 1997; Figure 12.2).

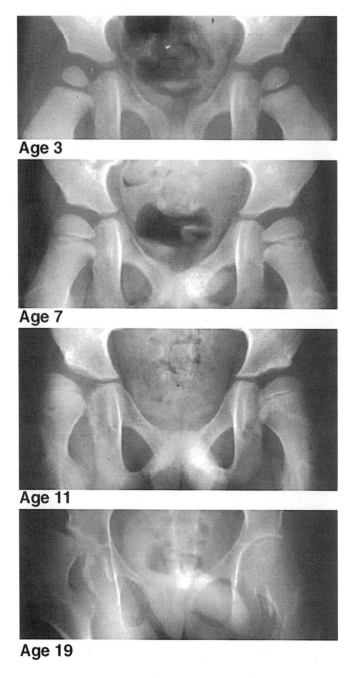

Age 3

Age 7

Age 11

Age 19

Fig. 12.2   The pathology in the lower limbs in children with cerebral palsy is progressive as this sequence of hip X-rays shows. At 3 years of age, the hip X-ray is normal. At age 7 there is a very mild uncovering of the right hip. At age 11, the hip is subluxed and more than 50% is outside the acetabulum. At age 19, there is painful degenerative arthritis with few management options remaining.

Measuring spasticity in children: clinical

The Ashworth scale

There are few useful clinical measures of spasticity and none validated for use in children. The Ashworth and modified Ashworth scales are blunt and unresponsive tools in the assessment of the child with cerebral palsy (Ashworth, 1964; Bohannon & Smith, 1987). These tools are subjective and reliability between investigators may be a problem. Most muscles in most children are Grade 1+ to Grade 3. Most useful clinical responses to spasticity management are within, not across a single Ashworth grade. Of much greater utility is the measurement of dynamic joint range, which can be used across most major joints as a quantitative measure of spasticity (Tardieu et al., 1954; Boyd et al., 2000).

The dynamic and static joint range of motion

The range of motion of joints in both the upper and lower limbs is classically used as a proxy measure of the length of muscles crossing that joint. In the upper limb the range of elbow extension is taken to be a measure of the length of the elbow flexors, the biceps and brachialis. Loss of elbow extension (fixed flexion deformity) is taken to mean shortening of the elbow flexors although it should be noted that other factors such as intrinsic joint contractures must be excluded. In the lower limb the range of dorsiflexion at the ankle is considered to be a measure of the calf muscle length. A further refinement is that the range of ankle dorsiflexion with the knee flexed is a measure of soleus length and the range of ankle dorsiflexion with the knee extended is a measure of gastrocnemius length (Silfverskiold, 1924). This is the basis for the Silfverskiold test and although it may be only completely reliable under anaesthesia, it is of great value as a simple test to differentiate between gastrocnemius versus gastrocnemius and soleus contracture. Typically, in hemiplegia there is usually shortening of both the gastrocnemius and soleus but in diplegia, isolated gastrocnemius shortening is common. The criticism of the Silfverskiold test (Silfverskiold, 1924) by Perry has in our view led to an unwarranted devaluation of this most useful clinical test (Perry et al., 1974, 1976, 1978).

In children with spasticity, joint range of motion measurements are performed slowly in order to avoid provoking a stretch reflex that might invalidate the measurement. The joint range and muscle length estimation performed slowly approximates to that determined under anaesthesia and is a measure of true muscle length or contracture. Because this measurement is performed slowly with the patient on an examination couch, we refer to this as the 'static muscle length' or R2.

Dynamic joint range of motion is measured by performing the same type of examination much more quickly. The aim is to deliberately provoke a stretch reflex, if it is present. Typically this first catch or R1 comes in at a repeatable joint angular position. This is usually 20°–50° prior to R2, the static muscle length (Tardieu et al., 1954). The variation is due to the proportion of the deformity, which is dynamic, as opposed to fixed. R2 approximates to the degree of 'myostatic contracture' or fixed shortening, and R1 the degree of spasticity or dynamic shortening. These simple clinical tests of R1 and R2, static and dynamic muscle length can be performed to assess the length of the adductors of the hip, the hamstrings, quadriceps and the calf muscles, some of the most important lower limb muscle groups to be affected by spasticity.

The measurement of R2 and R1 are of great practical relevance in the management of spasticity because they help to:
- differentiate between spasticity and contracture;
- quantify the degree of spasticity present;
- select which muscles might respond to spasticity management;
- serve to monitor the response to spasticity management.

R2 measures the static muscle length or contracture, which may require tendon lengthening. R1 reflects the degree of spasticity or dynamic shortening, which may respond to spasticity management.

Example 1

A three-year-old child with spastic diplegia has an equinus gait affecting both lower limbs equally.
R1: negative 35° (35° of equinus);
R2: positive 5° (5° of dorsiflexion);
R2 minus R1: 40°.
Spasticity management is likely to be beneficial because there are 40° of dynamic shortening to be exploited by spasticity management. Surgical lengthening of the heel cord is contraindicated because the degree of fixed contracture is so small.

Example 2

A 10-year-old boy with hemiplegia walks with an equinus gait on the affected side.
R1: negative 30° (30° of equinus);
R2: negative 20° (20° of equinus);
R2 minus R1: 10°.
Surgical lengthening of the Achilles tendon is indicated because R2 minus R1 = 10°. This is not enough dynamic shortening for spasticity management and there would be too much residual contracture.

Measuring spasticity in children: instrumented

Although we believe that dynamic joint range of motion is a useful clinical tool in the measurement of spasticity in children, there is a clear need for objective measurements with a greater degree of validity and repeatability. A number of techniques have been described and although most are useful within research settings, none have become popular in clinical practice.

Electromyography (EMG) can be considered to be the most direct technique because it measures the electrophysiological component of spasticity. Dynamic EMG, whereby the EMG is recorded as part of gait analysis during walking, is preferred to EMG recordings on the examination couch. EMG recorded during active or passive joint motion on the examination couch may indicate the presence of an abnormal stretch reflex but it is difficult to quantify and may not relate to what happens when the child walks (Perry, 1992). EMG during gait may delineate a variety of abnormal patterns of activity in muscle including activity which is premature, prolonged or out of phase (Perry, 1992).

Measurements of muscle stiffness address the biomechanical rather than the neurophysiological components of spasticity. These measurements may also be obtained on the examination couch or during walking. Static measurements include measurements of muscle torque and resonant frequency (Walsh, 1988; Corry et al., 1998; McLaughlin et al., 1998). In a placebo controlled, clinical trial, resonant frequency was found to be an objective means to quantify muscle stiffness in the hemiplegic upper limb. Reductions in resonant frequency were recorded after injecting the forearm muscles with BTXA (Corry et al., 1998).

Video recording of gait and aspects of the static, couch examination are very useful in clinical practice. Utility is further enhanced by split screen, two-dimensional recording with freeze-frame facilities. Careful editing and archiving of patient records is also important.

Various scoring systems or 'physician rating scales' have been devised to increase the sensitivity and objectivity of information gained from video recordings of children's gait (Koman et al., 1993, 1994; Corry, 1994; Boyd & Graham, 1999). Although some have been tested for repeatability, none have been tested for validity (Corry, 1994).

Three-dimensional gait analysis, including kinematics and kinetics, provide the clinician with valuable information regarding the effects of spasticity, contractures and other manifestations of the UMN syndrome on gait (Gage, 1995; Gage et al., 1995). Typical kinematic and kinetic patterns can be recognized and interpreted in the light of the patient's history and clinical examination. The downward slope of the sagittal plane ankle kinematic is indicative of a stiff gastrosoleus (Boyd et al., 2000). Measuring gastrosoleus R1 and R2 on the examination couch should help differentiate between spasticity and contracture. After intervention such as injecting the gastrosoleus with BTXA, repeat gait analysis can be used to quantify the magnitude of the response (Corry, 1994).

Three-dimensional kinetics have recently been shown to be of value in characterizing the muscle stiffness of younger children with cerebral palsy and give further insight into the benefits and limitations of spasticity management (Boyd et al., 2000).

The current dilemma is that only instrumented gait analysis gives valid, repeatable and accurate measures of the effects of spasticity and associated limb pathology on gait. Instrumented gait analysis, however, is limited in clinical utility because of cost and availability. Furthermore, many of the children who may need and benefit most from spasticity management are too small and lacking in co-operation for instrumented gait analysis using available techniques and hardware. Our current system requires the child to be at least 95 cm tall, over 20 kg in weight and walk independently and co-operatively along a walkway, especially for kinetic studies. There is an urgent need for new tools to measure spasticity directly in an objective, valid and repeatable manner.

Managing spasticity in children

Spasticity management has entered a new era because of developments in methods of assessment and the introduction of new and effective methods of management (Sussman, 1992; Dormans & Pellegrino, 1998). Selecting the appropriate child and the appropriate method of spasticity management requires careful judgement and experience. Clinicians, who only have a hammer, tend to see a lot of nails!

In our preliminary open-label study into the use of BTXA in the lower limbs of children with cerebral palsy, we defined our entry criteria as:

'Children with dynamic deformities which were interfering with function, in the absence of fixed, myostatic deformities' (Cosgrove et al., 1994).

Although we believe that this statement remains valid, we increasingly recognize the twin difficulties in differentiating between dynamic and fixed deformities and in measuring functional outcomes in motor disabled children. Spasticity should not be treated just because it is present. The natural history of spasticity in children is not sufficiently well known nor are our present methods of management sufficiently safe and effective to warrant such an approach. Children with severe, 'whole body' involvement frequently use spasticity in functional activities. A total extensor pattern may aid standing transfers. In this scenario, 'successful' spasticity management, if measured by reduction in tone and improved range of motion, might reduce rather than enhance function. Hence the prime goal of spasticity management must be improved function.

How can we differentiate dynamic from fixed deformities? The dynamic range of motion measures described above are a useful starting point, supplemented with appropriate instrumented measures of spasticity and its effects on function, such as motion analysis.

An understanding of motor development and methods of assessing function in children is also crucial. A major characteristic of children who have cerebral palsy is the delayed acquisition of motor skills. Given that spasticity management must often be undertaken against a background of growth and motor development, it is clear that only controlled clinical trials can reliably separate the effects of spasticity management on function from gains made as part of normal motor development. It is relatively straightforward to demonstrate reduction in tone, improved joint range of motion and improved muscle length after spasticity management but evidence of functional gains is much more demanding. The gross motor function measure (GMFM) is a most useful, validated tool, which is being increasingly used to measure functional outcomes (Russell et al., 1989; Boyce et al., 1995; Palisano et al., 1997). However, administration of this test is time consuming and it is not always sensitive to subtle changes in young children (Reddihough, 1999, personal communication). It does represent a significant step forward in measuring function in cerebral palsy.

The best candidates for spasticity management are children who share the following features:
- mild to moderate spasticity;
- good cognitive ability;
- no fixed contractures or deformities;
- good selective motor control;
- good general health;
- stable supportive home environment;
- access to appropriate physiotherapy;
- access to appropriate orthotics.

Spasticity management may fail for a variety of reasons, including:
- spasticity, too severe and generalized;
- poor cognitive ability;
- fixed deformity;
- poor selective motor control;
- associated medical disease;
- inadequate home support;
- no access to appropriate physiotherapy or orthotics.

Children in the latter group may have a much greater need for spasticity management, but failure is more likely. Good results are harder to achieve and sustain. Most of the criteria suggested above can be measured or assessed in some agreed manner, apart from the nebulous concept of 'home support'. We have included this as an observation based on extensive experience, although we have not been able to measure this in any convincing manner. Bringing up children is hard work and caring for disabled children adds immeasurably to parental stress. Many parents of

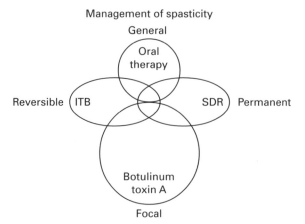

Fig. 12.3   The four-way compass of spasticity management with general versus focal (north and south) and reversible versus permanent (west versus east). ITB: intrathecal baclofen; SDR: selective dorsal rhizotomy.

disabled children are living at the edge of coping, with a range of financial and social difficulties. The extra stress of invasive treatment which requires active participation by them in the overall management or rehabilitation may be the last straw.

Methods of spasticity management can be classified on a four-way compass (Figure 12.3), according to whether they are focal or general in effect and as to whether the effects are permanent or temporary. Within this four-way matrix permanent–temporary, focal–general, practical clinical guidelines may be derived. The child with acquired spasticity from focal traumatic brain injury may have a relatively short period of severe spasticity in a hemiplegic distribution. This could be managed by a programme that may include intramuscular BTXA to large muscle groups on the affected side including the elbow flexors, the forearm muscles and the gastrosoleus. In this scenario the focal and temporary nature of BTXA may be advantageous. Selective dorsal rhizotomy (SDR) would be contraindicated because it is permanent and usually bilateral.

A child with spastic diplegia who demonstrates lower limb spasticity may respond favourably to SDR, the permanence and generalized effects on the lower limbs may be advantageous. Multiple, repeated injections of BTXA would be less effective and risk systemic side-effects.

The spasticity team and the spasticity clinic

Successful spasticity management in children depends as much on teamwork as it does on techniques and technology. Given that options in spasticity management in children include administration of drugs by oral and intrathecal routes, neuro-surgical procedures and orthopaedic surgery, it should be self-evident that spasticity management is a multidisciplinary exercise. In many centres, the concept of a spasticity team and a spasticity clinic are well developed. At the Royal Children's Hospital in Melbourne, the members of the team are drawn from the following backgrounds:

- child development and rehabilitation;
- physiotherapy;
- orthotics;
- neurosurgery;
- orthopaedic surgery;
- motion analysis laboratory.

Many children are managed successfully by individual clinicians. However, there are a sufficient number of very difficult management problems to justify a monthly spasticity clinic where the management of a small number of problem children is discussed in detail. Often investigations such as gait analysis or examination under anaesthesia are requested to aid decision making. We find the multidisciplinary discussions stimulating and the communication between specialties invaluable. Management is frequently altered, with benefit to our patients. The most frequent management issue is the interplay between spasticity management and orthopaedic surgery for deformity correction. Are the deformities dynamic or fixed? To resolve this common dilemma, an examination under the full relaxation of a general anaesthetic may be invaluable. We have avoided subjecting children to the invasiveness of selective dorsal rhizotomy and our budget to the expense of funding an intrathecal baclofen pump by examination under anaesthesia.

Oral medications: generalized–temporary

Although there are new invasive means for the management of spasticity in children such as selective dorsal rhizotomy and intrathecal baclofen, oral medications are probably used in a much larger number of children (Figure 12.3). The paradox is that oral medications have received much less attention in terms of clinical trials in recent years. There is a paucity of good evidence on which to base the management decisions of the spasticity in children with orally administered medication. Anecdotal evidence suggests that these medications are widely used in children who have spasticity despite very limited evidence regarding efficacy, safety, pharmacokinetics and mechanism of action (Ried et al., 1998).

A basic aim of oral medication is to reduce spasticity with a minimum of side-effects. This may be achieved by such mechanisms as reducing afferent input, inhibition or blocking of the excitation of intraspinal neurones, reducing motor neurone output or by directly relaxing muscle. Whilst evidence exists regarding efficacy in reducing spasticity, evidence for improved function is still largely lacking.

Oral medications for the management of spasticity in children are in the temporary-generalized category of the treatment compass (Figure 12.3). The agents most frequently used are diazepam (Valium), baclofen (Lioresal) and dantrolene sodium (Dantrium). In general, oral medications have a rather narrow therapeutic window between efficacy and side-effects. Individual responses vary greatly and a careful clinical trial is necessary for many children to determine the individual response/side-effect profile. The advantages and disadvantages of oral agents have recently been discussed (Ried et al., 1998).

Diazepam

Most clinicians are familiar with the role of diazepam as an anxiolytic agent. However evidence from animal work suggests that it possesses both a muscle relaxant and spinal reflex blocking property. The spinal actions of diazepam are the result of potentiation of the presynaptic inhibitory effects of gamma aminobutyric acid (GABA) at $GABA_A$ receptors on spinal afferent presynaptic terminals. Central effects in the brainstem reticular formation result in sedation (Costa & Guidoffi, 1979; Young & Delwaide, 1981a,b; Davidoff, 1989; Blackman et al., 1992).

Diazepam is rapidly and almost completely absorbed following oral or rectal administration. Intravenous administration is occasionally used to gain rapid control of muscle spasms in a child who is excessively anxious and in pain after orthopaedic procedures but there is a risk of respiratory depression and this route is not recommended for routine use. Intramuscular injections are painful, rarely required and erratic in their absorption profile. Rectal administration is ideal when children are fasting, nauseated or unable to take medication orally. The half-life in children is shorter than in adults but is still quite long at 18 hours. There tends to be a cumulative effect of diazepam and it may take some time to reach the appropriate levels in body tissues and to reach optimal clinical effect. The drug's volume of distribution is large reflecting its extensive tissue penetration within the body. It is metabolized by the liver to pharmacologically active metabolites including nordiazepam and oxazepam (Greenblatt et al., 1980). The most common side-effects are excessive sedation, respiratory depression, fatigue and ataxia. Paradoxical effects may occur including hallucinations and increased spasticity. These must be recognized and not managed by increasing the dose.

Many children with cerebral palsy and other forms of spasticity demonstrate increased spasticity when they are anxious and especially when they are in pain. Anxiety and pain seem to interact in a vicious circle to increase muscle tone after painful interventions such as orthopaedic surgery (Barwood et al., 2000). The central tranquillizing effects and peripheral tone reducing effects of diazepam are extremely useful in this situation (Binder & Eng, 1989). However, this means also that there is a very small threshold between effective reduction in spasticity and sedation, invalidating diazepam for chronic spasticity management in the vast majority of children. We use diazepam almost routinely in children with cerebral palsy who are facing painful invasive procedures including orthopaedic surgery, SDR, etc.

Addiction and withdrawal symptoms are reported in patients who use diazepam in the long-term (Young & Delwaide, 1981a,b). We have noted a 'rebound' phenomenon in children who have high doses of diazepam postoperatively, if it is stopped suddenly. We routinely recommend that children be 'weaned' slowly from diazepam use after short-term/high dose use.

Clinical trials in the use of diazepam are limited in the number of patients, outcome measures and in trial design. Phelps (1963) reported on 19 patients with athetoid cerebral palsy managed by diazepam. He felt that there was a positive effect on the emotional status of the children as well as a reduction in muscle tone. Although there were only two patients with predominantly spastic-type cerebral palsy in his study group, he felt that the response to diazepam was better in children with athetoid-type cerebral palsy (Phelps, 1963). Keats et al. (1963) also commented on a better response in children with athetoid-type cerebral palsy.

Nogen (1979) studied spasticity and activities of daily living, reporting that 20 out of 22 patients showed an improvement in comparison with placebo. However, in the second part of the study when diazepam was compared to dantrolene, he found that dantrolene was more effective in nine patients and diazepam and dantrolene were equally effective in four patients (Nogen, 1979). Diazepam is thought to be roughly equipotent with dantrolene for generalized spasticity. It may not be as effective as baclofen in the management of painful, intermittent flexor spasms (Young & Delwaide, 1981b).

Dantrolene

Dantrolene is known to physicians and surgeons because of its undoubted value in the treatment and prevention of malignant hyperthermia (Arens & McKinnon, 1971; Waterman et al., 1980). The main effect on skeletal muscle appears to be direct muscle relaxation rather than a central or a spinal level of action. Dantrolene inhibits the release of calcium from the sarcoplasmic reticulum of muscle cells (Hainaut & Desmedt, 1974; VanWinkle, 1976; Desmedt & Hainaut, 1979; Molnar & Kathirithamby, 1979). All muscles, both spastic and normal, tend to be affected, ranging from relaxation through to weakness. Dantrolene is rapidly and extensively absorbed but there is a lack of pharmacokinetic data in children and especially in children who have spasticity (Lietman et al., 1974; Young & Delwaide, 1981a; Lerman et al., 1989).

The utility of dantrolene (Dantrium®) has been limited by the potential for hepatotoxicity (Utili et al., 1977; Wilkinson et al., 1979; Chan, 1990). Fatal dantrolene induced hepatitis has been reported in adults but not in children. In children, transaminase levels may rise, leading to a withdrawal of therapy. Liver function should be assessed prior to starting dantrolene therapy and at frequent intervals thereafter (Ried et al., 1998).

A number of studies have been reviewed by Blackman et al. (1992) who note that within the published literature, the numbers of patients are small and the outcome measures are not particularly objective. However, most studies do report that in comparison with placebo, dantrolene has a positive effect in reducing muscle tone, but not necessarily in improving function.

Baclofen

Baclofen was introduced in the mid-1970s and appears to act as a GABA agonist on the $GABA_B$ receptors (Rice, 1987). Baclofen inhibits transmitter release by competitive inhibition of excitatory neurotransmitters at the spinal level. There may be actions in the spinal cord or more centrally which are not yet fully described or understood (Pedersen et al., 1974; Calta & Santomauro, 1976; Milla & Jackson, 1977; McKinlay et al., 1980; Young & Delwaide, 1981a,b; Dolphin & Scott, 1986; Fromm & Terrence, 1987). Pharmacokinetic data in respect of baclofen children is lacking. Although baclofen is rapidly absorbed after oral administration, cerebrospinal fluid levels are low because of its low lipid solubility and 30% binding to plasma proteins. This limits its transport across the blood–brain barrier (Knutson et al., 1974; Gilman et al., 1990). It can be administered orally or intrathecally but not parenterally. The response to baclofen in children varies widely (Milla & Jackson, 1977). In general, the threshold between effective reduction in spasticity or muscle tone and side-effects such as dizziness, weakness and fatigue is rather small. However, individual children can respond well, and a careful trial of various dose levels is worthwhile, although the majority will have their medication discontinued because of side-effects. Hallucinations and seizures may occur with abrupt withdrawal of baclofen, therefore, as with diazepam, children who have become habituated to larger doses should be weaned slowly off the drug. A double-blind cross-over trial of oral baclofen administration in children documented a decrease in spasticity with little change in functional abilities, such as ambulation and the performance of ADLs (activities of daily living) (Milla & Jackson, 1977; Molnar & Kathirithamby, 1979).

Much interest has been raised by the intrathecal administration of baclofen (Knutson et al., 1974; Penn & Kroin, 1985; Albright et al., 1991). Using this technique, the low lipid solubility and binding to plasma proteins is avoided by administration of the drug directly to the target tissues. As will be seen in a later section, this introduces a new 'risk–benefit' profile with specific advantages and disadvantages.

Casting and orthoses: temporary–focal

The use of casting and orthoses can be classified as focal–temporary. The concept of 'tone reducing' or 'inhibitory' casting became popular in the 1970s and both treatment modalities are now widely used in the management of spasticity in children (Sussman & Cusick, 1979; Duncan & Mott, 1983). The theoretical basis for casting and orthoses are that positioning the limb in a more anatomic, tone reducing posture would increase the base of support, decrease tone and improve joint range of motion and function (Law et al., 1991). Both biomechanical and neurophysiological explanations have been offered with limited supporting evidence (Ried et al., 1998). Neurophysiological explanations involve the reduction in sensory feedback from the plantar surface of the foot which might otherwise increase or maintain spasticity (Sussman & Cusick, 1979). Biomechanical mechanisms are more plausible and better supported by the available evidence. In children who have cerebral palsy and are 'toe walking', serial casting results in a temporary improvement in gait, as evidenced by sagittal plane ankle kinematics, consistent with lengthening of the gastrosoleus muscle–tendon unit (Corry et al., 1998). The efficacy and duration of casting are related to the proportions of dynamic and fixed contracture before treatment and the responsiveness to the connective tissue to stretching forces. Many clinicians combine casting with intramuscular injections of BTX or phenol. The combined effect of injection and casting may be better than either intervention on its own (Boyd & Graham, 1997). However, the evidence remains anecdotal.

Spasticity of the gastrosoleus, resulting in dynamic equinus, is usually treated by serial below knee casting for periods of one to four weeks. Given the very widespread utilization of the technique by physiotherapists, there have been very few outcome studies, little objective measurement and only one clinical trial published (Corry et al., 1998). Proponents claim either a 'tone-reducing' effect (Sussman & Cusick, 1979) or simply describe the use of serial casting (Westin & Dye, 1983). The former hypothesize that the pressure under certain plantar areas inhibits dynamic equinus and has led to the use of the term 'tone-reducing ankle–foot orthoses' (TRAFOs) (Jordan, 1984). In general, this has been a poorly researched intervention for spasticity in children (Sussman, 1983; Hinderer et al., 1988). In a randomized, clinical trial Corry et al. (1998) compared serial casting with injection of BTX, in the management of dynamic equinus in children with cerebral palsy. They concluded that both interventions were effective but that the effects of BTX lasted longer (Corry et al., 1998).

Orthoses such as the ankle–foot orthosis (AFO) are widely used in the management of younger children who have calf spasticity. The effects of AFOs are difficult to study in younger children but there are definite biomechanical benefits, confirmed by motion analysis (Rose et al., 1991; Ounpuu et al., 1993, 1996). Functional benefits are more difficult to demonstrate. It is unclear if 'TRAFOs' offer any advantages over the more conventional designs.

Intramuscular injections: chemoneurolysis – temporary–focal

Intramuscular injections are focal in nature. The duration depends on the agent, the concentration used and the site of injection. Chemoneurolysis refers to a nerve block resulting in impaired neuromuscular conduction, by the destruction of neural tissue, either temporarily or permanently. Injection can be performed at many levels in the peripheral nervous system from nerve root to motor end plate (Glenn, 1990). The more proximal the injection site, the more general and prolonged the effect. Sciatic nerve block results in a variable degree of weakness of all of the muscles supplied by the sciatic nerve in the distal thigh and leg. Injection of the gastrocnemius muscle affects small local motor nerves and for this reason is classified as a motor point block (Bankheit et al., 1996).

Local anaesthetic blocks are used for a short-term effect, usually as a diagnostic test rather than for therapeutic effects. The duration can be varied according to the agent used – e.g. lignocaine, bupivacaine.

Ethylalcohol and phenol have been used for many years and are both cheap and easily available. Phenol denatures proteins in the myelin sheath and is capable of destroying axons of all sizes (Fischer et al., 1970; Felsenthal, 1974; Beckerman et al., 1996). Electrical stimulation is required to localize the optimum injection site. This can be at the level of the peripheral nerve (Khalili & Benton, 1966; Spira, 1971; Petrillo et al., 1980), the large motor branch (Easton et al., 1979; Carpenter 1983) or the endplate (DeLateur, 1972). The younger child poorly tolerates this localization technique. O'Hanlan and associates used an intramuscular ethanol wash technique that does not require electrical guidance, however it gives the least consistent effect (O'Hanlan et al., 1969; Carpenter & Sietz, 1980). Although quicker, an anaesthetic was still required. Higher concentrations of both agents may cause severe pain at the site of injection, dysaesthesia and tissue necrosis (Easton et al., 1979; Petrillo et al., 1980). Sedation or general anaesthesia is required in younger children (Griffiths & Melampy, 1977). Pure motor nerves are better targets for these agents than mixed motor and sensory nerves. We use phenol injections for the management of adductor spasticity by injecting the obturator nerve. In the hemiplegic upper limb, injection of the musculo-cutaneous nerve can be useful in the management of elbow flexor spasticity. Although both the obturator and musculo-cutaneous nerves have a sensory component, dysaesthesias are rarely a problem.

These type of blocks produce muscular relaxation in the target area, providing a 'window of opportunity' for a focused programme of splinting, casting, gait training and strengthening of antagonist muscles. Children with mild spasticity do better than those with more severe spasticity. Repeat blocks appear to have little effect and little is achieved by injections in isolation (Mazur et al., 1992). The response to these injections has been well described in clinical terms but there are no studies utilizing motion analysis. Children with severe spasticity or those with a recurrence of spasticity after an initial block are not good candidates for repeated injection.

With the introduction of BTXA, injections of phenol and alcohol have largely been superceded, especially when injection of a mixed sensory and motor nerve would pose a risk of painful dysaesthesias – e.g. sciatic nerve, posterior tibial nerve and median nerve.

Peripheral neurectomy: permanent–focal

Peripheral nerve surgery has a limited role in spasticity management. It can be classified as permanent–focal intervention. The most widely used technique in the management of adductor spasticity and hip subluxation, both in a historical context and current practice, is neurectomy of the anterior branch of the obturator nerve. Children who exhibit spastic cerebral palsy in a quadriplegic or 'whole body' pattern of involvement have a very high incidence of adductor spasticity and hip migration (Letts et al., 1984; Kalen & Bleck, 1985; Cooperman, 1987; Scrutton, 1989).

Careful assessment of these children is necessary to determine the contribution of contractures of the adductor muscles as opposed to spasticity of these muscles. This assessment requires serial radiological examinations of the hips, to determine 'at risk' signs, as well as clinical examination, both in the clinic and under the relaxation afforded by a general anaesthetic (Scrutton & Baird, 1997). The most appropriate management can then be selected. This includes various focal spasticity treatments and abduction-bracing in early cases, and surgery for more advanced cases when they manifest hip subluxation. The benefits of lengthening of the contracted adductor muscles can be enhanced by selective use of anterior branch obturator nerve neurectomy (Stoffel, 1913).

The role of obturator neurectomy is controversial. Its indiscriminate use can undoubtedly lead to poor outcomes, including the reverse deformity (abduction contracture), windswept hips and excessive weakening. It should never be employed in the ambulant child. When used cautiously, the benefits in preventing hip displacement, improving seating and making nursing care less burdensome can be striking. When there is uncertainty regarding the indication for obturator neurectomy, a reasonable simulation can be achieved by the injection of BTXA. This simulation was used in nine children in our clinic. Seven of the nine sets of parents elected to proceed with surgical neurectomy and two preferred to continue with repeated injections of BTXA.

The only other peripheral nerve surgery which is occasionally used in our clinic is section of the suprascapular nerve or musculo-cutaneous nerve for intractable shoulder or elbow flexor spasticity. A trial of BTXA chemodenervation is advisable in all cases before permanent, surgical denervation.

Selective dorsal rhizotomy: permanent–generalized

SDR is a neurosurgical procedure in which a percentage of the dorsal rootlets that make up the roots of the lumbo-sacral plexus are divided to reduce spasticity in the lower limbs. This is a permanent procedure with selectivity for the lower limbs (Peacock & Arens, 1982). Some reduction in spasticity and occasionally improved function has been reported in the upper limbs after SDR by a mechanism, which has neither been fully investigated nor satisfactorily explained (Oppenheim et al., 1992).

SDR has a long and interesting history but can be considered to have been refined and introduced as a reliable procedure in present spasticity management by the South African group, especially Warwick Peacock, the neurosurgeon responsible for refining the procedure (Peacock & Arens, 1982; Peacock et al., 1987; Peacock & Staudt, 1990, 1991).

The ideal candidate for SDR is a child with moderately severe spastic diplegia, good cognitive abilities, no fixed contractures, good underlying muscle strength and good voluntary muscle control. The optimum age is between four and eight years – i.e. old enough to participate in a rigorous rehabilitation programme and young enough not to have fixed deformities.

The key features of a successful SDR programme would appear to include:
• Multidisciplinary approach to selection and management.
• Availability of motion analysis for selection and monitoring outcome.
• Good surgical programme, intra-operative monitoring.
• Rehabilitation programme.

Expected outcomes include permanently reduced muscle tone, reduced co-contraction, improved joint range of motion and reduction of dynamic deformities. Intuitively these improvements would be expected to improve function but as yet evidence from controlled clinical trials does not confirm this. There is convincing evidence for improvements in gait using kinematics, electromyography and energy studies. However, in three randomized controlled clinical trials, utilizing GMFM (gross motor function measure) as the principal outcome measure, in the largest trial, function was not significantly better in children managed by SDR combined with physiotherapy compared with physiotherapy alone (Wright et al., 1988; Steinbok et al., 1997; McLaughlin et al., 1998).

The relationship between SDR and deformities is of great significance (Oppenheim, 1990). Fixed contractures and bony torsional problems are unaffected by SDR and require corrective orthopaedic surgery. Intuitively, SDR should be performed before the development of contractures and bony torsion for two reasons. Firstly, children with mainly dynamic deformities may benefit most and SDR may prevent the progression of deformity although no study has confirmed this (Vaughan et al., 1988, 1991; Arens et al., 1989). Unfortunately some deformities may be caused or may progress more rapidly after SDR including spinal deformity (lumbar lordosis, scoliosis), hip subluxation and foot deformities (Greene et al., 1991).

The longer-term effects of SDR are not clearly known. Although there are several good short- to medium-term outcome studies with objective measures, too few children have been followed through the adolescent growth spurt (Cahan et al., 1989; Perry et al., 1989; Peacock & Staudt, 1991; Vaughan et al., 1991). In children with cerebral palsy, the adolescent growth spurt may pose a great challenge. Deformities may increase and become more fixed, function may deteriorate and borderline ambulators may opt for wheelchair mobility. Residual weakness of large antigravity muscles and sensory impairment post rhizotomy may add to this already challenging natural history.

Intrathecal baclofen (ITB): semipermanent–generalized

There has been a substantial experience with the use of baclofen as an oral medication in spasticity management but the narrow therapeutic window between efficacy and side-effects has limited clinical utility. Delivering baclofen to the target tissue directly avoids this conflict (Penn & Kroin, 1985; Penn et al., 1989; Coffey et al., 1993). Using a programmable implanted pump, baclofen can be delivered intrathecally. The delivery of a relatively high concentration of the drug to the intra-spinal pathways can be achieved, avoiding systemic side-effects (Knutson et al., 1974; Dralle et al., 1985; Muller, 1992; Kroin et al., 1993). It is a form of semipermanent and generalized treatment.

The requirement of a delivery system places ITB therapy in the semipermanent category. The programmable pump offers considerable flexibility in dose control and the ability to modulate the clinical effects (Albright, 1996). The drug acts mainly on the lower limbs but there is some spread within the intrathecal space and there can be beneficial effects on the upper limbs (Ziegelgansberer et al., 1988; Muller, 1992; Albright et al., 1993). As the pumps become smaller and more reliable, younger children can be offered this spasticity management option.

The costs of ITB are a major disadvantage and are limiting clinical trials and patient access (Albright, 1996). These costs include the cost and maintenance of the pump and associated hardware, the surgical procedure and the drug itself.

There is reasonable evidence of efficacy in terms of short-term measures such as tone reduction and improved joint range of motion (Penn et al., 1989; Lazorthes et al., 1990; Penn, 1992; Albright et al., 1993). The evidence for functional improvements is lacking and controlled clinical trials with functional outcome measures are clearly needed.

Preliminary clinical experience suggests that ITB may be more suited to the management of spasticity of spinal rather than cranial origin (Albright, 1996). However, in cerebral palsy, ITB may have a role in the management of other movement disorders such as generalized dystonia.

BTXA: focal–temporary

BTXA is a reversible, focal agent which has been under evaluation since the early 1990s in the management of spasticity in children (Koman et al., 1993, 1994, 1996, 2000; Cosgrove et al., 1994; Corry et al., 1995, 1998). The toxin was first identified as the causative factor in some forms of food poisoning and then investigated as a potential biological weapon. The first therapeutic applications were in the management of strabismus and focal dystonias including blepharospasm, spasmodic torticollis and hemifacial spasm (Scott, 1980; Scott et al., 1990; Jankovic & Brin, 1991). In these early indications the target muscles were small skeletal muscles and both the clinical and economic profile of BTXA is more suited to these applications than to the management of spasticity in large skeletal muscles.

However, the focal and temporary nature of BTXA permit exploitation in spasticity management in a manner which no other available agent can be used (Graham, 1995; O'Brien, 1995). In children with cerebral palsy there is a need for a minimally invasive method of spasticity management which can be targeted to specific muscles and the effects varied by dose levels. BTXA meets a least some of these requirements (American Academy of Neurology, 1990; NIH Consensus Development Conference, 1990; O'Brien, 1995). The pharmacology and pharmacokinetics of BTXA have been covered in Chapter 9. There is no important pharmacological difference in the effects of BTXA in different muscles or in different conditions but there can be very different clinical effects and priorities.

Children with cerebral palsy rarely have deformities at birth, most are acquired during growth, especially during periods of rapid growth (Rang, 1990). Although orthopaedic surgery is the mainstay of deformity correction in older children, corrective surgery in the younger child is unpredictable and should be avoided whenever possible. The obvious exception to this principle is surgery to prevent spastic hip dislocation.

Since 1992 we have investigated a possible role for the use of BTXA in children with cerebral palsy (Figure 12.4). Our first study was a randomized controlled trial (RCT) in an animal model, the hereditary spastic mouse (Cosgrove & Graham, 1994). This strain of mice has a neurotransmitter deficiency, which is inherited in

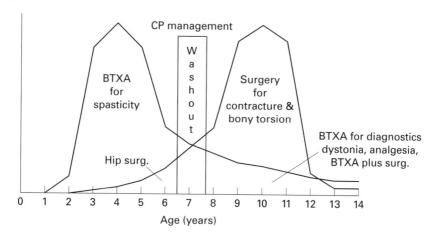

Fig. 12.4　The approximate time line for the use of botulinum toxin A (BTXA) as an agent for spasticity management in the lower limb, in children with cerebral palsy (CP). On the horizontal axis is the age in years. Note that the only early surgery is hip surgery to prevent dislocation when there are clinical and X-ray signs of the hips being 'at risk'. We reserve the use of botulinum toxin for younger children peaking at age 4. Surgery for fixed contractures and bony torsional problems is used in the age 8–12 years with a decreasing use in this age group of botulinum toxin for diagnostic purposes, postoperative analgesia and in the management of dystonia. (Reproduced with permission from Boyd & Graham, 1997, Blackwell Science Ltd, Osney Mead, Oxford)

an autosomal recessive fashion, and which has a number of features that mimic cerebral palsy. This model had been previously studied by Ziv and Rang who described the failure of longitudinal muscle growth in affected mice leading to musculo-tendinous contractures (Ziv et al., 1984).

We investigated muscle and tendon growth in a RCT in which the calf muscle was injected on day 6 of life with BTXA or normal saline. In summary, spastic mice injected with saline developed contractures in comparison with their normal litter-mates but those injected with BTXA did not. This seemed to confirm the Ziv & Rang 'muscle growth inhibition by spasticity' hypothesis and suggested a preventative role by BTXA.

Our first clinical trial was of necessity, an 'open-label' uncontrolled study (Cosgrove & Graham, 1994). No information was available at that time regarding dose, method of administration, frequency of injection, outcomes or side-effects. In effect, each injection was approached as an individual clinical trial. In order to reduce the risk to individual children and to gain the maximum information, we admitted each child to hospital for three to five days during which objective measurements including gait analysis were performed. We quickly learned to titrate the dose to achieve our desired effect and developed practical injection techniques for the principal target muscles in both the upper and lower limbs (Couper-Brash,

1955; Cosgrove et al., 1994; Corry et al., 1997). We used simple tests to confirm needle placement in target muscles, including manual palpation, freehand needle placement and confirmation by moving the distal joint through a range of motion prior to connecting the syringe containing the toxin.

We used a short inhalational general anaesthetic (GA) in this first study and continue to use GA much more than other groups. Using GA has a number of important advantages which may go some way to explain differences in the outcomes which we have achieved and reported in comparison with other groups. Firstly, GA provides the definitive method of distinguishing dynamic from fixed contractures. Sometimes we remain in doubt until the child is fully relaxed under GA and we are prepared to cancel the injection, advise supplementary casting or proceed to surgery according to the clinical findings under GA (Graham, 1995; Boyd & Graham, 1997). It is pointless to proceed with injecting a contracted muscle. Secondly, the control afforded by GA permits us to inject target muscles in an accurate relaxed manner, using multiple injection sites. Multiple injection sites are probably safer and possibly more effective than fewer sites. Typically we inject four sites in the calf and two sites in the adductors and hamstrings. Although it is reasonably easy to target the calf under sedation or local anaesthesia, the same cannot be said for the adductors and hamstrings. In the diplegic child who is receiving multiple injections in multiple muscles, we believe that GA is mandatory.

The conclusions from our first clinical trial were that large doses of BTXA in children were safe and that reduction in tone was reasonably predictable but short lived. Some improvements in the kinematics of gait were noted and in some children, these improvements persisted after the pharmacological effects of toxin would have been expected to wear off. Function was assessed crudely by the Hoffer classification of ambulatory status (Hoffer et al., 1973) and was noted to improve in some children. No matter which outcome parameter we studied, there was an exponential decrease in benefit with age – i.e. older children responded less well than did younger children. This observation confirmed our clinical impression that the primary cause of clinical unresponsiveness was fixed contracture, which becomes increasingly prevalent as the children become older.

This study raised more questions than it answered, but provided a reasonable basis for our second phase of investigation, three controlled clinical trials.

RCT 1: hemiplegic upper limb

We felt very strongly that BTXA should be investigated in a placebo-controlled trial and we selected the hemiplegic upper limb. Many of the parents of children who had received lower limb spasticity management asked for upper limb treatment in addition. These were mostly older children with spastic hemiplegia who could co-operate with injection under local anaesthesia or sedation. This was at a time when most of our multiple lower limb injections were performed under general anaesthesia, precluding randomization to receive placebo.

The aims of the study were to determine if the effects of BTXA were consistent in a RCT/placebo-controlled environment by both subjective and objective means (Corry et al., 1997). The subjective assessment was obtained by canvassing the opinion of the parents and therapist as to whether the child's condition after injection was improved/unchanged/worse compared to pre-injection status. The results were very positive; the effects of BTXA in producing relaxation of spastic upper limb were easily and consistently recognized.

We also introduced an objective means of measuring muscle stiffness by using resonant frequency by a modification of the method and techniques described by Walsh (Walsh, 1988). The resonant frequency of the forearm muscle in the hemiplegic upper limb was significantly greater than that in the normal limb. This increased resonant frequency, reflecting increased stiffness, was significantly decreased by injection of BTXA.

Functional outcomes were equivocal. Improvements in range of motion were sometimes offset by decreased grip strength. As with other interventions in the upper limb, the improvements in cosmesis, related to decreased hemiplegic posturing, were more appreciated by our patients than the functional gains which were achieved.

We believe that there is much more research to be done in the upper limb including combining BTXA injection with surgery and exploiting the muscular relaxation achieved by BTXA with targeted splinting and therapy programmes. Not all muscles make the transition from dynamic to fixed contacture at the same speed. In the hemiplegic upper limb the pronator teres is almost always the first muscle to develop a contracture and this can be a principal cause of failure after BTXA injection. In the younger child we sometimes combine release or re-routing of pronator teres with BTXA injections to the wrist and finger flexors. Other uses of BTXA in the hemiplegic upper limb include pain relief and protection of upper limb tendon transfers from postoperative spasm.

RCT 2: BTXA vs casting for dynamic equinus

In this study we compared the effects of BTXA and casting in the management of dynamic equinus (Figure 12.5) in a group of younger children with cerebral palsy (Corry et al., 1998). Casting is a popular management option for the younger child who exhibits dynamic equinus but despite its popularity and widespread utilization there are few studies with objective outcome measures and no clinical trials which have demonstrated efficacy.

The entry criterion for our study was 'the intention to treat dynamic equinus'. Children were then randomized to receive serial casting or BTXA. Outcome

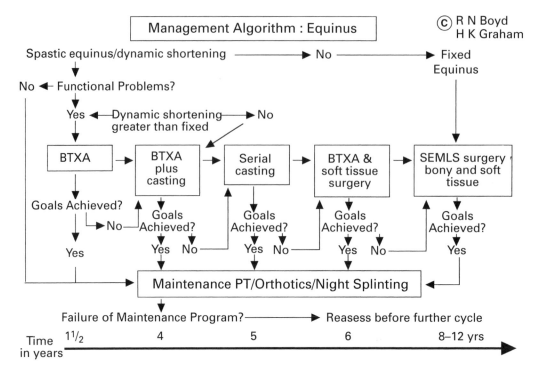

Fig. 12.5   A 'stepped' approach to the management of equinus in the child with cerebral palsy
commencing with botulinum toxin (BTXA) injections to the gastrosoleus for the younger
child, with a purely dynamic problem. It progresses through botulinum toxin plus casting,
serial casting or toxin plus limited surgery. Finally there is multilevel surgery for those
children who may benefit, between the ages of 8 and 12 years. (Reproduced with
permission from Boyd & Graham, 1997, Blackwell Science Ltd, Osney Mead, Oxford)

measures included clinical measures and gait analysis. Younger/less co-operative
children had a two-dimensional video recording of gait and from this the physician
rating scale was applied by experienced observers, blinded to the form of treatment.
Older/more co-operative children had instrumented gait analysis, concentrating
on sagittal plane kinematics.

Both interventions were equally effective in terms of correcting equinus gait but
the effects of BTXA were more prolonged. Given that both interventions were comparable in terms of cost, BTXA was at least as cost effective as casting and was preferred by the majority of parents. A longer-term study is required to address
cost–benefit issues more rigorously.

Similar results have been obtained recently by Flett et al. (1999). They performed
prospective, randomized, single-blind controlled study comparing BTXA injections with fixed plaster cast stretching in the management of dynamic calf tightness. They concluded that BTXA injections were of similar efficacy to serial fixed
plaster casting in improving calf tightness in ambulant or partially ambulant

children with cerebral palsy. It was also noted that parents consistently favoured BTXA, highlighting the inconvenience of serial casting (Flett et al., 1999).

Cost comparisons in both trials were attempted. Superficially it appears that BTXA therapy is more expensive when a single limb is treated with BTXA as compared with fixed plaster cast stretching. When both lower limbs were treated the costs appear similar. However, a comprehensive economic analysis including the costs incurred by parents in terms of absence from work, travel time, etc. is required prior to a firm conclusion.

RCT 3: hamstring injection

In this trial children with flexed knee gait were managed by injections of BTXA to the hamstrings (Cosgrove et al., 1994; Corry et al., 1999). Children were randomly assigned to immediate injection or injection after a period of observation. The main outcome measures were kinematics and energy studies. The results were inconclusive. Popliteal angle measurements showed significant reductions but only some of the patients had improvements in their gait. Some who had a good correction of crouch gait, also had reduced energy expenditure. Our conclusions were that individual improvements were worthwhile for some children but selection needed to be more rigorous and that injections of other levels needed to be considered.

BTXA doses in children: all doses are for Botox® (Allergan, Inc)

In large skeletal muscles (calf, hamstrings, adductors) predictable responses occur at about 4 U/kg, especially if the dose is spread over multiple sites. Some responses are seen at 2 U/kg but these are neither so predictable nor long lasting. It is rarely beneficial to exceed 6 U/kg. A muscle, which does not respond at a dose of 6 U/kg, will usually have a fixed contracture.

We use a standard dilution of 100 Units of the Allergan preparation Botox® in 1 ml of normal saline. Allergan is the manufacturer of the US product Botox®. The British product, Dysport®, and Botox®, are not of equivalent dosage. Care must be taken in following the dosage guidelines of clinical papers. No convincing data exists from animal or clinical studies to confirm the optimum dilution.

We follow empirical guidelines, established by detailed observations in toxin administration including:

Maximum dose at one site, 50 Units.

Maximum dose per muscle, 6 U/kg.

Maximum dose per child, 12 U/kg or 300 Units, whichever is lower.

A muscle will respond to BTXA at a dose of 4 U/kg if there is $>30°$ difference between R2 and R1 – i.e. more spasticity than contracture. This does not mean however that the child will automatically benefit in terms of achieving the desired functional goal.

Sutherland et al. (1995) in an open-label trial have further demonstrated the efficacy of BTXA in the treatment of dynamic equinus. In a group of children with dynamic equinus, there were improvements in stance phase dorsiflexion, swing phase dorsiflexion and foot rotation post injection. Most of the patients who had exhibited low level EMG activity in the tibialis anterior throughout stance in their baseline study, also exhibited a normal firing pattern of their tibialis anterior after injection (Sutherland et al., 1995). The improvements in peak ankle dorsiflexion in stance and swing were also confirmed in their RCT/placebo-controlled trial (Sutherland et al., 1999).

In a recent randomized double blind, placebo-controlled trial Koman and colleagues have also demonstrated a significant improvement in gait, as measured on the physician rating scale. However, there were mild, adverse effects in 17% of the study population (Koman et al., 2000).

Management of equinus can be simple or remarkably difficult. In younger children with hemiplegia, assessment of equinus is straightforward and management planning similarly simple. Dynamic equinus deformity will usually respond well to BTXA. If the response is incomplete, a short period of casting will usually help achieve the required correction, which can then be sustained by the use of an AFO and physiotherapy.

In diplegia the situation is often much more complicated. The easiest scenario is a bilateral, symmetrical, equinus gait with little proximal involvement. This can be managed in a similar manner to hemiplegia.

However, when there is proximal spasticity and hip and knee flexion as well as equinus, good judgement and a sound appreciation of biomechanics is required to plan logical and effective management. We find that many clinicians treat all equinus by calf injection, forgetting that 'apparent equinus' secondary to hamstring and/or psoas spasticity is very common in diplegia.

If the equinus is secondary to hamstring spasticity, calf injection may achieve 'foot flat' and apparent correction, but at the high cost of increased 'crouch' gait. A better strategy may be to inject the psoas and hamstrings and use AFOs.

We do not advocate or practice long-term spasticity management with BTXA in children with cerebral palsy. Neither safety nor efficacy has been established. We use BTXA for the younger child as part of a management plan, which includes physiotherapy, and the use of orthotics with a view to definitive surgical correction at the age of 6–12 years. The use of BTXA in the younger child appears to have the following advantages:

• Improved motor ability.
• Reduced dynamic deformity.
• Delayed progress to fixed deformity.
• Later age at first surgery.
• Less repeat surgery.
• Simplified surgery.

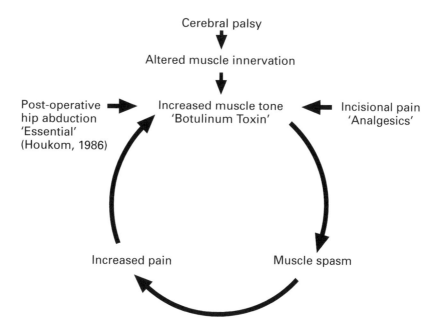

Fig. 12.6   The pain/spasm vicious circle in the child with celebral palsy after hip release surgery. Muscle tone increases postoperatively because of the combination of incisional pain and postoperative hip abduction in plasters or splints. The incisional pain is managed by a various combination of analgesics and the hip abduction is considered to be essential. The cycle of spasm increasing pain which produces further spasms can be broken by preoperative chemodenervation by intramuscular adductor injection of BTXA.

The use of BTXA in other forms of childhood spasticity is less well defined than in cerebral palsy. There do not appear to be any intrinsic differences between the responses of large skeletal muscles to BTXA in relation to the underlying cause of the spasticity but the natural history of the spasticity is of great importance. BTXA has been of great value in the management of spasticity secondary to traumatic brain injury, cerebrovascular accident and following surgery for arteriovenous malformation or tumour. BTXA is more applicable to short- or medium-term spasticity management in a restricted number of target muscles. Severe, generalized, long-term spasticity should be managed by other means.

Finally, an emerging application for the use of BTXA is in the management of pain associated with muscle spasm (Figure 12.6). Soft tissue injury and surgery in children who have spastic cerebral palsy can be associated with pain, which is disproportionately severe and prolonged. Relatively minor orthopaedic procedures such as adductor release surgery can be overshadowed by inadequate pain control. Musculoskeletal pain in spastic cerebral palsy responds poorly to standard analgesic regimens.

Narcotic analgesics even in large doses seem to leave painful spasms untouched but are associated with side-effects including nausea, vomiting and constipation.

We observed that when injections of BTX were combined with orthopaedic surgery, children appeared to have a significant reduction in their pain, spasms and analgesic requirements (Barwood et al., 2000). We decided to investigate this further in a double-blind, randomized, placebo-controlled trial. We chose to investigate pain and analgesic requirements after adductor releases in children with cerebral palsy who had both clinical and radiological evidence of hip subluxation (Figure 12.6). When the decision to perform adductor surgery had been reached, the children were randomly allocated to have an injection of BTXA at a dose of 4 U/kg to each adductor muscle group, or normal saline of an equal volume. Injections were performed in the outpatient department between five and ten days before the scheduled date of surgery. All aspects of the perioperative care were standardized. Postoperative pain and analgesic consumption was carefully monitored. When the code was broken, it became evident that children who had received BTX chemodenervation prior to surgery had lower pain scores, reduced analgesic consumption and earlier discharge from hospital than those in the placebo group. We feel that these findings confirmed our hypothesis that BTX would break the postoperative cycle of pain and spasm. There are potentially many other applications for the use of BTX in the perioperative period including tendon transfers in the upper limb and tendon lengthenings and transfers in the lower limb.

Orthopaedic surgery: permanent–focal

Orthopaedic surgery for children with spasticity due to cerebral palsy can be conveniently classified as soft tissue surgery or bony surgery. This is a form of focal and permanent treatment. Soft tissue operations include surgery on muscles and tendons. Tendons can be released, lengthened or transferred and muscle bellies can be recessed or detached from underlying fascia or their tendons (Dormans & Copley, 1998).

Tenotomies, or complete division of tendon, are reserved for the management of contractures and spasticity in muscle units whose effect is considered to be harmful. When a tendon is completely severed, it probably reattaches to its original insertion point with scar tissue. This occurs over a period of time. Subsequently, it may begin to function with a possible reduction in its strength (Moseley, 1992).

Controlled lengthening of muscle bellies and tendons, to correct the deformities often seen in children with cerebral palsy, is the preferred option. This includes lengthening of the hip flexors, the knee flexors and the ankle plantar flexors. Complete loss of muscle function could be very harmful as muscles are the important 'motors' working on the skeletal levers to produce movement. The controlled lengthening, usually required to retain useful function of individual muscle tendon units on bony levers, translates into an improved gait pattern. Such surgery is best performed following a careful analysis of walking patterns with three-dimensional gait analysis (Gage et al., 1995; Boyd & Graham, 1997).

Lengthening of muscles and tendons has a profound effect on the physiology and biomechanics of muscle (Miller et al., 1995). It is widely accepted that lengthening muscles produces a weakening effect (Moseley, 1992). This may be true in a narrow sense. However, careful restoration of muscle–tendon unit relationship, which allows the joint to work in its most functional position, may actually increase power generation, as measured by a force plate.

Lengthening muscles has significant effects on the underlying component of spasticity. In the initial postoperative period, when children have pain and anxiety, muscle tone remote from the site of surgery is frequently increased. If this periop-erative increase in spasticity is not managed appropriately, undesirable posture may result. There may be a resultant progression of deformities at other sites.

In the muscle–tendon units which have been lengthened, clonus is frequently abolished and the deep tendon reflexes are reduced for a variable period of time. This may be the result of both biological and biomechanical effects of lengthening, including changes in the proprioceptive and muscle spindle inputs to the reflex arc. Part of the explanation may also lie in the servo-mechanism theory proposed by Moseley in which the brain is described as part of the servo-mechanism whose activities are dependent on the perceived results of any of the activities in the feed-back loop (Moseley, 1992). The relationship between brain and muscle is consid-ered not to be unidirectional such as that between a rifle and a bullet, but more similar to that between a thermostat and a heating furnace. There has been little investigation of the magnitude of the reduction in spasticity by soft tissue surgery, its duration and its benefits.

A second important component of orthopaedic surgery for deformity correction is osteotomy and joint stabilization. Osteotomies in the management of children with cerebral palsy are usually rotational in nature. Typically medial femoral torsion (Lewis et al., 1964; Staheli et al., 1968; Beals, 1969; Bleck, 1979) is corrected by an external rotation osteotomy of the femur (Eilert & MacEwen, 1977; Root & Siegel, 1980; Tylkowski et al., 1980; Canale & Holland, 1983; Beauchense et al., 1992; Brunner & Baumann, 1997). Lateral tibial torsion (Staheli et al., 1968; Nicol & Menelaus, 1983; King & Staheli, 1984) is corrected by an internal rotation osteo-tomy of the tibia (McNichol et al., 1983; Dodgin et al., 1998; Stefko et al., 1998). Rotational osteotomies can be helpful in the management of gait disturbance but the effects on muscle can also be very significant. An osteotomy of the femur in the intertrochanteric region will change the effective line of pull of muscle whose origins and insertion points cross the line of the osteotomy. These include iliopsoas, the hip adductors and the hamstrings. Computer modelling indicates that some of these muscles may be relaxed by the rotational osteotomy but others may have their tension increased. As described above, spasticity may increase, in the postoperative period in children with cerebral palsy, because of pain and anxiety. In addition, we must now add the potential for increased muscle tension due to the rotational osteotomy. Such increased muscle tone and spasticity should be anticipated and managed appropriately by acute spasticity management and when necessary associated prophylactic lengthening of muscle–tendon units. As outlined earlier, the use of diazepam can be very effective in the perioperative period.

The main role of orthopaedic surgery, for children with cerebral palsy and other forms of spasticity, is the management of fixed deformities. However, the correction of these deformities by both soft tissue and bony surgical procedures may have a very significant acute effect in the postoperative period, and a more gradual, longer-term effect on the associated spasticity. These effects must be anticipated and included in an overall management plan. Much basic research remains to be done on these effects in both animal models and in children with spasticity.

Conclusion

The management of spasticity in children is best achieved by a multidisciplinary team approach. Spasticity, muscle imbalance and restricted weight bearing may initiate a chain of events which lead to progressive fixed contractures, torsional deformities in long bones and eventually joint instability and even frank degenerative arthritis. Because spasticity seems to play a key role in the development of deformity, spasticity management is very important in the growing child. There is now a range of options from which the clinician can choose in order to manage spasticity as safely and as effectively as possible. By considering whether the intervention is focal or general in its effects and as to whether it is permanent or temporary, appropriate choices can be made. By utilizing a range of clinical and objective measures, the clinician has an ability to measure spasticity and monitor the effects of intervention. Outcome studies, with objective measures including gait analysis and appropriate measures of functional activity, should be the focus of our efforts in spasticity management research in children.

REFERENCES

Adams, J., Cahan, L. D., Perry, J. & Beeler, L. M. (1995). Foot contact pattern following selective dorsal rhizotomy. *Pediatr Neurosurg*, **23**: 76–81.

Albright, A. L. (1995). Spastic cerebral palsy: approaches to drug treatment. *CNS Drugs*, **4**: 17–27.

Albright, A. L. (1996). Baclofen in the treatment of cerebral palsy. *J Child Neurol*, **11**: 77–83.

Albright, A. L., Barron, W. B., Fasick, M. P., Polinko, P. & Janosky, J. (1993). Continuos intrathecal baclofen infusion for spasticity of cerebral origin. *JAMA*, **270**: 2475–7.

Albright, A. L., Cervi, A., Singletary, J. (1991). Intrathecal baclofen for spasticity in cerebral palsy. *JAMA*, **265**: 1418–22.

American Academy of Neurology (1990). Assessment: the clinical usefulness of botulinum toxin-A in treating neurologic disorders. Report of the therapeutics and technology assessment subcommittee of the American Academy of Neurology. *Neurology*, **40**: 1332–6.

Arens, J. F. & McKinnon, W. M. P. (1971). Malignant hyperpyrexia during anaesthesia. *JAMA*, **215**: 919–22.

Arens, L. J., Peacock, W. J. & Peter, J. (1989). Selective posterior rhizotomy: a long-term follow-up study. *Child's Nerv Syst*, **5**: 148–52.

Ashworth, B. (1964). Preliminary trial of cardisoprodol in multiple sclerosis. *Practitioner*, **192**: 540–2.

Bankheit, A. M. O., Badwan, D. A. H. & McLellan, D. L. (1996). The effectiveness of chemical neurolysis in the treatment of lower limb spasticity. *Clin Rehabil*, **10**: 40–3.

Barwood, S., Baillieu, C., Boyd, R., Brereton, K., Low, J., Nattrass, G. & Graham, H. K. (2000). Analgesic effects of botulinum toxin A: a randomized placebo-controlled clinical trial. *Dev Med Child Neurol*, **42**: 116–21.

Beals, R. K. (1969). Developmental changes in the femur and acetabulum in spastic paraplegia and diplegia. *Dev Med Child Neurol*, **11**: 303–13.

Beauchense, R. B., Miller, F. & Moseley, C. (1992). Proximal femoral osteotomy using the AO fixed-angle blade plate. *J Pediatr Orthop*, **12**: 735–40.

Beckerman, H., Becker, J., Lankhorst, G. J. & Verbeek, A. L. M. (1996). Walking ability of stroke patients – efficacy of tibial nerve blocking and a polypropylene ankle–foot orthosis. *Arch Phys Med*, **77**: 1144–51.

Binder, H. & Eng, G. D. (1989). Rehabilitation management of children with spastic diplegic cerebral palsy. *Arch Phys Med Rehabil*, **70**: 481–9.

Blackman, J. A., Reed, M. D. & Roberts, C. D. (1992). Muscle relaxant drugs for children with cerebral palsy. In *The Diplegic Child Evaluation and Management*, ed. M. D. Sussman, pp. 229–240. Rosemont: American Academy of Orthopedic Surgeons.

Bleck, E. E. (1979). *Orthopaedic Management of Cerebral Palsy*. Philadelphia: Saunders.

Bohannon, R. W. & Smith M. B. (1987). Interrater reliability of a modified Ashworth scale of muscle spasticity. *Phys Ther*, **67**: 206–7.

Boyce, W., Gowland, C., Rosenbaum, P., Lane, M., Plews, N., Goldsmith, C., Russell, D., Wright, V., Zdrobov, S. & Harding, D. (1995). The gross motor performance measure: validity and responsiveness of a measure of quality of movement. *Phys Ther*, **75**: 603–13.

Boyd, R. N. & Graham, H. K. (1997). Botulinum toxin A in the management of children with cerebral palsy: indications and outcomes. *Eur J Neurol*, **4**(Suppl. 2): S15–S22.

Boyd, R. N. & Graham, H. K. (1999). Objective measurement of clinical findings in the use of botulinum toxin type A for the management of children with cerebral palsy. *Eur J Neurol*, **6** (Suppl 4): S23–S35.

Boyd, R. N., Pliatsios, V., Starr, R., Nattrass, G. & Graham, H. K. (2000). Biomechanical transformation of the gastrocsoleus muscle by injection of botulinum toxin A in children with cerebral palsy. *Dev Med Child Neurol*, **42**: 32–41.

Brunner, R. & Baumann, J. U. (1997). Long-term effects of intertrochanteric varus-derotation osteotomy on femur and acetabulum in spastic cerebral palsy: an 11- to 18-year follow-up study. *J Pediatr Orthop*, **17**: 585–91.

Cahan, L. D., Adams, J. M., Beeler, L. & Perry, J. (1989). Clinical electrophysiologic and kinesiologic observations in selective dorsal rhizotomy in cerebral palsy. *Neurosurg State Art Rev*, **4**: 477–84.

Calta, R. G. & Santomauro, E. T. (1976). The use of baclofen in children with cerebral palsy. *Folia Med*, **73**: 199.

Canale, A. T. & Holland, R. W. (1983). Coventry screw fixation of osteotomies about the paediatric hip. *J Pediatr Orthop*, **3**: 592–600.

Carpenter, E. B. (1983). Role of nerve blocks in the foot and ankle in cerebral palsy: therapeutic and diagnostic. *Foot Ankle*, **4**: 164–6.

Carpenter, E. B. & Seitz, D. G. (1980). Intramuscular alcohol as an aid in management of spastic cerebral palsy. *Rev Med Child Neurol*, **22**: 497–501.

Chan, C. H. (1990). Dantrolene sodium and hepatic injury. *Neurology*, **40**: 1427–32.

Coffey, R. J., Cahill, D., Steers, W. et al. (1993). Intrathecal baclofen for severe spasticity of spinal origin: results of a long-term multicenter study. *J Neurosurg*, **78**: 226–32.

Cooperman, D. R. (1987). Hip dislocation in spastic cerebral palsy: long-term consequences. *J Pediatr Orthop*, **7**: 268–276.

Corry, I. S. (1994). *Use of a Motion Analysis Laboratory in Assessing the Effects of Botulinum Toxin A in Cerebral Palsy*. Thesis for Doctor of Medicine in the Faculty of Medicine, Queen's University, Belfast.

Corry, I. S., Cosgrove, A. P., Duffy, C. M., McNeill, S., Eames, N., Taylor, T. C. & Graham, H. K. (1995). Botulinum toxin A as an alternative to serial casting in the conservative management of equinus in cerebral palsy. *Dev Med Child Neurol*, **37**: 20–1.

Corry, I. S., Cosgrove, A. P., Duffy, C. M., McNeill, S., Eames, N., Taylor, T. C. & Graham, H. K. (1998). Botulinum toxin A compared with stretching casts in the treatment of spastic equinus: a randomized prospective trial. *J Pediatr Orthop*, **18**: 304–11.

Corry, I. S., Cosgrove, A. P., Duffy, C. M., Taylor, T. C. & Graham, H. K. (1999). Botulinum toxin A in hamstring spasticity: gait posture. *Dev Med Child Neurol*, **10**: 206–13.

Corry, I. S., Cosgrove, A. P., Walsh, E. G., McClean, D. & Graham, H. K. (1997). Botulinum toxin A in the hemiplegic upper limb: a double blind trial. *Dev Med Child Neurol*, **39**: 185–93.

Cosgrove, A. P., Corry, I. S. & Graham, H. K. (1994). Botulinum toxin in the management of the lower limb in cerebral palsy. *Dev Med Child Neurol*, **36**: 386–96.

Cosgrove, A. P. & Graham, H. K. (1994). Botulinum toxin A prevents the development of contractures in the hereditary spastic mouse. *Dev Med Child Neurol*, **36**: 379–85.

Costa, E. & Guidoffi, A. (1979). Molecular mechanisms in the receptor action of benzodiazepines. *Ann Rev Pharmacol Toxicol*, **19**: 531–45.

Couper-Brash, J. (1955). *Neurovascular Hila of Limb Muscles*. Edinburgh: E. and S. Livingstone.

Davidoff, R. A. (1989). Mode of action of antispasticity drugs. *Neurosurg State Art Rev*, **4**: 315–24.

DeLateur, B. (1972). A new technique of intramuscular phenol neurolysis. *Arch Phys. Med Rehabil*, **53**: 179–85.

Desmedt, J. E. & Hainaut, K. (1979). Dantrolene and A23187 ionophore: specific action on calcium channels revealed by the aequorin method. *Biochem Pharmacol*, **28**: 957–64.

Dodgin, D. A., De Swart, R. J., Stefko, R. M., Wenger, D. R. & Ko, J-Y. (1998). Distal tibial/fibular derotation osteotomy for correction of tibial torsion: review of technique and results in 63 cases. *J Pediatr Orthop*, **18**: 95–101.

Dolphin, A. C. & Scott, R. Y. (1986). Inhibition of calcium currents in cultured rat dorsal root ganglion neurons by baclofen. *Br J Pharmacol*, **88**: 213–20.

Dormans, J. P. & Copley, L. A. (1998). Orthopedic approaches to treatment. In *Caring for Children with Cerebral Palsy: A Team Approach*, ed. J. P. Dormans & L. Pellegrino. Baltimore: Brookes Publishing Co.

Dormans, J. P. & Pellegrino, L. (Eds.) (1998). *Caring for Children with Cerebral Palsy: A Team Approach*. Baltimore: Brookes Publishing Co.

Dralle, D., Muller, H., Zierski, J. & Klug, N. (1985). Intrathecal baclofen for spasticity. *Lancet*, **2**: 1003.

Duncan, W. & Mott, D. (1983). Foot reflexes and the use of the 'inhibitive cast'. *Foot Ankle*, **4**: 145–8.

Eames, N. W. A., Barker, R., Hill, N., Graham, K., Taylor, T. & Cosgrove, A. (1999). The effect of botulinum toxin A on gastrocnemius length. The magnitude and duration of the response. *Dev Med Child Neurol*, **41**: 226–32.

Easton, J., Ozel, T. & Halpern, D. (1979). Intramuscular neurolysis for spasticity in children. *Arch Phys Med Rehabil*, **60**: 155–8.

Eilert, R. E. & MacEwen, G. D. (1977). Varus derotational osteotomy of the femur in cerebral palsy. *Clin Orthop*, **125**: 168–72.

Felsenthal., G. (1974). Pharmacology of phenol in peripheral nerve blocks: a review. *Arch Phys Med Rehabil*, **55**: 13–16.

Fischer, E., Cress, R. H., Haines, G., Pannin, N. & Paul, B. J. (1970). Evoked nerve conduction after nerve block by chemical means. *Am J Phys Med*, **49**: 333–47.

Flett, P. J., Stern, L. M., Waddy, H., Connell, T. M., Seeger, J. D. & Gibson, S. K. (1999). Botulinum toxin A versus fixed cast stretching for dynamic calf tightness in cerebral palsy. *J Pediatr Child Health*, **35**: 71–7.

Fromm, F. G. & Terrence, C. F. (1987). Comparison of L-baclofen and racemic baclofen in trigeminal neuralgia. *Neurology*, **37**: 1725–8.

Gage, J. R. (1995). The clinical use of kinetics for evaluation of pathological gait in cerebral palsy. (Instructional course lectures). *J Bone Joint Surg Am*, **44**: 507–15.

Gage, J. R., Deluca, P. A. & Renshaw, T. (1995). Gait analysis: principles and applications. Emphasis on its use in cerebral palsy. (Instructional Course Lectures). *J Bone Joint Surg Am*, 1607–23.

Gans, B. M. & Glenn, M. B. (1982). Introduction. In *The Practical Management of Spasticity in Children and Adults*, ed. B. M. Glenn & J. Whyte, 1982, pp. 1–7. Philadelphia: Lea & Febiger.

Gilman, A. G., Goodman, L. S. & Gilman, A. (1990). *Goodman and Gilman's The Pharmaceutical Basis of Therapeutics*, 8th edn. New York: MacMillan Publishing.

Glasgow, J. F. T. & Graham, H. K. (1997). *Management of Injuries in Children*, pp. 345–78. Plymouth: BMJ Publishing Group.

Glenn, M. B. (1990). Nerve blocks. In *The Practical Management of Spasticity in Children and Adults*, ed. M. B. Glen & J. Whyte, pp.227–258. Philadelphia: Lea & Febiger.

Graham, H. K. (1995). Management of spasticity associated with cerebral palsy. In *Management of Spasticity with Botulinum Toxin: A Clinical Monograph*, ed. C. O'Brien & S. Yablon, pp. 17–23. Colorado: Colorado Postgraduate Institute for Medicine.

Greene, W. B., Dietz, F. R., Goldberg, M. J., Gross, R. H., Miller, F. & Sussman, M. D. (1991). Rapid progression of hip subluxation in cerebral palsy after selective posterior rhizotomy. *J Pediatr Orthop*, **11**: 494–7.

Greenblatt, D. J., Allen, M. D., Harmatz, J. S. & Shader, R. J. (1980). Diazepam disposition determinants. *Clin Pharmacol Ther*, **27**: 301–12.

Griffiths, E. & Melampy, C. (1977). General anaesthesia use in phenol intramuscular neurosis in children with spasticity. *Arch Phys Med Rehabil*, **58**: 154–7.

Hainaut, K. & Desmedt, J. E. (1974). Effect of dantrolene sodium on calcium movements in single muscle fibres. *Nature*, **252**: 728–30.

Hinderer, K. A., Harris, S. R., Purdy, A. H., Chew, D. E., Staheli, L. T., McLaughlin, J. F. & Jaffe, K. M. (1988). Effects of tone-reducing vs standard plaster casts on gait improvement of children with cerebral palsy. *Dev Med Child Neurol*, **30**: 370–7.

Hoffer, M .M., Felwell, E., Perry, R., Perry, J. & Bonnet, C. (1973). Functional ambulation in children with myelomeningocoele. *J Bone Joint Surg Am*, **55**: 137–48.

Houkom, J. A., Roach, J. W., Wenger, D. R., Speck, G., Herring, J. A. & Norris, E. N. (1986). Treatment of acquired hip subluxation in cerebral palsy. *J Pediatr Orthop*, **6**: 285–90.

Jankovic, J. & Brin, M. F. (1991). Therapeutic use of botulinum toxin. *New Eng J Med*, **324**: 1186–94.

Jordan, R. P. (1984). Therapeutic considerations of the feet and lower extremities in the cerebral palsied child. *Clin Podiatry*, **1**: 547–51.

Kalen, V. & Bleck, E. E. (1985). Prevention of spastic paraplegic dislocation of the hip. *Dev Med Child Neurol*, **27**: 17–24.

Keats, S., Morgese, A. & Nordland, T. (1963). Role of diazepam in the comprehensive treatment of cerebral palsied children. *Western Med*, **4**(Supp. 1): S22.

Khalili, A. A. & Benton, J. G. (1966). A physiologic approach to the evaluation and the management of spasticity with procaine and phenol nerve block: including a review of the physiology of the stretch reflex. *CORR*, **47**: 97–104.

King, H. A. & Staheli, L. T. (1984). Torsional problems in cerebral palsy. *Foot Ankle*, **4**: 180–4.

Knutson, E., Lindblom, U. & Martensson, A. (1974). Plasma and cerebrospinal fluid levels of baclofen (lioresal) at optimal therapeutic responses in spastic paresis. *J Neurol Sci*, **23**: 473–84.

Koman, L. A., Mooney, J. F. & Smith, B. P. (1996). Neuromuscular blockade in the management of cerebral palsy. *J Child Neurol*, **11**(Suppl. 1): S23–S28.

Koman, L. A., Mooney, J. F., Smith, B., Goodman, A. & Mulvaney, T. (1993). Management of cerebral palsy with botulinum-A toxin: preliminary investigation. *J Pediatr Orthop*, **13**: 489–95.

Koman, L. A., Mooney, J. F., Smith, B. P., Goodman, A. & Mulvaney T. (1994). Management of spasticity in cerebral palsy with botulinum-A toxin: report of a preliminary, randomized, double-blind trial. *J Pediatr Orthop*, **14**: 299–303.

Koman, L. A., Mooney, J. F., Smith, B. P., Walker, F. & Leon, J. M. (2000). Botulinum toxin type A neuromuscular blockade in the treatment of lower extremity spasticity in cerebral palsy: a randomized, double blind, placebo controlled trial. BOTOX study group. *J Pediatr Orthop*, **20**: 108–15.

Kroin, J. S., Ali, A., York, M. & Penn, R. D. (1993). The distribution of medication along the spinal canal after chronic intrathecal administration. *Neurosurgery*, **33**: 226–30.

Lance, J. W. (1980). Symposium synopsis. In *Spasticity: Disordered Motor Control*, ed. R. G. Feldman, R. R. Young & W. P. Koella, pp. 485–94. Chicago: Year Book Medical Publishers.

Law, M., Cadman, D., Rosenbaum, P., Walter, S., Russell, D. & DeMatter, C. (1991). Neurodevelopmental therapy and upper-extremity inhibitive casting for children with cerebral palsy. *Dev Med Child Neurol*, **33**: 379–87.

Lazorthes, Y., Sallerin-Caute, B., Versie, J. C., Bastide, R. & Carillo, J. P. (1990). Chronic intrathecal baclofen administration for control of severe spasticity. *J Neurosurg*, **72**: 393–402.

Lerman, J., McLeod, M. E. & Strong, H. A. (1989). Pharmacokinetics and intravenous dantrolene in children. *Anaesthesiology*, **70**: 625–9.

Letts, M., Shapiro, L., Muider, K. & Klassen, O. (1984). The windblown hip syndrome in total body cerebral plasy. *J Pediatr Orthop*, **4**: 55–62.

Lewis, F. R., Samilson, R. R. & Lucas, D. B. (1964). Femoral torsion and coxa valga: a preliminary report. *Dev Med Child Neurol*, **6**: 591.

Lietman, P. S., Haslam, R. H. A. & Walcher, J. R. (1974). Pharmacology of dantrolene sodium in children. *Arch Phys Med Rehabil*, **55**: 388–92.

Massagli, T. L. (1991). Spasticity and its management in children. *Phys Med Rehabil Clin N A*, **2**: 867–89.

Mazur, J. M., Shanks, D. E., Cummings, R. J., McCluskey, W. P., Federico, L. & Goins, M. (1992). Nonsurgical treatment of tight achilles tendon. In *The Diplegic Child, Evaluation and Management*, ed. M. D. Sussman, pp. 343–54. Rosemont: American Academy of Orthopedic Surgeons.

McKinlay, I., Hyde, E. & Gordon, N. (1980). Baclofen: a team approach to drug evaluation of spasticity in childhood. *Scot Med J*, **25**: 526–8.

McLaughlin, J. F., Bjornson, K. F., Astley, S. J., Graubert, C., Hays, R. M., Roberts, T. S., Price, R. & Temkin, N. (1998). Selective dorsal rhizotomy: efficacy and safety in an investigator-masked randomized clinical trial. *Dev Med Child Neurol*, **40**: 220–32.

McNichol, D., Leong, J. C. Y. & Hsu, L. C. S. (1983). Supramalleolar derotation osteotomy for lateral tibial torsion and associated equinovarus deformity of the foot. *J Bone Joint Surg BR*, **65**: 166–70.

Milla, P. J. & Jackson, A. D. (1977). A controlled trial of baclofen in children with cerebral palsy. *J Int Med Res*, **5**: 398–404.

Miller, F., Dabney, K. W. & Rang, M. (1995). Complications in cerebral palsy treatment. In *Complications in Pediatric Orthopaedic Surgery*, ed. C. H. Epps & J. R. Bowen, pp. 477–544. Philadelphia: Lippincott.

Molnar, G. E. & Kathirithamby, R. (1979). Lioresal in the treatment of cerebral palsy. *Arch Phys Med Rehab*, **60**: 540.

Moseley, C. (1992). Physiologic effects of soft-tissue surgery. In *The Diplegic Child, Evaluation and Management*, ed. M. D. Sussman. Rosemont: American Academy of Orthopedic Surgeons.

Muller, H. (1992). Treatment of severe spasticity: results of a multicenter trial conducted in Germany involving the intrathecal infusion of baclofen by an implantable drug delivery system. *Dev Med Child Neurol*, **34**: 739–45.

National Institutes of Health Consensus Developmental Conference (1990). Consensus statement. Clinical use of botulinum toxin. *NIH Consensus Dev Conf*, **8**: 12–14.

Nicol, R. O. & Menelaus, M. B. (1983). Correction of combined tibial torsion and valgus deformity of the foot. *J Bone Joint Surg Br*, **65**: 641–5.

Nogen, A. G. (1979). Effect of dantrolene sodium on the incidence of seizures in children with spasticity. *Child's Brain*, **5**: 420–5.

O'Brien, C. (1995). Clinical pharmacology of botulinum toxin. In *Management of Spasticity with Botulinum Toxin: A Clinical Monograph*, ed. C. O'Brien & S. Yablon, pp. 3–6. Colorado: Colorado Postgraduate Institute for Medicine.

O'Hanlan, J., Galford, H. & Bosley, J. (1969). The use of 45% alcohol to control spasticity. *Va Med Mo*, **96**: 429–36.

Oppenheim, W. L. (1990). Selective posterior rhizotomy for spastic cerebral palsy: a review. *Clin Orthop*, **253**: 20–9.

Oppenheim, W. L., Standt, L. A. & Peacock, W. J. (1992). The rationale for rhizotomy. In *The Diplegic Child, Evaluation and Management*, ed. M. D. Sussman. Rosemont: American Academy of Orthopedic Surgeons.

Ounpuu, S., Bell, K. J., Davis, R. B. & DeLuca, P. A. (1993). An evaluation of the posterior leaf spring orthosis using gait analysis. *Dev Med Child Neurol*, **35**(Suppl. 69): S8.

Ounpuu, S., Bell, K. J., Davis, R. B. & DeLuca, P. A. (1996). An evaluation of the posterior leaf spring orthosis using joint kinematics and kinetics. *J Pediatr Orthop*, **16**: 378–84.

Palisano, R., Rosenbaum, P., Walker, S., Russell, D., Wood, E. & Galuppi, B. (1997). Development and reliability of a system to classify gross motor function in children with cerebral palsy. *Dev Med Child Neurol*, **39**: 214–23.

Peacock, W. J. & Arens, L. J. (1982). Selective posterior rhizotomy for the relief of spasticity in cerebral palsy. *S Afr Med J*, **62**: 119–24.

Peacock, W. J., Arens, L. J. & Berman, B. (1987). Cerebral palsy spasticity: selective posterior rhizotomy. *Paedtr Neurosurg*, **13**: 61–6.

Peacock, W. J. & Staudt, L. A. (1990). Spasticity in cerebral palsy and the selective posterior rhizotomy procedure. *J Child Neurol*, **5**: 179–85.

Peacock, W. J., Staudt, L. A. (1991). Functional outcomes following selective posterior rhizotomy in children with cerebral palsy. *J Neurosurg*, **74**: 380–5.

Pedersen, E., Arlien-Soborg, P. & Mai, J. (1974). The mode of action of the GABA derivative baclofen in human spasticity. *Acta Neurol Scand*, **50**: 665–80.

Pellegrino, L. & Dormans, J.P. (1998). Definitions, etiology and epidemiology of cerebral palsy. In *Caring for Children with Cerebral Palsy: A Team Approach*, ed. J. P. Dormans & L. Pellegrino, pp. 3–30. Baltimore: Brookes Publishing Co.

Penn, R. D. (1992). Intrathecal baclofen for spasticity of spinal origin: seven years of experience. *J Neurosurg*, **77**: 236–40.

Penn, R. D. & Kroin, J. S. (1985). Continuous intrathecal baclofen for severe spasticity. *Lancet*, **2**: 125–7.

Penn, R. D., Savoy, S. M., Corcos, D., Latash, M., Gottlieb, G., Parke, B. & Kroin, J. S. (1989). Intrathecal baclofen for severe spinal spasticity. *New Eng J M*, **320**: 1517–21.

Perry, J. (1985). Normal and pathological gait. *Atlas of Orthotics*, 2nd edn., pp. 76–111. St.Louis: C. V. Mosby.

Perry, J. (1992). '*Phases of Gait*', *Gait Analysis: Normal and Pathological Function*. New Jersey: Slack.

Perry, J., Adams, J. & Cahan, L.D. (1989). Foot-floor contact patterns following selective dorsal rhizotomy, abstract. *Dev Med Neurol*, **31** (suppl. 59): S19.

Perry, J., Giovan, P., Harris, L. J., Montgomery, R. P. T. & Azaria, M. (1978). The determinants of muscle action in the hemiplegic lower extremity and their effect on the examination procedure. *Clin Orthop*, **131**: 71–89.

Perry J., Hoffer M. M., Antonelli, D., Plut, J., Lewis, G. & Greenberg, R. (1976). Electromyography before and after surgery for hip deformity in children with cerebral palsy. *J Bone Joint Surg Am*, **58**: 201–8.

Perry, J., Hoffer, M.M., Giovan, P., Antonelli, D. & Greenberg, R. (1974). Gait analysis of the triceps surae in cerebral palsy: a preoperative and postoperative clinical and electromyographic study. *J Bone Joint Surg Am*, **56**: 511–20.

Petrillo, C., Chu, D. & Sanders, W. (1980). Phenol block of the tibial nerve in the hemiplegic patient. *Orthopaedics*, **3**: 871–4.

Petterson, B., Nelson, K. B., Watson L. & Stanley F. J. (1993a). Twins, triplets, and cerebral palsy in births in Western Australia in the 1980s. *BMJ*, **307**: 1239–43.

Petterson, B., Stanley, F. J. & Garner, B. J. (1993b). Spastic quadriplegia in Western Australia: II Pedigrees and family patterns of birthweight and gestational age. *Dev Med Child Neurol*, **35**: 202–15.

Phelps, W. M. (1963). Observations of a new drug in cerebral palsy. *Western Med*, **4**(Suppl. 1): S5.

Rang, M. (1990). Cerebral palsy. In *Lovell and Winter's Pediatric Orthopedics*, 3rd edn., vol.1, ed. R. T. Morrissy, pp. 465–506. Philadelphia: J. B. Lippincott.

Rice, G. P. A. (1987). Pharmacotherapy of spasticity: some theoretical and practical considerations. *Can J Neurol Sci*, **14** (Suppl. 3): S510–S512.

Ried, S., Pellegrino, L., Albinson-Scull, S. & Dormans, J. P. (1998). The management of spasticity. In *Caring for Children with Cerebral Palsy*, ed. J. P. Dormans & L. Pellegrino, pp. 99–123. Baltimore: Brookes Publishing Co.

Root, L. & Siegel, T. (1980). Ostetomy of the hip in children: posterior approach. *J Bone Joint Surg Am*, **62**: 571–5.

Rose, S. A., Ounpuu, S. & DeLuca, P. A. (1991). Strategies for the assessment of paediatric gait in the clinical setting. *Phys Ther*, **71**: 961–80.

Russell, D., Rosenbaum, P., Cadman, D., Gowland, C., Hardy, S. & Jarvis, S. (1989). The gross motor function measure: a means to evaluate the effects of physical therapy. *Dev Med Child Neurol*, **31**: 341–52.

Rymer, W. Z. & Powers, R. K. (1989). Pathophysiology of muscular hypertonia in spasticity. *Neurosurg State Art Rev*, **4**: 291–301.

Scott, A. B. (1980). Botulinum toxin injection into extraocular muscles as an alternative to strabismus surgery. *Ophthalmology*, **87**: 1044–9.

Scott, A. B., Magoon, E. H., McNeer, K. W. & Stager, D. R. (1990). Botulinum treatment for childhood strabismus. *Ophthalmology*, **97**: 1434–8.

Scrutton, D. (1989). The early management of hips in cerebral palsy. *Dev Med Child Neurol*, **31**: 108–16.

Scrutton, D. & Baird, G. (1997). Surveillance measures of the hips of children with bilateral cerebral palsy. *Arch Disease Child*, **76**: 381–4.

Silfverskiold, N. (1924). Reduction of the uncrossed two-joint muscles of the leg to one-joint muscles in spastic conditions. *Acta Chir Scand*, **56**: 315–30.

Spira, R. (1971). Management of spasticity in cerebral palsied children by peripheral nerve block with phenol. *Dev Med Child Neurol*, **13**: 164–73.

Staheli, L. T., Duncan, W. R. & Schaefer, E. (1968). Growth alterations in the hemiplegic child. *Clin Orthop*, **60**: 205–12.

Stanley, F. J. & Alberman, E. (1984). *The Epidemiology of the Cerebral Palsies*. Philadelphia: J. B. Lippincott.

Stefko, R. M., De Swart, R. J., Dodgin, D. A., Wyatt, M. P., Kaufman, K. R., Sutherland, D. H. & Chambers, H. G. (1998). Kinematic and kinetic analysis of distal derotation osteotomy of the leg in children with cerebral palsy. *J Pediatr Orthop*, **18**: 81–7.

Steinbok, P., Armstrong, R. W. & Cochrane, D. D. (1997). A randomized clinical trial to compare selective posterior rhizotomy plus physiotherapy and physiotherapy alone in children with spastic diplegic cerebral palsy. *Dev Med Child Neurol*, **39**: 178–84.

Stoffel, A. (1913). The treatment of spastic contractures. *Am J Orthop Surg*, **10**: 611–44.

Sussman, M. D. (1983). Casting as an adjunct to neurodevelopmental therapy for cerebral palsy. *Dev Med Child Neurol*, **25**: 804–5.

Sussman, M. D. (Ed.) (1992). *The Diplegic Child, Evaluation and Management.* Rosemont: American Academy of Orthopedic Surgeons.

Sussman, M. & Cusick, B. (1979). Preliminary report: the role of short-leg tone-reducing casts as an adjunct to physical therapy of patients with cerebral palsy. *Johns Hopkins Med J*, **145**: 112–14.

Sutherland, D. H., Kaufman, K. R., Wyatt, M. P. & Mubarak, S. J. (1995). Effects of botulinum toxin on gait of patients with cerebral palsy: an open-label study. *Gait Posture*, **3**: 2.

Sutherland, D. H., Kaufman, K. R., Wyatt, M. P., Chambers, H. G. & Mubarak, S. J. (1999). Double-blind study of botulinum A toxin injections into the gastrocnemius muscle in patients with cerebral palsy. *Gait Posture*, **10**: 1–9.

Tardieu, G., Centaur, S. & Delarue, R. (1954). A la recherche d'une technique de mesure de la spasticite 'imprime' avec le periodique. *Rev Neurol*, **91**: 143–4.

Tippets, R. H., Walker, M. L. & Liddel, K. L. (1989). Long-term follow-up of selective dorsal rhizotomy for relief of spasticity in cerebral-palsied children, abstract. *Dev Med Neurol*, **31**(Suppl. 59): S19.

Tylkowski, C. M., Rosenthal, R. K. & Simon, S. R. (1980). Proximal femoral osteotomy in cerebral palsy. *Clin Orthop*, **151**: 183–92.

Utili, R., Boitnott, J. K. & Zimmerman, H. J. (1977). Dantrolene-associated hepatic injury: incidence and character. *Gastroenterology*, **72**: 610–16.

VanWinkle, W. B. (1976). Calcium release from skeletal muscle sarcoplasmic reticulum: site of action of dantrolene sodium? *Science*, **193**: 1130–1.

Vaughan, C. L., Berman, B. & Peacock, W. J. (1988). Gait analysis of spastic children before and after selective lumbar rhizotomy. *Paedtr Neurosci*, **14**: 297–300.

Vaughan, C. L. Berman, B. & Peacock, W. J. (1991). Cerebral palsy and rhizotomy. A three-year follow-up and evaluation with gait analysis. *J Neurosurg*, **74**: 178–84.

Walsh, E. G. (1988). Assessment of human hemiplegic spasticity by a resonant frequency method. *Clin Biomechan*, **3**: 173–8.

Waterman, P. M., Albin, M. S. & Smith, R. B. (1980). Malignant hyperthermia: a case report. *Anesth Analg*, **59**: 220–1.

Westin, G. W. & Dye, S. (1983). Conservative management of cerebral palsy in the growing child. *Foot Ankle*, 4: 160–3.

Wilkinson, S. P., Portman, B. & Williams, R. (1979). Hepatitis from dantrolene sodium. *Gut*, **20**: 33–6.

Wright, F. V., Sheil, E. M. H., Drake, J. M., Wedge, J. H. & Naumann, S. (1988). Evaluation of selective dorsal rhizotomy for the reduction of spasticity in cerebral palsy: a randomized control trial. *Dev Med Child Neurol*, **40**: 239–47.

Young, R. R. & Delwaide, P. J. (1981a). Drug therapy: spasticity (first of two parts). *New Eng J Med*, **304**: 28–33.

Young, R. R. & Delwaide, P. J. (1981b). Drug therapy: spasticity (second of two parts). *New Eng J Med*, **304**: 96–9.

Ziegelgansberger, W., Howe, J. R. & Sutor, B. (1988). The neuropharmacology of baclofen. In *Local-Spinal Therapy of Spasticity*, ed. H. Muller, J. Zierski & R. D. Penn, pp. 37–49. New York: Springer-Verlag.

Ziv, I., Blackburn, N., Rang, M. & Koreska, J. (1984). Muscle growth in normal and spastic mice. *Dev Med Child Neurol*, **26**: 941–84.

Index

Note: page numbers in *italics* refer to figures and tables